MOSBY'S
MASSAGE THERAPY REVIEW

evolve

MOSBY'S
MASSAGE THERAPY REVIEW

second edition

2

SANDY FRITZ, MS, NCTMB

Founder, Owner, Director, and Head Instructor
Health Enrichment Center
School of Therapeutic Massage and Bodywork
Lapeer, Michigan

With 48 illustrations

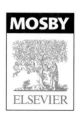

11830 Westline Industrial Drive
St. Louis, Missouri 63146

MOSBY'S MASSAGE THERAPY REVIEW, EDITION 2

Notice

Neither the Publisher nor the Author assume any responsibility for any loss or injury and/or damage to persons or property arising out of or related to any use of the material contained in this book. It is the responsibility of the treating practitioner, relying on independent expertise and knowledge of the patient, to determine the best treatment and method of application for the patient.

The Publisher

Previous edition copyrighted 2002

ISBN-13: 978-0-323-03751-8
ISBN-10: 0-323-03751-8

Publishing Director: Linda Duncan
Acquisitions Editor: Kellie White
Developmental Editor: Jennifer Watrous
Publishing Services Manager: Melissa Lastarria
Project Manager: Rich Barber
Design Coordinator: Teresa McBryan

Printed in the United States of America

Last digit is the print number: 9 8 7 6 5 4 3

*This review guide is dedicated
to those who study—not just for tests,
but to achieve excellence.*

Preface

The second edition of *Mosby's Massage Therapy Review* has been revised and updated to assist those preparing for various licensing and certification exams achieve successful outcomes.

Based on the success of the first edition and input from those who have used the text during preparation for various exams, the following additions have been made to the second edition:

- Information about how questions are developed and strategies for identifying wrong answers
- Study suggestions for content areas such as musculoskeletal anatomy, assessment, and treatment plan development
- Additional questions in each content area with rationales designed to help the reader understand the question pattern and how to identify the correct answer
- Study aids such as a comprehensive glossary, muscle location and function, pathology, and Asian theory and practice
- Expanded practice exams and CD support

Two exams are currently available from the National Certification Board for Therapeutic Massage and Bodywork (NCBTMB). One exam targets massage therapy as well as other bodywork methods, including Asian bodywork approaches and energy-based methods.

This exam structure is the original exam content since the process began. Recently, based on industry demand, an exam that only targets therapeutic massage content has also been offered. This second exam is essentially the same as the original exam, minus the questions relating to the Asian and energetic bodywork approaches. The content removed has been replaced with more anatomy, physiology, kinesiology, pathology, and massage therapy theory and practice.

The choice of which exam to take would depend on the content of your specific education and any requirements of your state or local government. *Mosby's Massage Therapy Review* addresses content found in both exams and allows readers to target which exam they are preparing to take.

This book continues to support a clinical reasoning model for both successful test-taking and increased excellence in professional practice and development. I am confident that if you use this book in the manner suggested in the first section and throughout the text (paying special attention to the rationales at the end of each chapter), your commitment to effective study will be productive.

SANDY FRITZ

Acknowledgments

Writing a book is a team effort. Many thanks to my team:

My assistant—Amy Husted

Laura Cochran (my daughter) for proofreading

My editors—Kellie Fitzpatrick, Jennifer Watrous, Elizabeth Clark, and Rich Barber

My designer—Teresa McBryan

My marketing representative—Julie Burchett, and all the sales representatives

Contents

Learning Styles, Study Tips, and Test-Taking Habits

This study guide has been created to support the therapeutic massage student and graduate through a review process; preparing them for various educational evaluations such as midterm and final exams; and local, state, and national licensing or certification exams. The questions are based on *Mosby's Essential Sciences for Therapeutic Massage* and *Mosby's Fundamentals of Therapeutic Massage*.

Information presented in most educational curriculums and information required to function as a massage professional can be divided into four areas. These categories form the basis of most licensing and certifying examinations. The four categories are the following:
- Human anatomy, physiology, and kinesiology
- Clinical pathology and indications and contraindications for massage application
- Massage therapy and bodywork
- Professional standards, ethics, and business practices

Four Content Areas of Preparation

1. Human anatomy, physiology, and kinesiology
   The general education in human anatomy, physiology, and kinesiology prepares the student to understand the benefits of massage and lays the foundation for the following area.
2. Clinical pathology and indications and contraindications for massage application
   Human anatomy, physiology, kinesiology, clinical pathology, and indications and contraindications for

massage application cover half of the content on most exams. The focus is to provide sufficient information to support safe and beneficial professional practice.

Usually these two categories are studied most effectively in an integrated format. For example, discussion of the anatomy of the nervous system leads to understanding the functions of the nervous system. Subsequently, understanding how massage affects the nervous system leads to identification of indications for massage and the nervous system, pathologic conditions of the nervous system, and contraindications for applications of massage, including cautions for use of massage when pathologic conditions are present.

Many find the sciences a more difficult study area. The terminology can seem overwhelming—almost like learning another language. If we can agree that the various methods and theoretical base of the many different bodywork modalities provide diversity, then the sciences provide commonality. The human body in structure and function remains consistent; therefore it makes sense that an understanding of the sciences is essential and relevant to massage.

Non-Western science content is focused primarily on traditional Chinese medicine but also covers other energy systems such as shiatsu, polarity therapy, and Ayurveda.

3. Massage therapy and bodywork: theory and application
   Competency in this area indicates that the massage professional is able to appropriately apply methods in a safe and beneficial way. A commonality exists in

most bodywork approaches. The content in this area covers methods used to obtain a database about the client and proper methods usage.

In addition to therapeutic massage, general knowledge about complementary bodywork modalities such as hydrotherapy, Asian theory, and applications such as acupressure, trigger points, and connective tissue massage often is measured.

4. Professional ethics and business practices

The professional standards, ethics, and business practices area develops the professional abilities needed to conduct oneself in a manner that reflects decision making to support ethical standards and sound business practices.

National Certification Examination (NCE) and National Certification Examination for Therapeutic Massage and Bodywork (NCETMB)

Credentialing is an important process. About two thirds of the states have licensing for massage therapy, and most of these states use the National Certification Examination as the written portion of the licensing exam. For states that have developed their own exam, the content and question styles are similar, so using this review guide helps you prepare for both types of exams.

In states that are not licensed or that use their own exams, massage therapists have the opportunity to become nationally certified by an independent, non-profit, private organization, the National Certification Board for Therapeutic Massage and Bodywork (NCBTMB). This board was first established in 1992. The goals when established were to give massage professionals a way to demonstrate their desire for excellence in massage practice by establishing a credential beyond their education and experience and to provide consumers proof that they are receiving care from a massage professional who is committed to a high level of practice standards and ethical behavior.

The current goals of the NCBTMB are as follows:

Establish National Certification as a recognized credential of professional and ethical standards; to promote the worth of National Certification to health, therapeutic massage and bodywork professionals, public policy makers and the general public; to assure and maintain the integrity, stability and quality of the National Certification Program; and to periodically update the program to reflect state-of-the-art practices in therapeutic massage and bodywork.

Currently there are close to 80,000 certified massage professionals in the United States. The NCBTMB has been accredited by the National Commission for Certifying Agencies since 1993 and is a member of the American National Standards Institute and the Coalition for Professional Certification.

To become a certified massage practitioner, one must pass an exam and qualify to sit for this exam by meeting one of the following criteria:
- A certificate of achievement with a minimum of 500 in-class supervised hours from a qualified school
- A portfolio that shows training and experience that is equivalent to a formal 500-hour program

All information to become a certified massage therapist and the most current requirements to sit for the exam can be obtained from visiting the NCBTMB web site. Those who graduated from a qualified program should request the candidate handbook, and those seeking portfolio approval should ask for the portfolio review handbook.

Contact information is as follows:

NCBTMB, 8201 Greensboro Dr., Suite 300, McLean, VA 22102

Phone: 1-800-296-0664; or web site: www.ncbtmb.com

Sample Questions in Relation to the Four Areas of Study

On an exam the four content areas are addressed specifically within a test question, or the content is mixed to develop combination test questions. For example, a pure science question may appear as follows: "The largest of the fontanels in the infant skull is _____?" An example of a question combining content may appear as follows: "During infant massage, it is important to apply only light pressure to the anterior fontanel for which of the following reasons?"

ANALYZING THE QUESTION

A good multiple-choice question presents sufficient facts so that you can identify the correct answer. You need to analyze the four possible answers based on the facts presented in the question and your knowledge to determine the best correct answer. All possible answers should be plausible, and the incorrect answers should not be evident. Analyzing the possible answers requires a comprehensive factual base provided during your education and found in the textbooks so that you can eliminate wrong answers and then identify and justify the correct answer.

In this review guide each sample question embodies a chunk of essential knowledge and is a representation of how that knowledge can be addressed in a multiple-choice exam. Each of the four possible answers also identifies important information. When using the questions to study for an exam, you should identify the information in all of the possible answers, the one correct answer, and the three incorrect answers in the textbooks and reference material you are used to studying. The correct answer should stand out clearly, and the reasons why incorrect answers are false should be apparent. Many of the questions are framed in mini case studies because this is a more relevant format for massage practitioners as they use the information in the context of the client population they serve.

TYPES OF MULTIPLE-CHOICE QUESTIONS

The three basic types of multiple-choice questions are factual recall and comprehension, application and concept identification, and clinical reasoning and synthesis. Examples of the three types of questions follow.

1. Factual recall and comprehension

The information necessary to answer this type of question can be found in various textbooks and reference material in the form of descriptions and definitions. Memorization of data is a method you can use to prepare to answer these types of questions. An example of this type of question follows:

1. Which bone makes up the heel of the foot?

   a. Navicular
   b. Calcaneus
   c. Hamate
   d. Xyphoid

   1. The answer is b.

2. Application and concept identification

This type of question requires that you understand the language posed in the question or be able to identify simple concepts and patterns. In addition, this type of question measures one's ability to understand language as it relates to contextual frameworks. Application and concept identification questions also address concrete information that can be described in terms, definitions, rules, laws, and other forms of structure. This information can be found directly in the textbooks and reference material. An example of this type of question follows:

1. Which method would be most appropriate if the client desires to remain passive during the massage?

   a. Pulsed muscle energy
   b. Reciprocal inhibition
   c. Approximation
   d. Post-isometric relaxation

   1. The answer is c.

3. Clinical reasoning and synthesis

Clinical reasoning and synthesis questions require you to analyze information and make appropriate professional decisions. Identifying the answer to this type of question requires that you use the information in a contextual manner. The case study scenario is a common approach to this question design. The answer is not found directly in any textbook or reference material; only the language and concepts would be in the books. An example of this type of question follows:

1. A client is taking an aspirin for osteoarthritis of the left knee. What precautions are needed for massage intervention?

   a. Avoid any type of massage to the affected knee.
   b. Avoid the use of compression above and below the knee.
   c. Reduce pressure level around the knee only.
   d. Monitor pressure levels of the massage to reduce potential bruising.

   1. The answer is d.

COMMON WRONG ANSWER STRATEGIES

Developing plausible wrong answers is the most difficult aspect of writing multiple choice questions. The wrong answers need to be clearly wrong but also need to seem plausible.

Good wrong answers are developed by misusing terminology. This is one of the reasons why studying glossaries, key terms in textbooks, and labeled illustrations is important.

Often, conflicting terms are used together to make an answer wrong.

Examples:

Compression is a massage application that glides and kneads.

This is a wrong answer because compression by definition does not glide or knead. Gliding and kneading may have compression qualities. This combination of words would be wrong usage.

Sanitation supersedes standard precautions.

This is a wrong answer because sanitation is an aspect of standard precautions, not something seperate.

The prone positioning of the client limits the ability to bolster and drape for modesty and warmth.

This is a wrong answer because positioning does not affect maintaining modesty and warmth.

Another strategy for developing wrong answers is to use opposite concepts.

Examples:

Flexion straightens the elbow.

This is incorrect. Flexion bends the elbow.

Lymphatic drainage follows a proximal to distal massage direction.

This is incorrect because the direction is distal to proximal even though the strokes begin close to the torso.

Cross-fiber friction is applied with the direction of the muscle fibers.

This is incorrect because cross-fiber friction is applied perpendicular to the muscle fibers.

Another strategy is to combine two or more unrelated types of information in the wrong answer.

Examples:

Geriatric massage treats sport injury.

These two concepts are not congruent with each other.

Body mechanics describes various draping protocols.

These two areas are not interrelated.

The gastrocnemius attaches on the venous lateral condyle.

Muscles do not attach to veins, and there is no such structure as the venous lateral condyle.

Use these examples to analyze the wrong answer in the sample questions to determine why the answer is incorrect. This is an effective study strategy. When you are actually taking an exam, it should be easier to determine the incorrect answers.

Make the Textbooks and Reference Material Work for You

It is best to study for exams using accepted textbooks and references. Most exams use standardized textbooks to reference the questions written for the exam. It may not be prudent to invest in study guides that "rewrite" textbook content because the content has not been actually referenced to the exams. The purpose of a study help such as this book is to guide the review process and assist in using problem-solving methods to identify correct answers.

The questions in the next two sections of this review guide are presented sequentially, chapter by chapter, following the outlines of *Mosby's Essential Sciences for Therapeutic Massage* and *Mosby's Fundamentals of Therapeutic Massage*, two of the most used and widely accepted therapeutic massage textbooks. Using this format, specific content areas are grouped together, such as the nervous system, assessment, ethics, and massage methods. Readers can determine which content they are proficient and in which areas they need more study.

The answers and rationales are located at the end of each chapter. You can use other textbooks as resources as well by looking up the content in the index. In an actual exam, the content will be mixed up. Section III

of this Review Guide provides questions that overlap knowledge with application, theory, ethics, and sciences because this represents how knowledge acquired for formal massage training and self-study is used in professional practice. The labeling exercises in Section IV, although not found on an exam, are an effective study tool.

Using the Mosby Textbook

The Mosby textbooks are designed as interactive work texts, making them excellent for self-study. Space is provided within the text for completion of activities, exercises, and workbook sections. If you resist writing in the book, do the exercises on pages copied from the textbooks.

Each chapter covers a large piece of knowledge. Chapter objectives reflect suggested competencies for the content. The chapters are relatively large, so each chapter is divided into sections. These sections also have objectives. Subheadings divide sections into smaller bits of information that can be processed in about 15 minutes of reading. This supports most individuals' sustained attention span.

An activity or exercise corresponds with the various subheadings. For memory retention, manipulation of the information in some way is important. Various strategies are used to support this information retention, such as paraphrasing, metaphors, drawings, practical applications, relationship to personal experiences, and movement. Use these activities and exercises as points of study. Each chapter ends with a workbook section. The workbook is designed to summarize the chapter. At the end of the workbook is an answer key. The answer key is like a chapter summary (e.g., Cliff's Notes). There is also some sort of problem-solving activity in each workbook section. These activities take the form of professional application exercises, problem-solving activities, or research for further study. This type of activity helps you develop clinical reasoning skills necessary to address the clinical reasoning and synthesis type of exam questions successfully. After you have studied the chapter in the textbook, then challenge yourself with the questions in this study guide that relate to the chapter content.

Completing all of the interactive exercises, activities, and self-study using this study guide should be adequate preparation for educational exams used during school and the licensing and certification exams currently being used. Recommended textbook lists for exam preparation are usually available from those that administer the various exams. It is prudent to obtain these lists and compare the information to be prepared confidently for the challenge of an exam.

Using this Review Guide

Accompanying this review guide is a CD-ROM. Two testing features are available on this CD to aid you in studying for massage exams. The Tutorial mode serves questions by category and provides instant feedback, including rationales. The Test mode randomly serves questions and allows for review after a test has been completed.

Many test questions and answers from Sections I and II in the review guide are included. Although questions in the review guide are arranged by content area, the CD randomizes the questions, which provides a more realistic representation of electronic exams. Each practice exam consists of 200 questions. A scoring matrix is provided after each and presents the overall number of attempted and correct questions, as well as the percentage of correct answers. The matrix also provides information regarding the four categories emphasized in the review guide (human anatomy, physiology, and kinesiology; clinical pathology and indications and contraindications for massage application; massage therapy and bodywork; and professional standards, ethics, and business practice) and indicating the student's score in each category. Following the categories is a breakdown of the chapters from the review guide, again showing the number of attempted questions, the number of correct answers, and the percentage of correct answers.

Once you have reviewed the scoring matrix, you can use the Tutorial mode to emphasize areas of weakness that have been identified. For example, if you scored a low percentage in clinical pathology and indications and contraindications for massage application, you can bring up the tutorial and practice questions in that category only.

RECOMMENDATIONS FOR STUDYING FOR AN EXAM

Important Note: One of the biggest errors readers make when using study guides, such as this text, is to concentrate on making sure they know the answers to the questions in the study guide. *Do not do this.* The questions in this study guide, as well as any of the others available, will not appear on the various exams. Those who administer the exams routinely screen and remove questions from the exams that appear in various review guides. *Memorizing the answers to the questions in any of the review guides is a waste of precious study time.*

This study guide has been developed to help you understand how to take an exam. The various questions are examples of how content may appear in an exam question. Each sample question and all of the possible answers contain the terminology you will encounter. Each sample question also teaches you how to address the various question styles found on exams.

This study tool does not replace your textbooks; instead it assists you in preparing to take exams successfully and become comfortable with how textbook content may appear on exams. This study guide is designed to enhance your understanding of textbook material.

When you study, you should have your textbooks, a medical dictionary, and an anatomy atlas of some sort available for reference. The study tool resources in this guide—the comprehensive glossary, the various charts and review content, the labeling exercises—do not replace the textbooks but are available for your convenience.

Rationales for the sample/example questions in this text are structured to teach you how to find the right answer to a test question, not to restate information found in the textbooks. If a rationale tells you to look up the definitions for the terminology used in the questions and possible answers, then that is the best method to use for study. In concept identification questions there is some sort of relationship among the terminology, and that can be explained in the rationale. In clinical reasoning and synthesis questions the rationales describe the clinical reasoning process used to solve the problem posed by the question.

The following list of suggestions should enhance your study process:

1. Relax. Anxiety interferes with the ability to integrate and recall information.
2. Have fun and be silly. Things learned with laughter are more easily retained.
3. Study in short bursts. Thirty minutes at a time is ideal.
4. Generally read a chapter and then study one small section at a time.
5. Know the meaning of any words displayed in key terms lists, in bold or italics print, and in the glossary and be able to use the words correctly in a sentence.
6. Study the illustrations and diagrams, paying attention to the labeling.
7. Manipulate the information. The interactive exercises and workbook segments of *Mosby's Fundamentals of Therapeutic Massage* and *Mosby's Essential Sciences for Therapeutic Massage* are designed to integrate information from short-term to long-term memory. Other textbooks often offer similar features.
8. Seek to understand the information. Do not anticipate the test. Paraphrase and reword the information presented in the text.

9. Use the questions in this study guide as a study strategy. The questions are organized sequentially chapter by chapter in each of the textbooks. Write your own exam questions. The most difficult task is developing plausible wrong answers. (Use the questions in this book as examples.)
10. Work together in study groups by sharing information, by taking turns "teaching," or by taking each other's tests from the questions you wrote.

Recommendations for Taking an Exam

1. Get plenty of rest before the exam.
2. Arrive at the exam location in plenty of time to settle into the environment.
3. Ask questions about the exam process so that you clearly understand how to take the exam.
4. Acknowledge that you are nervous, relax as much as you can, and put the exam in perspective. The worst that can happen is that you might not pass. This only means more study and another attempt. The best that can happen is that you pass.
5. Begin at the beginning of the exam and answer questions sequentially.
6. If the answer to a question is not apparent to you, mark the question and return to it after the exam is completed. Often other questions on the exam will provide information to help you answer the question you skipped.

7. When you finish the exam, go back and answer the skipped questions. If you still do not know the answer, guess and let intuition work. Do not leave a space blank. A blank is wrong and a guess is possible.
8. Do not second-guess your answers. Only change an answer if you are sure that you were wrong with your first choice.
9. Review the exam to make sure you answered all the questions and that basic information such as your name is completed.
10. Turn in the exam as instructed and breathe. The exam is over. There is no sense in worrying. Remember perspective, and go do something fun.

The questions found in this guide will not appear on any exam. Instead, they are written to reflect the type of questions encountered on educational and certification and licensing exams and as a sequential study through the sciences, theory, business, and ethics of the practice of therapeutic massage and related bodywork modalities. The questions have been thought out carefully so that if you study the question and all the possible answers (correct and incorrect), you should have the factual knowledge and the critical thinking skills to approach an exam confidently. Just because you can answer all the questions in this study guide does not mean that you will pass an exam. The ability to be confident in one's knowledge and problem-solving skills will assure success, not memorization of the questions and answers in this book or any other textbook or study guide.

Success to you!

SECTION

1
The Body as a Whole

Review Tips

The content concerning the body as a whole typically creates a platform for understanding the design of the body and how the body functions. The sciences are described in essentially a foreign language. To be able to understand this content, you need to learn the language. The science studies in general, not only in this chapter, have a heavy emphasis on terminology.

This content usually is tested in the factual recall type of question relying on correct use of terminology. The best study skill is rote memorization of the terminology. In the answer key at the end of this chapter, many of the rationales indicate that the correct answer is the definition of the term.

You must know the definition of the terms and must be able to use the terms correctly. More complex questions use the terminology in the question and possible answers, and unless you decipher the language, you will not know what the question or the provided answers mean. There is no easy way to study terminology. Using flash cards, reading glossaries, and doing labeling exercises reinforce the definitions of the various terms. Use the study resources in this guide, and make sure when you read the textbooks that you know what the words mean. Also make sure that you understand the meaning of general language used to write the questions. If you are not sure of the meaning of a word, look it up in the dictionary.

Questions

1. Adenosine triphosphate (ATP) releases energy in muscles by what process?

   a. Mitosis
   b. Interphase
   c. Catabolism
   d. Anabolism

2. The substance between cell tissues made up of ground substance and fibers is called _____.

   a. Matrix
   b. Nucleic acids
   c. Basement membrane
   d. Meiosis

3. In the relationship of anatomy and physiology, the phrase "structure and function" means _____.

   a. Gross anatomy translates to regional anatomy
   b. Anatomy guides physiology and is modified by function
   c. Systemic physiology involves organizational anatomy
   d. Duality of wholeness represented in catabolism and anabolism

4. The complementary relationship of opposites is described by _____.

   a. Organ and system organization
   b. Responsiveness and metabolism
   c. Yin and yang
   d. Qi and shen

Correct answers are on pages 15-17.

5. How do we use physiology in the application of massage?

    a. Location of structures to be manipulated
    b. Specific positioning of the client for assessment
    c. Decision making relating to projected outcomes
    d. Directional communication in charting

6. Characteristics of life involve _____.

    a. Physiology
    b. Yin
    c. Anatomy
    d. Tissue

7. The chemical reaction that occurs in cells to effect transformation, production, or consumption of energy is _____.

    a. Absorption
    b. Digestion
    c. Responsiveness
    d. Metabolism

8. The process of homeostasis is a logical, well-coordinated pattern of balance. When balance is disrupted, patterns of dysfunction occur. Often homeostasis begins at what level of body organization?

    a. Chemical
    b. Cellular
    c. Tissue
    d. Organ

9. The concept of yang as compared with atomic structure is _____.

    a. Nucleus
    b. Protons
    c. Electrons
    d. Neutrons

10. Atomic bonding to form molecules occurs because of the action among _____.

    a. Nuclei
    b. Protons
    c. Electrons
    d. Neutrons

11. The most stable of atomic bonds is the _____.

    a. Ionic bond
    b. Covalent bond
    c. Polar covalent bond
    d. Catabolic bond

12. Which type of atomic bond holds together DNA?

    a. Ionic bond
    b. Covalent bond
    c. Polar covalent bond
    d. Catabolic bond

13. When chemical bonds are broken and new ones are formed, what has occurred?

    a. Mitochondrial reactivity
    b. Hydrolysis response
    c. Conductivity interaction
    d. Chemical reaction

14. The physiologic process that converts food and air into energy is called _____.

    a. Metabolism
    b. Homeostasis
    c. Responsiveness
    d. Dehydration

15. Massage creates chemical reactions in what way?

    a. Generates a stimulus
    b. Encourages interphase
    c. Supports hypertrophy
    d. Disrupts differentiation

16. In which of the following chemical reactions are complex compounds formed?

    a. Anabolism
    b. Metabolism
    c. Catabolism
    d. Mitosis

17. The study of chemical actions in the body is of what importance to the massage professional?

    a. Charting depends upon these interactions.
    b. Many massage benefits are derived from chemical reactions.
    c. Validation of subtle energy will be atomic.
    d. Chemical reactions are responsible for all pathologic conditions.

18. Which of the following organelles is involved in manufacture of proteins?

    a. Spindle cells
    b. Mitochondria
    c. Lysosomes
    d. Ribosomes

19. The most abundant component in cells is _____.

    a. Water
    b. Protein
    c. Lipids
    d. Carbohydrates

20. Cell division is the reproductive process of cells called _____.

    a. Interphase
    b. Mitosis
    c. Cytosol
    d. Catabolism

21. When a cell is able to perform a specialized function, the structure of the cell is modified. This is called _____.

    a. Hypertrophy
    b. Atrophy
    c. Differentiation
    d. Meiosis

22. Basement membrane connects epithelial tissue to _____.

    a. Muscle tissue
    b. Nervous tissue
    c. Neutrophil tissue
    d. Connective tissue

23. Which of the following is considered a cutaneous membrane?

    a. Skin
    b. Mucous membrane
    c. Serous membrane
    d. Collagen

24. Which of the following membranes lines cavities not open to the external environments and many organs?

    a. Basement membranes
    b. Mucous membranes
    c. Serous membranes
    d. Cutaneous membranes

25. Which of the following tissues are the most abundant in the body?

    a. Epithelial tissue
    b. Connective tissue
    c. Muscle tissue
    d. Nervous tissue

26. Specialization of connective tissue is focused to _____.

    a. Support
    b. Contractility
    c. Excitability
    d. Hypertrophy

27. The diverse forms of connective tissue are attributed to _____.

    a. Properties of cells and composition of matrix
    b. Extensive distribution of blood vessels
    c. The distribution of chondroblasts in the matrix
    d. The collagen formation of ground substance

28. The connective tissue type with the most blood flow is _____.

    a. Cartilage
    b. Dense irregular
    c. Areolar
    d. Dense regular

Correct answers are on pages 15-17.

29. The type of connective tissue most often found in ligaments and tendons is _____.

    a. Dense regular
    b. Dense irregular
    c. Areolar
    d. Adipose

30. Which following cell type is found in the connective tissue matrix that secretes bone?

    a. Fibroblast
    b. Chondroblast
    c. Osteoblast
    d. Hemocytoblast

31. Which of the following cartilage types is most likely to be damaged from wear and tear of the hip or knee joint?

    a. Hyaline cartilage
    b. Fibrocartilage
    c. Elastic cartilage
    d. Reticular cartilage

32. Massage methods applied to connective tissue have benefit because of the thixotropic properties of the tissue. This means _____.

    a. Massage stimulates mast cells to release histamine to reduce inflammation
    b. Massage separates the desmosomes and gap junctions to allow flexibility
    c. Massage increases the secretion of synovial fluid to increase joint mobility
    d. Massage acts to agitate ground substance and encourages a softer, more pliable tissue texture

33. What property of collagen may make it viable in the generation of body energy?

    a. Resistance to deformation
    b. Piezoelectric aspects
    c. Colloid formation
    d. Macrophagic activity

34. The Asian healing theory of the law of five elements relates best to _____.

    a. Muscle tissue structures
    b. Nervous tissue structures
    c. Organs
    d. Prana

35. Which of the following would be considered yin?

    a. Heart
    b. Stomach
    c. Body systems
    d. Qi

36. A massage practitioner is charting the location of a bruise. If the bruise is charted as located on the thigh, which of the following is correct to describe where the bruise is located?

    a. Systems anatomy
    b. Regional anatomy
    c. Pathophysiology
    d. Collagenous fibers

37. A massage therapist notices that a client's heart rate has decreased and the client's breathing has become slower and deeper. Which of the following best describes this outcome from the massage?

    a. Characteristics of life
    b. Organizational physiology
    c. Change in physiology
    d. Change in anatomy

38. The terms basement membrane and reticular fibers relate to which of the following?

    a. Epithelial and connective tissue
    b. Nervous tissue and neural tissue
    c. Cardiac and smooth muscle
    d. Cytoplasm and filtration

39. If the benefits of a relaxing hot bath with Epsom salt dissolved in the bath water is described as osmosis, which of the following is most correct?

    a. Hydrostatic pressure forces water across a semipermeable membrane
    b. Diffusion of water across an impermeable membrane
    c. Active transport of substances across the cell membrane
    d. The diffusion of water from a lower solution concentration to higher concentration through a semipermeable membrane

40. A client reports that he or she has some hormonal imbalances relating to a diet low in lipids. Which of the following is most correct?

    a. The diet is acid and high in fat.
    b. The diet is low in amino acids.
    c. The diet is excessively low in fat.
    d. The carbohydrates are insufficient.

Correct answers are on pages 15-17.

Exercise

Using the foregoing questions as examples, now write at least three more questions—one of each type: factual recall and comprehension, application and concept identification, and clinical reasoning and synthesis. Make sure to develop plausible wrong answers, and be sure that the correct answer is clearly correct. Then write a rationale for each question. The more questions you write, the better you will understand the material.

Answers and Discussion

1. **c**
   Factual recall
   Rationale: Adenosine triphosphate is a compound that stores energy in muscle. This energy is released during the chemical process of catabolism.

2. **a**
   Factual recall
   Rationale: The question is the definition of matrix.

3. **b**
   Application and concept identification
   Rationale: Anatomy is the study of the structure of the body, and physiology is the study of the function of the body. This question asks for the relationship of the two.

4. **c**
   Factual recall
   Rationale: This question is asking for a definition of Asian terminology, specifically yin and yang.

5. **c**
   Application and concept identification
   Rationale: The question asks for an application of the study of physiology to massage and bodywork. Most benefits from massage are the result of physiologic changes. The potential of these changes is a determinate of what will be the outcome of the massage.

6. **a**
   Application and concept identification
   Rationale: The question is asking for the relationship between two concepts that define life. Although anatomy can be studied on cadavers, physiology is apparent when life is manifested.

7. **d**
   Factual recall
   Rationale: The question is a definition of metabolism.

8. **a**
   Application and concept identification
   Rationale: The question asks for an understanding of homeostasis and the relationship to the development of disease. The chemical level of the organizational structure of the body is often where homeostasis begins to break down and disease begins.

9. **b**
   Application and concept identification
   Rationale: Yang is considered positive energy flow, and protons are the positively charged particles in an atom.

10. **c**
    Factual recall
    Rationale: The question describes a function of electrons.

11. **b**
    Factual recall
    Rationale: Ionic, covalent, and polar covalent are types of atomic bonds. Catabolic bond does not exist, so this is an incorrect word usage. Of the three, the covalent bond is most stable.

12. **c**
    Application and concept identification
    Rationale: DNA represents a type of molecule formed by a type of atomic bond. DNA is formed by polar covalent bonds.

13. **d**
    Factual recall
    Rationale: The question is the definition of a chemical reaction.

14. **a**
    Factual recall
    Rationale: The question is a definition of metabolism.

15. **a**
    Application and concept identification
    Rationale: The question asks for the interaction between the physiologic response to massage as a stimulus to chemical reactions.

16. **a**
    Factual recall
    Rationale: The question is the definition of anabolism.

17. **b**
    Application and concept identification
    Rationale: The question asks why the massage professional needs to understand chemical actions. The best answer is related to understanding the benefit of massage.

18. **d**
    Factual recall
    Rationale: The question describes an organelle function. Ribosomes manufacture proteins. An understanding of all organelle function is necessary to identify the correct answer.

19. **a**
    Factual recall
    Rationale: Of the four listed components that make up cells, water is the most abundant.

20. **b**
Factual recall
Rationale: Mitosis is the reproductive process of cells.

21. **c**
Factual recall
Rationale: The question is the definition of differentiation.

22. **d**
Factual recall
Rationale: The question describes a function of basement membrane.

23. **a**
Factual recall
Rationale: Skin is the largest cutaneous membrane.

24. **c**
Factual recall
Rationale: The question is the definition of serous membranes.

25. **b**
Factual recall
Rationale: Of the four tissue types, connective tissue is the most abundant in the body.

26. **a**
Factual recall
Rationale: Support is a major function of connective tissue.

27. **a**
Application and concept identification
Rationale: The only answer provided that correctly described connective tissue is related to the properties of the cells and composition of the matrix. The other three answers incorrectly describe connective tissue.

28. **c**
Factual recall
Rationale: Areolar connective tissue has a high vascularity, unlike the other types mentioned, which have limited blood flow.

29. **a**
Factual recall
Rationale: The question describes the location of dense regular connective tissue.

30. **c**
Factual recall
Rationale: The question is the definition of an osteoblast.

31. **a**
Application and concept identification
Rationale: The question asks for the relationship between a type of cartilage and the function of a joint. Hyaline cartilage is found at the ends of bones in synovial joints such as the hip and knee and is subject to damage from repetitive movement.

32. **d**
Application and concept identification
Rationale: The question asks for the relationship between a massage application and a physiologic outcome of connective tissue. You must understand the terminology in the question and the answers to identify the correct answer. The incorrect answers describe wrong physiologic processes or do not address the facts of the question. The only correct response is answer d.

33. **b**
Factual recall
Rationale: Deforming collagen creates a piezoelectric current.

34. **c**
Application and concept identification
Rationale: The law of five elements is correlated most directly with the organs. Muscle and nerve tissue is too limited an answer, and *prana* is a term used to describe life energy.

35. **a**
Factual recall
Rationale: Understanding the terminology and definition of yin organ functions is necessary to identify the heart with yin.

36. **b**
Factual recall
Rationale: This question is answered by knowing the definition of the words. The thigh is a regional location. Physiology is about function, not location. Systems anatomy describes the body systems such as the digestive system and muscular system. Collagenous fibers are connective tissue, not a body location.

37. **c**
Concept identification
Rationale: The question describes changes in body function. This is physiology. Organizational physiology targets physiologic organizational function, and the question describes two different physiologic functions Function is physiology not anatomy, and characteristics of life are not relevant to the question.

38. **a**

    Factual recall
    Rationale: This is a terminology question.
    Basement membrane relates to epithelial tissue,
    and reticular fibers relate to connective tissue.

39. **d**

    Concept identification
    Rationale: This question is all about the
    terminology. The correct answer is the definition
    of osmosis. Answer a is wrong because
    hydrostatic pressure is not a factor. Answer b is
    wrong because the term *impermeable* means
    that nothing can cross the membrane. Answer c
    is incorrect because the content of the question
    does not describe cell membrane activity.

40. **c**

    Concept identification
    Rationale: The term *lipid* relates to fat. Answer a
    is wrong because it indicates a diet high in fat.
    Answer b is incorrect because amino acids relate
    to protein. Carbohydrates are sugars and
    starches, not fats.

2

Mechanisms of Health and Disease

Review Tips

The content concerning mechanisms of health and disease is targeted to physiology and anatomy. The content can be tested with all three question types, although typically the factual recall question is most common because language is still the main focus. The rationales in the answers and discussion section usually tell you to define all the terms in the question and possible answers.

The information in this content area often is used when creating case study type of questions combining massage application with physiologic outcomes. These questions are based on the clinical reasoning/synthesis model. Be aware of this in future chapters when the content becomes more complex.

As previously explained, you must know the definition of the terms and be able to use the terms correctly. More complex questions use the terminology in the question and possible answers, and unless you can decipher the language, you will not know what the question or the provided answers mean. There is no easy way to study terminology. Using flash cards, reading glossaries, and doing labeling exercises reinforce the definitions of the various terms. Use the study tools in this guide, and make sure that when you read your textbooks, you know what the words mean. Also make sure that you understand the meaning of the general language used to write the questions. If you are not sure of the meaning of a word, look it up in a glossary or dictionary. One of the challenges of any entry-level study is learning the ABCs of the system. It does not matter what you are studying—massage, computers, cooking, carpentry—you have to learn the names and meanings of the materials and equipment. For massage, this means anatomy and physiology medical terminology.

Questions

1. The common relationship between yin/yang, the five-element theory, and Ayurvedic dosha is _____.

    a. Entrainment
    b. Somatic
    c. Homeostasis
    d. Etiology

2. Ayurvedic theory classifies physiologic functions by _____.

    a. Elements
    b. Visceral function
    c. Feedback
    d. Doshas

3. Which of the following represents principles of movement?

    a. Pitta
    b. Vata
    c. Kappa
    d. Ether

4. Feedback is an essential aspect of homeostasis because of _____.

    a. Afferent discharge
    b. Effector response
    c. Information exchange
    d. Efferent signaling

5. Any stimulus that disrupts internal homeostasis is _____.

    a. Consciousness
    b. Negative feedback
    c. Stress
    d. Pathology

6. A sensor mechanism, integration/control center, and effector mechanism are part of a _____.

    a. Stress response
    b. Post-isometric relaxation
    c. Stimulus response
    d. Feedback loop

7. Feedback that reverses the original stimulus, stabilizing physiologic function, is _____.

    a. Positive feedback
    b. Negative feedback
    c. Stimulus response feedback
    d. Regulatory response

8. Massage is part of a feedback loop in the _____.

    a. Controlled condition
    b. Control center
    c. Response
    d. Stress stimulus

9. Many benefits of massage are a result of _____.

    a. Nonspecific stress stimulus that encourages feedback response to more optimum function
    b. Precise application of selected stimulus-creating positive feedback
    c. Positive feedback response to return function to homeostasis
    d. Afferent transmission to the sensory mechanism with the disrupted homeostasis reduced by the control center

10. Biologic rhythms are related to _____.

    a. Circadian patterns
    b. Pathogenesis rhythm
    c. Negative feedback
    d. Positive feedback

11. Relaxed mood states are experienced by persons when _____.

    a. Biologic rhythms are entrained to sympathetic patterns
    b. Biologic rhythms are oscillated independently
    c. Biologic rhythms are entrained to the chakra system
    d. Biologic rhythms are entrained to parasympathetic patterns

12. Relaxed ordered entrainment is produced by massage in response to _____.

    a. The practitioner's direct application of methods
    b. The practitioner's calm presence and rhythmic application
    c. The practitioner's emotional state
    d. The practitioner's specific choice of methods that address the chakra system

13. Relaxation methods that focus on breathing produce entrainment because _____.

    a. Cortisol increases during parasympathetic response
    b. Respiration rate is a major biologic oscillator
    c. Sympathetic mechanisms are generated
    d. Baroreceptors are inhibited

14. An interesting similarity between the traditional chakra system and biologic oscillators is _____.

    a. Rhythm patterns
    b. Vibratory rate
    c. Shared location
    d. Size comparison

15. Evidence of a healthy state includes _____.

    a. Adaptive capacity to stress
    b. Strain in response to stress
    c. Susceptibility to bacterial infection
    d. Stress exceeds adaptive capacity

16. A massage professional needs an understanding of disease processes. This study of disease processes is called _____.

    a. Pathogenesis
    b. Pathology
    c. Epidemiology
    d. Pharmacology

17. A group of signs and symptoms that identify a pathologic condition linked to a common cause is called a(n) _____.

    a. Disease
    b. Diagnosis
    c. Etiology
    d. Syndrome

18. A disease with a vague onset that develops slowly and remains active for a long time is considered _____.

    a. Acute
    b. Communicable
    c. Chronic
    d. Idiopathic

19. Susceptibility to the disruption of homeostasis extensive enough to cause disease could be due to which of the following factors?

    a. Hyperplasia
    b. Malnutrition
    c. Antineoplastics
    d. Pathogenesis

20. Pathogenic organisms are considered to be _____.

    a. Parasites
    b. Chemical agents
    c. Allergy
    d. Neoplasm

21. A neoplasm resulting from hyperplasia that is contained and encapsulated is considered _____.

    a. Acute
    b. Chronic
    c. Benign
    d. Malignant

22. Cancer cells' reproduction of undifferentiated cells without boundary recognition is called _____.

    a. Replacement
    b. Carcinogens
    c. Metastasis
    d. Anaplasia

23. Heat, redness, swelling, and pain are signs of _____.

    a. Cancer
    b. Degeneration
    c. Counterirritation
    d. Inflammation

24. Inflammatory exudate that accumulates during an inflammatory process _____.

    a. Reduces swelling
    b. Dilutes irritants
    c. Inhibits tissue repair
    d. Causes the release of mediators of inflammation

25. An inflammatory mediator that dilates blood vessels is _____.

    a. Histamine
    b. Prostaglandins
    c. Inflammatory exudates
    d. Neutrophils

26. The purpose of increased tissue fluid volume during inflammation is _____

    a. To allow parenchymal cells to regenerate the area of injury
    b. To allow immune cells to travel quickly to destroy pathogens
    c. To support the activity of labile cells during tissue repair
    d. To increase the activity of histamine and kinins during tissue repair

27. Tissue repair for regeneration of functional cells is accomplished by _____.

    a. Stromal cells
    b. Labile cells
    c. Parenchymal cells
    d. Fibrin cells

28. Tissue repair that results in a scar is called _____.

    a. Stroma
    b. Replacement
    c. Regeneration
    d. Idiopathic

29. A major component of scar tissue is _____.

    a. Epidermis
    b. Epithelium
    c. Fibroblasts
    d. Collagen

30. Inflammation that persists beyond beneficial healing is considered an inflammatory disease. This chronic form of inflammation may be helped with what form of massage?

    a. Extensive application of deep transverse friction
    b. Light surface stroking
    c. Controlled use of friction, stretching, and pulling
    d. Brisk beating and pounding

31. Systemic inflammatory responses and fibromyalgia are _____.

    a. Indicated for massage that causes inflammation
    b. Indicated for massage that involves extensive stretching and pulling techniques
    c. Contraindicated for massage that causes inflammation
    d. Contraindicated for massage only in the area of the joints

32. Genetics, age, lifestyles, stress, environment, and preexisting conditions are _____.

    a. Determinants of immune hypersensitivity
    b. Predisposing risk factors for development of disease
    c. Potential distribution routes for pathogens
    d. Warning signs of cancer

33. The No. 1 complaint of persons to their health care professional is _____.

    a. Decreased circulation
    b. Joint stiffness
    c. Breathing difficulties
    d. Pain

34. Potential tissue damage is signaled by _____.

    a. Pain
    b. Inflammation
    c. Steroids
    d. Moxibustion

35. The sensory mechanisms for pain are called _____.

    a. Intractable
    b. Hyperalgesia
    c. Nociceptors
    d. Bradykinin

36. Pain that is poorly localized, nauseating, and associated with sweating and blood pressure changes is _____.

    a. Superficial somatic pain
    b. Burning pain
    c. Aching pain
    d. Deep pain

37. Pain that may be a symptom of an organ disorder is _____.

    a. Superficial somatic pain
    b. Burning pain
    c. Aching pain
    d. Deep pain

38. Pain that arises from stimulation of receptors in the skin or from stimulation of receptors in skeletal muscles, joints, tendons, and fascia is called _____.

    a. Visceral pain
    b. Phantom pain
    c. Somatic pain
    d. Referred pain

39. A massage application that creates superficial somatic pain that blocks transmission of deep somatic or visceral pain is called _____.

    a. Counterirritation
    b. Pain-spasm-pain cycle
    c. Reflex contraction
    d. Cutaneous stimulation

40. When pain is felt in a surface area away from the stimulated receptors, particularly in organs, it is called _____.

    a. Visceral pain
    b. Phantom pain
    c. Somatic pain
    d. Referred pain

41. A client comes to you complaining of an aching pain just under the ribs right of the midline, under the right scapula, and in the right neck and shoulder area. The pain has been occurring more frequently and is now almost constant. The referred pain pattern might indicate problems with what organ?

    a. Bladder
    b. Kidney
    c. Stomach
    d. Gallbladder

42. A client's low back pain returns within 3 hours of receiving massage. What organ may be the cause of referred back pain?

    a. Bladder
    b. Kidney
    c. Stomach
    d. Gallbladder

43. A massage client does not provide effective feedback about the amount of pressure requested for massage. The client asks for very deep pressure. As the massage professional, you keep asking if the pressure is causing pain and the client says no. It seems that any deeper pressure may cause bruising and other tissue damage.
    This client may be exhibiting _____.

    a. Counterirritation
    b. Reduced influence of beta endorphins
    c. High pain tolerance
    d. Hyperstimulation analgesia

44. Massage used as a pain management strategy is a form of _____.

    a. Stimulus-induced analgesia
    b. Acupuncture
    c. Dermatomal inhibition
    d. Prostaglandin stimulation

45. Aspirin is used in pain management because its effects include _____.

    a. Increased inflammation
    b. Inhibiting enkephalins
    c. Inhibiting prostaglandins
    d. Stimulating A delta nerve fibers

46. If a pathologic condition occurs because of a state of "too much" or "not enough," then health would occur because of _____.

    a. Increased immune activity
    b. Decreased sympathetic arousal response
    c. Effective feedback and adaptive capacity
    d. Tolerance and hardiness

Correct answers are on pages 26-29.

47. According to Hans Selye, the response of the body to stress is called the _____.

    a. Fight-or-flight response
    b. Resistance reaction
    c. Exhaustion phase
    d. General adaptation syndrome

48. Persons who perceive an event as a threat activate the alarm reaction. What is the first response?

    a. The sympathetic centers activate.
    b. The hypothalamus is stimulated.
    c. The adrenal cortex releases glucocorticoid.
    d. The adrenal medulla releases epinephrine.

49. A common breathing disturbance in excessive or long-term stress is _____.

    a. Hyperventilation syndrome
    b. Immune suppression
    c. Gastritis
    d. Tetany

50. Many aspects of ancient healing wisdom are being shown as valid stress management strategies because of _____.

    a. Support of increased heart rate
    b. Reduction in sympathetic arousal
    c. Increase in glucocorticoids
    d. Increase in blood glucose levels

51. At which life stage are we best able to maintain effective homeostasis?

    a. Birth to 3 years old
    b. 4 years old to 12 years old
    c. Adolescence to midlife
    d. 65 years old and older

52. The massage outcome is determined to be a reduction in blood pressure. Which of the following is most correct?

    a. This is a positive feedback response.
    b. This is a virulent response.
    c. This would be a feedback loop.
    d. This would be reduction of a fistula.

53. Massage that simulates sensory receptors to create a response to stimulate the homeostatic mechanism is best described as which of the following?

    a. Entrainment
    b. Feedback loop
    c. General adaptation syndrome
    d. Threshold and tolerance

54. What do all the following terms have in common: biofeedback, massage aromatherapy, medication, and hypnosis?

    a. Strategies for pain management
    b. Methods of massage
    c. Risk factors for pain
    d. Methods of controlling inflammation

55. A client has had to deal with multiple stressors, including a family death and having a car stolen. The client is not sleeping well. The client is 69 and tells the massage therapist about not feeling able to deal with it all. Which of the following most logically explains this response?

    a. The client has reduced stress threshold, straining the cortisol enhancement of the immune system.
    b. The client's ability to adapt to the multiple stressors also is challenged by increased age.
    c. The client's adaptive capacity is adequate, but the family death is enough to increase mental strain.
    d. The client's stress response is increasing adaptive capacity that is challenged by age-related immune suppression.

56. A client informs the massage practitioner about noticing hair loss, mouth ulcers, and bladder urgency. How are the symptoms related?

    a. They are examples of inflammatory stress.
    b. They are stress/pain modulators.
    c. They are genetic disease risk factors.
    d. They are stress-related disease symptoms.

Exercise

Using the foregoing questions as examples, now write at least three more questions—one of each type: factual recall and comprehension, application and concept identification, and clinical reasoning and synthesis. Make sure to develop plausible wrong answers, and be sure that the correct answer is clearly correct. Then write a rationale for each question. The more questions you write, the better you will understand the material.

Correct answers are on pages 26-29.

Answers and Discussion

1. **c**
Factual recall
Rationale: Eastern bodywork theory has homeostasis as a primary philosophy. The ability to define the words in the question and the four possible answers is necessary.

2. **d**
Factual recall
Rationale: The question is a definition of dosha.

3. **b**
Factual recall
Rationale: The question asks for a function of vata.

4. **c**
Application and concept identification
Rationale: Information exchange is necessary for a feedback loop, and feedback loops support homeostasis.

5. **c**
Factual recall
Rationale: The question is a definition of stress.

6. **d**
Factual recall
Rationale: The question lists the parts of a feedback loop.

7. **b**
Factual recall
Rationale: The question gives a definition of negative feedback.

8. **d**
Application and concept identification
Rationale: The question is asking for a connection between massage and feedback loops. To understand the question requires understanding the definitions of the terms and the physiologic response to massage stimuli. Massage and bodywork methods initially are processed as a stress stimulus.

9. **a**
Application and concept identification
Rationale: The three incorrect answers misuse the terminology. The correct answer identifies how massage begins a feedback process.

10. **a**
Factual recall
Rationale: Definition of the terms in the question and answers is necessary to analyze for the correct answer. Circadian patterns keep body rhythms organized.

11. **d**
Application and concept identification
Rationale: Three concepts are correlated: biologic rhythms, entrainment, and autonomic nervous system functions. All three must be connected correctly. Only answer d is correct.

12. **b**
Application and concept identification
Rationale: The question asks for justification of physiologic outcome of massage. The terms need to be defined correctly to answer the question. Two processes take place to provide the outcome described in the question, and only answer b identifies both.

13. **b**
Application and concept identification
Rationale: Four concepts are described in the question and correct answer. All four concepts must be correlated correctly: relaxation, breathing, entrainment, and respiration as a biologic oscillator. Only answer b connects the concepts correctly.

14. **c**
Factual recall
Rationale: The Eastern thought justifying bodywork modalities often corresponds with anatomy and physiology described in Western science. This question describes this type of relationship.

15. **a**
Factual recall
Rationale: The question gives a definition of health.

16. **b**
Factual recall
Rationale: The question gives a definition of pathology. All the terms need to be defined to answer the question correctly and identify wrong answers.

17. **d**
Factual recall
Rationale: The question gives a definition of a syndrome. All the terms need to be defined to answer the question correctly and identify wrong answers.

18. **c**
Factual recall
Rationale: The question gives a definition of chronic. All the terms need to be defined to answer the question correctly and identify wrong answers.

19. **b**
Factual recall
Rationale: Malnutrition is the only possible answer that would describe disease susceptibility. All the terms need to be defined to answer the question correctly and identify wrong answers.

20. **a**
Factual recall
Rationale: "Parasites" is the only answer that fits the criteria of being a pathogenic organism.

21. **c**
Factual recall
Rationale: All the terms need to be defined to answer the question correctly and identify wrong answers. A neoplasm is abnormal tissue growth, hyperplasia is an uncontrolled increase in cell number, and the definition of benign includes growths that are contained and encapsulated as opposed to malignant, which is a nonencapsulated mass.

22. **d**
Factual recall
Rationale: The question gives a definition of anaplasia. All the terms need to be defined to answer the question correctly and identify wrong answers.

23. **d**
Factual recall
Rationale: The question gives a definition of inflammation. All the terms need to be defined to answer the question correctly and identify wrong answers.

24. **b**
Factual recall
Rationale: The question asks for the function of exudates, which is to dilute irritants causing inflammation.

25. **a**
Factual recall
Rationale: Histamine is a vasodilator. All the terms need to be defined to answer the question correctly and identify wrong answers.

26. **b**
Factual recall
Rationale: The correct answer describes the function of increased fluid volume during inflammation. All the terms need to be defined to answer the question correctly and identify wrong answers.

27. **c**
Factual recall
Rationale: The terms need to be defined correctly to answer the question. When this is done, the only correct answer is answer c.

28. **b**
Factual recall
Rationale: The terms need to be defined correctly to answer the question. Tissue repair resulting in a scar is replacement.

29. **d**
Factual recall
Rationale: The terms need to be defined correctly to answer the question indicating that collagen is the major component of scar tissue.

30. **c**
Application and concept identification
Rationale: The question asks for the physiologic outcome of certain massage methods to resolve a type of chronic inflammation. This is done by creating a controlled therapeutic inflammation, and friction, stretching, and pulling tissue are the best methods to accomplish this.

31. **c**
Application and concept identification
Rationale: The conditions described in the question represent contraindications to the use of therapeutic inflammation because the body is unable to resolve inflammatory processes.

32. **b**
Factual recall
Rationale: The correct answer describes risk factors appropriately, whereas the incorrect answers are not correlated to the information in the question.

33. **d**
Factual recall
Rationale: Pain is the chief complaint over the other three listed.

34. **a**
Factual recall
Rationale: The question describes a function of pain.

35. **c**
Factual recall
Rationale: Nociceptors are the sensory mechanisms for pain perception. The other terms are incorrect.

36. **d**
Factual recall
Rationale: The question is the definition of deep pain.

37. **c**
    Factual recall
    Rationale: Organ pain is perceived as an aching. Differentiation of the types of pain is important so that appropriate referral can be made to the physician.

38. **c**
    Factual recall
    Rationale: The soma relates to the soft tissue elements described in the question.

39. **a**
    Factual recall
    Rationale: The question is a definition of counterirritation.

40. **d**
    Factual recall
    Rationale: The question is a definition of referred pain.

41. **d**
    Clinical reasoning and synthesis
    Rationale: To answer this question, use factual information of referred pain patterns to make a decision about what the information might mean. The facts of the question describe the referred pain pattern of the gallbladder.

42. **b**
    Application and concept identification
    Rationale: The question asks for a correlation between symptoms and referred pain patterns. The kidney most often refers pain to the lumbar area.

43. **c**
    Clinical reasoning and synthesis
    Rationale: The question is asking for an explanation for a client behavior, in this instance high pain tolerance. The other answers describe a massage outcome or a response that is contradictory (i.e., if endorphin levels drop, then the client would be more aware of pain, not less aware of pain).

44. **a**
    Application and concept identification
    Rationale: You must understand the terms to answer the question. The only answer that makes sense in relationship to the question is answer a.

45. **c**
    Factual recall
    Rationale: Effect of aspirin on pain perception is through effects on prostaglandins.

46. **c**
    Application and concept identification
    Rationale: The question uses a comparison or contrast structure to define health as the ability to use feedback mechanisms allowing the body to adapt to stress and to restore itself.

47. **d**
    Factual recall
    Rationale: The question is a definition of the general adaptation syndrome.

48. **b**
    Application and concept identification
    Rationale: The hypothalamus is the first responder to the perception of threat, and then the hypothalamus releases corticotropin-releasing hormones.

49. **a**
    Factual recall
    Rationale: The only term listed in the answer that relates to breathing is hyperventilation syndrome, which is a common functional disturbance of the stress response.

50. **b**
    Application and concept identification
    Rationale: All of the answers except b indicate an increase in the stress response instead of a method to manage stress.

51. **c**
    Factual recall
    Rationale: The very young and the old are not as able to maintain homeostasis, whereas young adults and those in the middle of life are the most able to stay healthy.

52. **c**
    Concept identification
    Rationale: If massage caused a decrease in blood pressure, it would be a negative feedback response. Virulence relates to pathogens, not blood pressure. A fistula is a result of chronic inflammation.

53. **b**
    Concept identification
    Rationale: Entrainment concerns body rhythms, general adaptation syndrome relates to the stress response, and *threshold* and *tolerance* are terms that describe aspects of pain. Only feedback loop addresses the information in the question.

54. **a**

    Concept identification
    Rationale: Specifically, hypnosis and medication are not within the scope of practice of massage, and none of the terms is a risk factor. These methods are not specific for treating inflammation.

55. **b**

    Clinical reasoning and synthesis
    Rationale: The main strategy for creating the wrong answers is to misuse the terminology or combine unrelated information or to reverse the meaning. Answer a: There is no such thing as a stress threshold straining, and cortisol is usually an immune suppressant. Answer c: The client's adaptive capacity is inadequate, and the client's stress levels, including age, decrease adaptive capacity.

56. **d**

    Concept identification
    Rationale: The listed terms are symptoms. They do not necessarily involve inflammation, and they are not necessarily genetic.

CHAPTER

3
Medical Terminology

Review Tips

The content about medical terminology is all about language. When studying, you must memorize all of the lists of prefixes, root words, and suffixes that combine to make medical terms—just like sounding out words using phonics. If you know what the parts mean, you can decipher what the word means. The textbook *Mosby's Essential Sciences for Therapeutic Massage* also includes Eastern and Asian terminology in the content area. Chapter 3 in *Mosby's Essential Sciences for Therapeutic Massage* and *Mosby's Fundamentals of Therapeutic Massage* discusses medical terminology. This is another area where you just have to memorize the language. Again, use the study aids in this text, read glossaries, and look up words you do not understand. It may be helpful to obtain a medical terminology textbook and use it as a self-teaching tool.

Elsevier has many medical terminology and dictionaries from which to choose:
- LaFleur Brooks M: *Exploring medical language: a student-directed approach*, ed 6, St Louis, 2005, Mosby.
- Chabner DE: *The language of medicine*, ed 7, St Louis, 2004, WB Saunders.
- Jonas WB: *Mosby's dictionary of complementary and alternative medicine*, St Louis, 2005, Mosby.
- Miller-Keane O'Toole MT: *Miller-Keane encyclopedia & dictionary of medicine, nursing & allied health*—revised reprint, ed 7, Philadelphia, 2005, WB Saunders.
- *Mosby's medical, nursing, & allied health dictionary—revised reprint*, ed 6, St Louis, 2005, Mosby.

Questions

1. A prefix, root, or suffix is based on Latin or Greek _____.
   a. Grammar
   b. Basic word meaning
   c. Word elements
   d. Sentence structure

2. The prefix auto- means _____.
   a. Self
   b. Hear
   c. Against
   d. Both sides

3. The prefix meaning against or opposite is _____.
   a. Circum-
   b. Caud-
   c. Contra-
   d. Brach-

4. The prefix mal- means _____.
   a. Large
   b. One or single
   c. Form or shape
   d. Illness or disease

5. The prefix for hard is _____.
   a. Schist(o)-
   b. Sepsi-
   c. Scler(o)-
   d. Kyph(o)-

6. The root word pneum(o)- means _____.
   a. Vein
   b. Lung or gas
   c. Chest
   d. Breathing

7. The root word for kidney is _____.
   a. Nephr(o)-
   b. Neur(o)-
   c. Uro-
   d. Phleb(o)-

8. The suffix for pain is _____.
   a. -asis
   b. -ase
   c. -algia
   d. -emia

9. The suffix -pnea means _____.
   a. To breathe
   b. Paralysis
   c. Putrefaction
   d. Little

10. The use of abbreviations in charting _____.
   a. Is universally understood
   b. Is more time consuming
   c. Requires a deciphering key
   d. Clearly communicates information

11. The ability to think through and justify an intervention process is called _____.
   a. History taking
   b. Assessment
   c. Database collection
   d. Clinical reasoning

12. The history-taking interview provides data for which part of the SOAP note charting process?
   a. Subjective data
   b. Objective data
   c. Analysis
   d. Plan

13. The aspect of the physical assessment that identifies altered movement patterns is _____.
   a. Visual assessment
   b. Functional assessment
   c. Palpation assessment
   d. Objective assessment

14. Physical assessment provides data for which SOAP charting area?
   a. Subjective data
   b. Objective data
   c. Analysis
   d. Plan

15. For the data collected during the interview process and physical assessment to be focused to a particular outcome for the client, the information must be _____.
   a. Recorded in a SOAP note
   b. Communicated to the client
   c. Analyzed using a logical process
   d. Written in medical terminology

16. Referral to another health care professional is based on which part of the clinical reasoning process?
   a. Assessment of data
   b. Data collection
   c. Plan development
   d. History interview

17. The head, neck, trunk, and spinal cord are considered to be _____.
   a. Appendicular
   b. Thoracic
   c. Axial
   d. Ventral

18. The bladder is located in which region of the abdomen?

    a. Epigastric
    b. Umbilical
    c. Left iliac
    d. Hypogastric

19. The liver is located in which quadrant?

    a. Right upper
    b. Left upper
    c. Right lower
    d. Left lower

20. Which movement decreases the angle of a joint?

    a. Flexion
    b. Extension
    c. Retraction
    d. Adduction

21. The term meaning on the same side is _____.

    a. Lateral
    b. Contralateral
    c. Ipsilateral
    d. Dextral

22. The term meaning closer to the trunk or point of origin is _____.

    a. Anterior
    b. Posterior
    c. Distal
    d. Proximal

23. Many ancient healing practices were developed based on _____.

    a. Measurement of concrete functions
    b. Experiential observation
    c. Scientific methods
    d. Meridian system

24. A commonality of the point phenomena is _____.

    a. All points are located over motor points
    b. All refer pain patterns
    c. They are located over A delta and C afferent nerve fibers
    d. They are located in meridian pathways

25. The cutaneous/visceral reflexes are correlated with which Chinese medicine concept?

    a. Essential substances
    b. Pernicious influences
    c. Organ systems
    d. Five elements

26. What do the following have in common: circum-, andro-, and steno-?

    a. Root words
    b. Prefixes
    c. Suffixes
    d. Abbreviations

27. A massage therapist identified a tense muscle in the occipital area. Where is this location?

    a. Leg
    b. Ankle
    c. Neck
    d. Arm

28. During assessment, the client appears twisted. Which of the following would be the most accurate statement?

    a. The client has frontal plane distortion.
    b. The client is rotated in the transverse plane.
    c. The client cannot abduct in the sagittal plane.
    d. Flexion and extension are limited in the transverse plane.

29. A client has been treated for circulatory system dysfunction. Which of the following would be the correct term to use to describe this area?

    a. Jing
    b. Cun
    c. Si shi
    d. Xue

30. A client is crying easily and is grieving over the death of a pet. He is also anxious about a job change. Which of the five elements do these symptoms indicate as out of balance?

    a. Earth
    b. Metal
    c. Water
    d. Heart

Correct answers are on pages 35-36.

Exercise

Using the foregoing questions as examples, now write at least three more questions—one of each type: factual recall and comprehension, application and concept identification, and clinical reasoning and synthesis. Make sure to develop plausible wrong answers, and be sure that the correct answer is clearly correct. Then write a rationale for each question. The more questions you write, the better you will understand the material.

Answers and Discussion

1. **c**
   Factual recall
   Rationale: The question is a definition.

2. **a**
   Factual recall
   Rationale: The question is a definition and is representative of this type of question. Any of the word elements can appear in a question structure; therefore you need to understand all of them.

3. **c**
   Factual recall
   Rationale: The question is a definition and is representative of this type of question. Any of the word elements can appear in a question structure; therefore you need to understand all of them.

4. **d**
   Factual recall
   Rationale: The question is a definition and is representative of this type of question. Any of the word elements can appear in a question structure; therefore you need to understand all of them.

5. **c**
   Factual recall
   Rationale: The question is a definition and is representative of this type of question. Any of the word elements can appear in a question structure; therefore you need to understand all of them.

6. **b**
   Factual recall
   Rationale: The question is a definition and is representative of this type of question. Any of the word elements can appear in a question structure; therefore you need to understand all of them.

7. **a**
   Factual recall
   Rationale: The question is a definition and is representative of this type of question. Any of the word elements can appear in a question structure; therefore you need to understand all of them.

8. **c**
   Factual recall
   Rationale: The question is a definition and is representative of this type of question. Any of the word elements can appear in a question structure; therefore you need to understand all of them.

9. **a**
   Factual recall
   Rationale: The question is a definition and is representative of this type of question. Any of the word elements can appear in a question structure; therefore you need to understand all of them.

10. **c**
    Application and concept identification
    Rationale: Whenever nonstandard abbreviations are used, a deciphering key is necessary.

11. **d**
    Factual recall
    Rationale: The question is a definition of clinical reasoning.

12. **a**
    Factual recall
    Rationale: The question is a definition of subjective data.

13. **b**
    Factual recall
    Rationale: The question is a definition of functional assessment. As in all questions, it is important to define all terms to analyze information properly for the correct answer.

14. **b**
    Factual recall
    Rationale: The question is a definition of objective data.

15. **c**
    Factual recall
    Rationale: The question is a definition of analysis.

16. **c**
    Factual recall
    Rationale: The question is representative of information in a plan.

17. **c**
    Factual recall
    Rationale: The question is a list of structures in the axial area.

18. **d**
    Factual recall
    Rationale: The question is representative of information about the structural plan of the body.
19. **a**
    Factual recall
    Rationale: The question is representative of information about the structural plan of the body.
20. **a**
    Factual recall
    Rationale: The question is representative of information about the movement of the body.
21. **c**
    Factual recall
    Rationale: The question is representative of information about the directional terms.
22. **d**
    Factual recall
    Rationale: The question is representative of information about the directional terms.
23. **b**
    Application and concept identification
    Rationale: Accumulated experience provided the base for consistent patterns observed by ancient healers.
24. **c**
    Factual recall
    Rationale: The question is representative of information that correlates Eastern theory with Western science. Many different systems evolved a point theory, and the location of these points consistently falls over nerves and sensory receptors.

25. **c**
    Application and concept identification
    Rationale: The three incorrect answers describe Chinese concepts that are not related to the cutaneous/visceral reflexes. Only answer c is logical if the definitions of essential substances, pernicious influences, and five-elements theory are understood. This question is representative of usage of Eastern terminology.
26. **b**
    Factual recall
    Rationale: They are prefixes.
27. **c**
    Factual recall
    Rationale: The occipital area is where the head joins the neck.
28. **b**
    Concept identification
    Rationale: Twisted would be a rotation, and rotation occurs in the transverse plane. Abduction does not occur in the sagittal plane, and flexion and extension are sagittal plane movements.
29. **d**
    Factual recall
    Rationale: Xue means the blood. Jing is the yin essence of life, cun is a measurement, and si shi is the four seasons.
30. **b**
    Factual recall
    Rationale: The question describes the extreme emotions of the metal element. Heart is not an element.

4
Nervous System Basics and the Central Nervous System

Review Tips

Research is identifying many interactions between massage and the nervous system. To understand the physiologic mechanisms of massage benefit, you must understand not just the terminology that is always important but the physiology as well. This is a different sort of study. Comprehension is necessary to appreciate how various aspects of the nervous system work together and how these functions affect massage. Comprehension is different from language. Studying for terminology/word definitions is like the ABCs. Comprehension is about how you recognize how the ABCs go together or form words that are symbols for meaning.

An effective study strategy is to explain a concept in words different from those in the text or to give an example of what the text is talking about or to develop a metaphor about the content. A metaphor is different from an example. A metaphor is more of a comparison. An example of a metaphor follows: Myelin is like the insulation around an electrical cord.

As for the previous sections, look up any terminology you do not understand and make sure you know why the wrong answers are wrong.

Review the content in the textbook that lists pathologic conditions relating to the body system and the related indications and contraindications for massage. Massage exams tend to target safe practice content. As a result, there is an emphasis on the appropriateness of massage for various pathologic conditions.

Questions

1. Which of the following is a principle of quantum physics?

   a. Predicts events
   b. Can be pictured
   c. Describes statistical behavior of systems and groups
   d. Holds that we can observe something without changing it

2. The nervous system and the endocrine system reflect quantum properties because _____.

   a. Predictable physiologic outcomes are constant
   b. Feedback loops reliably effect outcomes
   c. Linear pathways of affect are constant
   d. Tendency for response is most accurate

3. A function of neuroglia is to _____.

   a. Transmit signals to the cell body
   b. Carry signals away from the cell body
   c. Conduct signals from one neuron to another
   d. Support and protect neurons

4. Neurilemma is formed by _____.

   a. Schwann cells
   b. Myelin
   c. Dendrites
   d. Axons

Correct answers are on pages 43-45.

5. Neurons that conduct signals to the central nervous system are _____.

   a. Sensory neurons
   b. Motor neurons
   c. Interneurons
   d. Nodes of Ranvier

6. Sensory stimulation of massage causes a chemical change in neurons called _____.

   a. Action potential
   b. Refractory period
   c. Depolarization
   d. Saltatory conduction

7. When a neuron is positively charged on the outside of the cell membrane and negatively charged on the inside, it has _____.

   a. Saltatory conduction
   b. Membrane potential
   c. Action potential
   d. Refractory potential

8. Which phase of nerve signal conduction is related to muscle energy methods of massage that use some sort of muscle contraction to prepare the muscle to relax and lengthen?

   a. Action potential
   b. Refractory period
   c. Depolarization
   d. Saltatory conduction

9. Nerve axon repair in the peripheral nervous system is produced by _____.

   a. Oligodendrocytes
   b. Synaptic vesicles
   c. Neurilemma
   d. Endoplasmic reticulum

10. Action potential between neurons occurs across the synaptic cleft because of _____.

    a. Neurotransmitters
    b. Post-synaptic membrane
    c. Anterograde transport
    d. Nodes of Ranvier

11. The neurotransmitter that primarily excites the skeletal muscles is _____.

    a. Dopamine
    b. Acetylcholine
    c. Cholecystokinin
    d. Somatostatin

12. A person is clumsy and has a dull or foggy mind in terms of understanding information and making decisions. Which of the following neurotransmitters may be involved?

    a. Norepinephrine
    b. Histamine
    c. Glutamate
    d. Dopamine

13. Neurotransmitters work in excitatory and inhibitory pairs. Which of the following would provide a balancing action for enkephalin?

    a. Somatostatin
    b. Substance P
    c. Serotonin
    d. GABA (gamma-aminobutyric acid)

14. A massage client reports that after the massage she had some itchy areas of skin. Her clothes felt rough against her skin. Which neurotransmitter may be involved?

    a. Histamine
    b. Acetylcholine
    c. Epinephrine
    d. Cholecystokinin

15. A client reports before the massage that his mind is agitated. He feels like he wants to scream. He is talking loudly and pacing. After the massage, he feels calmer and wants a nap. Which neurotransmitter is largely responsible for the mood change?

    a. Norepinephrine
    b. Dopamine
    c. Serotonin
    d. Substance P

16. The purpose of therapeutic (feel good) pain during massage to manage undesirable pain is to stimulate which neurotransmitters?

    a. Serotonin and endorphin
    b. Epinephrine and histamine
    c. Acetylcholine and dopamine
    d. Histamine and substance P

17. The portion of the brain that interprets sensory data and compares it against past memories and experiences is the _____.

    a. Ventricles
    b. Pineal body
    c. Cerebrum
    d. Temporal lobe

18. The structure that connects the right and left hemispheres of the cerebrum is the _____.

    a. Basal ganglia
    b. Sulcus
    c. Corpus callosum
    d. Longitudinal fissure

19. The primary area of the brain that would process the pain/pleasure aspect of massage is the _____.

    a. Frontal lobe
    b. Parietal lobe
    c. Temporal lobe
    d. Occipital lobe

20. Activities that occur in the cerebrum after sensory signals are received and before motor responses are sent are called _____.

    a. Integrative functions
    b. Convolutions
    c. Inhibitory functions
    d. Activating systems

21. Conscious awareness of our environment is related to what structural and functional area of the brain?

    a. Primary motor cortex
    b. Reticular activating system
    c. Sensory associate cortex
    d. Temporal pole

22. The area of the brain responsible for motor sequencing, posture in relationship to the environment, and processing spatial relations is the _____.

    a. Limbic lobes
    b. Temporal lobes
    c. Frontal lobes
    d. Parietal lobes

23. States of higher consciousness are related to _____.

    a. Alertness with relaxation
    b. Decreased health states
    c. Increased sympathetic arousal
    d. Depression with pain

24. Uncontrolled emotional display may indicate problems with what brain area?

    a. Basal ganglia
    b. Left hemisphere of the cerebrum
    c. Limbic system
    d. Primary motor area

25. Why do the primary motor and the primary somesthetic sensory areas of the brain interfere with the ability successfully to self-massage areas of the back and limbs?

    a. The largest sensory and motor awareness is in these areas.
    b. The distribution of sensory and motor function to the hands is too small to stimulate sensation.
    c. The distribution of sensory and motor function is larger to the hands than to the back and limbs.
    d. The back and limbs have a predominance of sensory distribution over the motor distribution of the hands.

26. Protein synthesis and physical brain changes in the temporal lobes support long-term memory with _____.

    a. State-dependent memory
    b. Engrams
    c. Pleasure states
    d. Entrainment

27. Which of the following drugs is a central nervous system depressant?

    a. Cocaine
    b. Caffeine
    c. Alcohol
    d. Amphetamines

28. Which brain area functions to regulate vital life functions such as heart rate, blood pressure, and breathing?

    a. Midbrain
    b. Pons
    c. Cerebellum
    d. Medulla oblongata

29. Pleasure states experienced during massage that support mind-body health are processed in what area of the diencephalon?

    a. Thalamus
    b. Pineal body
    c. Meninges
    d. Midbrain

30. A massage session that incorporates rocking affects the vestibular system, including labyrinthine righting reflexes. Which brain area also is stimulated to coordinate appropriate posture?

    a. Cerebellum
    b. Pons
    c. Motor descending tracts
    d. Sensory ascending tracts

31. The protective membrane that adheres to the brain is the _____.

    a. Dura mater
    b. Arachnoid mater
    c. Epidural mater
    d. Pia mater

32. Massage sensations travel on which spinal cord tracts?

    a. Sensory ascending tracts
    b. Motor descending tracts
    c. Corticospinal tracts
    d. Lateral reticulospinal tracts

33. In which pathologic process would massage be most beneficial in assisting in the movement of body fluids?

    a. Upper motor neuron injury
    b. Lower motor neuron injury
    c. Aneurysm
    d. Chorea

34. Research indicates that massage increases the availability of the following neurotransmitters: norepinephrine, serotonin, and dopamine. Which central nervous system disorder would be most benefited by massage?

    a. Stroke
    b. Cerebral palsy
    c. Depression
    d. Schizophrenia

35. A client has essential tremor. Which of the following is most correct?

    a. Stress reduction massage would have a significant effect.
    b. Massage will have little effect.
    c. Massage with medication should reverse the condition.
    d. The associated headache is reduced by massage.

36. A client has a spinal cord injury resulting in paralysis but can walk with difficulty. Which of the following is the most correct statement?

    a. The client has monoplegia.
    b. The client has paraplegia.
    c. The client has quadriplegia.
    d. Amyotrophic lateral sclerosis

37. A client fell and sustained a hit to the head. The client was a bit confused at the time and the next day had a headache. Which of the following is the most accurate description of the client's condition?

    a. An aneurysm
    b. A severe contusion
    c. A transient ischemic attack
    d. A mild concussion

38. Which of the following is most involved in pain mechanisms?

    a. Histamine
    b. Substance P
    c. Acetylcholine
    d. Cholecystokinin

39. A medication that would stimulate epinephrine also could result in _____?

    a. Enhanced sleep
    b. Weakening of skeletal muscles
    c. An increase in serotonin
    d. An increase in dopamine

Correct answers are on pages 43-45.

Exercise

Using the foregoing questions as examples, now write at least three more questions—one of each type: factual recall comprehension, application and concept identification, and clinical reasoning and synthesis. Make sure to develop plausible wrong answers, and be sure that the correct answer is clearly correct. Then write a rationale for each question. The more questions you write, the better you will understand the material.

Answers and Discussion

1. **c**
   Factual recall
   Rationale: The question is a definition of quantum physics.

2. **d**
   Application and concept identification
   Rationale: The physiology of these two systems of control is best described in view of quantum mechanics.

3. **d**
   Factual recall
   Rationale: The correct answer is a primary function of this specialized connective tissue. The three wrong answers describe other nervous system function.

4. **a**
   Factual recall
   Rationale: Myelin, dendrites, and axons do not form or secrete any substance. Only Schwann cells form myelin and its outer covering called the neurilemma.

5. **a**
   Factual recall
   Rationale: The question is a definition of sensory neurons. To answer this question, you must know the definitions of all of the terms.

6. **c**
   Application and concept identification
   Rationale: To answer the question, you need to understand how nerve conduction functions. Some of these functions are listed in the possible answers. The question asks how massage causes the neuron to transmit a signal. A stimulus such as the pressure of massage causes a change in the charge of one segment of a neuron. This is depolarization.

7. **b**
   Factual recall
   Rationale: The question is the definition of membrane potential when the nerve is at rest.

8. **b**
   Application and concept identification
   Rationale: The question is asking for a connection to the application of a bodywork method: muscle energy when a muscle uses contraction to initiate relaxation. The refractory period occurs after a nerve transmission. During this time, the nerve does not readily respond to stimuli, allowing the muscle it controls to be lengthened.

9. **c**
   Factual recall
   Rationale: The question describes a function of neurilemma. You must define all the terms in the question and answers to answer the question correctly.

10. **a**
    Factual recall
    Rationale: The question describes a function of neurotransmitters. You must define all the terms in the question and answers to answer the question correctly.

11. **b**
    Factual recall
    Rationale: The question describes a function of acetylcholine. You must define all the terms in the question and answers to answer the question correctly.

12. **d**
    Application and concept identification
    Rationale: The question describes a function of dopamine in relationship to behavior. You must define all the terms in the question and answers to answer the question correctly.

13. **b**
    Application and concept identification
    Rationale: The question provides half of a balancing pair of neurotransmitters. You must define all the terms in the question and answers to answer the question correctly. Enkephalin inhibits pain signals, and substance P transmits pain signals.

14. **a**
    Application and concept identification
    Rationale: The question describes a function of histamine in relationship to behavior. You must define all the terms in the question and answers to answer the question correctly.

15. **c**
    Application and concept identification
    Rationale: The question describes a function of serotonin in relationship to behavior and in response to massage. You must define all the terms in the question and answers to answer the question correctly.

16. **a**
Application and concept identification
Rationale: The question describes a function of serotonin and endorphin in relationship to massage applications. You must define all the terms in the question and answers to answer the question correctly.

17. **c**
Factual recall
Rationale: The question describes a function of the cerebrum. You must define all the terms in the question and answers to answer the question correctly.

18. **c**
Factual recall
Rationale: The question describes the location of the corpus callosum. You must define all the terms in the question and answers to answer the question correctly.

19. **b**
Factual recall
Rationale: The question describes a function of the parietal lobe. You must define all the terms in the question and answers to answer the question correctly.

20. **a**
Factual recall
Rationale: The question describes integrative functions of the cortex. You must define all the terms in the question and answers and know the function of the cerebrum to answer the question correctly.

21. **b**
Factual recall
Rationale: The question describes a function of the reticular activating system. You must define all the terms in the question and answers to answer the question correctly.

22. **d**
Factual recall
Rationale: The question describes a function of parietal lobes in the brain. You must define all the terms in the question and answers to answer the question correctly.

23. **a**
Application and concept identification
Rationale: The question asks for an application of central nervous system functions. Only the correct answer is reasonable in relation to the concept of higher consciousness.

24. **c**
Factual recall
Rationale: The question describes a function of the limbic system. You must define all the terms in the question and answers to answer the question correctly.

25. **c**
Application and concept identification
Rationale: The question asks for an application of central nervous system function and an interpretation of sensory perception based on sensory and motor distribution in these areas of the brain. Only the correct answer explains the reason for self-massage being less than successful.

26. **b**
Factual recall
Rationale: The question describes creation of long-term memory. You must define all the terms in the question and answers to answer the question correctly.

27. **c**
Factual recall
Rationale: The question describes substances that affect the central nervous system. You must define all the terms in the question and answers to answer the question correctly.

28. **d**
Factual recall
Rationale: The question describes a function of the medulla oblongata. You must define all the terms in the question and answers to answer the question correctly.

29. **a**
Factual recall
Rationale: The question describes a function of the thalamus. You must define all the terms in the question and answers to answer the question correctly.

30. **a**
Factual recall
Rationale: The question describes a function of the cerebellum. You must define all the terms in the question and answers to answer the question correctly.

31. **d**
Factual recall
Rationale: The question describes the location of the pia mater. You must define all the terms in the question and answers to answer the question correctly. The epidural mater is an incorrect use of terms and does not exist.

32. **a**
    Application and concept identification
    Rationale: The question is asking for an understanding of how sensory signals of massage are processed. You must define all the terms in the question and answers to answer the question correctly.

33. **b**
    Application and concept identification
    Rationale: The question is asking for an understanding of how massage may be indicated for pathologic conditions of the central nervous system. You must define all the terms in the question and answers to answer the question correctly. Once you understand the disease processes, then you can decide which one would require assistance in moving fluids in the body. Lower motor neuron injury results in flaccid muscles, and the pumping action of muscles to assist fluid movement is lost.

34. **c**
    Application and concept identification
    Rationale: The question is asking for an understanding of how massage may be indicated for pathologic conditions of the central nervous system. You must define all the terms in the question and answers to answer the question correctly. Once you understand the disease processes, then you can decide which one would respond best to a change in neurotransmitters. Depression may respond to an increase in the availability of the neurotransmitters described in the question. Schizophrenia may temporarily worsen. The other two are not linked directly to neurotransmitters.

35. **b**
    Concept identification
    Rationale: Essential tremor does not result from a pathologic condition and is not affected by massage.

36. **a**
    Concept identification
    Rationale: Because only one limb is effective in monoplegia, walking could be possible. Answers b and c would limit the ability to walk, and answer d is not a spinal cord injury.

37. **d**
    Concept identification
    Rationale: An aneurysm is a bulging artery. A contusion is a bruise that the client could have, but the symptoms indicate a concussion. Answer c is a stroke.

38. **b**
    Factual recall
    Rationale: Substance P increases pain transmission.

39. **d**
    Concept identification
    Rationale: Epinephrine is a central nervous system stimulant. So sleep would be disturbed, skeletal system would be tense, and there would be a decrease in serotonin. Dopamine is also a stimulant.

5
Peripheral Nervous System

Review Tips

The content concerning the peripheral nervous system is more concrete than the previous section. The terminology is important as always. Massage interacts extensively with the peripheral nervous system by introducing various stimuli that target sensory receptors. How these stimuli are introduced and how the body processes them through feedback mechanisms provide many of the benefits of massage. Because of this, the content may appear in questions that are about massage benefits or describe how massage methods are applied. Questions are often of the concept identification type. An effective study approach in addition to reading glossaries and looking up the definition of terms is to list each of the massage methods and techniques and then describe how they are used to influence the peripheral nervous system.

Review the content in your textbook that lists pathologic conditions relating to the body system and the related indications and contraindications for massage. Massage exams tend to target safe practice content. As a result, there is an emphasis on the appropriateness of massage for various pathologic conditions.

Questions

1. Peripheral nerves that innervate the muscles and skin are known as _____.

    a. Visceral
    b. Afferent
    c. Somatic
    d. Thermal

2. A bundle of axons and dendrites that carries sensory or motor signals is called a _____.

    a. Neuron
    b. Nerve
    c. Dermatome
    d. Plexus

3. The connective tissue covering that surrounds the fasciculus is called _____.

    a. Endoneurium
    b. Epineurium
    c. Perineurium
    d. Meninges

4. What cranial nerve affects visceral function?

    a. Vagus nerve
    b. Hypoglossal
    c. Trigeminal
    d. Trochlear

5. The dorsal root ganglion contains cell bodies of _____.

    a. Sensory neurons
    b. Motor neurons
    c. Mixed nerves
    d. Cranial nerves

6. The phrenic nerve is part of which plexus?

    a. Cervical
    b. Brachial
    c. Lumbar
    d. Sacral

7. If a client complains of pain in the skin areas of the buttocks and into the lateral side of the leg, which plexus is a potential site of nerve impingement?

    a. Cervical
    b. Brachial
    c. Lumbar
    d. Sacral

8. Pain, tingling, and numbness in the arm and hand may result from nerve damage in which plexus?

    a. Cervical
    b. Brachial
    c. Lumbar
    d. Sacral

9. The obturator nerve is found in which plexus?

    a. Cervical
    b. Brachial
    c. Lumbar
    d. Sacral

10. During massage, pain that is not related to specific symptoms radiates around the ear. This indicates excessive pressure on which nerve?

    a. Greater auricular
    b. Thoracodorsal
    c. Medial cutaneous
    d. Pudendal

11. A client complains of pain in the region of the low back and buttocks. Which dermatome nerve distribution might indicate where the nerve impingement is located?

    a. C7
    b. T2
    c. C6
    d. L2

12. During the history interview, a client reports that she almost fell down stairs but caught herself and was able to regain her balance. What type of reflex action was required to accomplish this?

    a. Monosynaptic
    b. Polysynaptic
    c. Patellar
    d. Pacinian

13. Changes in blood pressure are monitored by _____.

    a. Exteroceptors
    b. Proprioceptors
    c. Visceroceptors
    d. Nociceptors

14. Reflexes most often are processed in which part of the central nervous system?

    a. Cerebrum
    b. Ventricles
    c. Dura
    d. Spinal cord

15. A client is complaining of difficulty hitting a golf ball and describes a sense of timing being off. This could be a result of a disruption in what type of reflex?

    a. Conditioned reflex
    b. Tendon reflex
    c. Stretch reflex
    d. Mono reflex

16. A client is having difficulty being comfortable with the touch of draping material during the massage. He says that he cannot get used to the scratchy feeling. The client may be displaying a reduced ability of sensory receptors to _____.

    a. Send impulses
    b. Adapt to sensation
    c. Remain monosynaptic
    d. Initiate reciprocal inhibition

17. The sensory receptors most affected by deep compression and slow gliding strokes are _____.

    a. Pacinian corpuscles
    b. Root hair plexuses
    c. Merkel's disks
    d. Ruffini's end organs

18. Which of the following receptors is most likely to adapt and cease responding to the sustained compression during massage on one specific area of the body?

    a. Meissner's corpuscles
    b. Thermal receptors
    c. Intrafusal fibers
    d. Nociceptors

19. Mechanical receptors that provide us with information about position and movement are _____.

    a. Reciprocal inhibition
    b. Thermal receptors
    c. Proprioceptors
    d. Externoreceptors

20. A compressive massage method is applied to the belly of a muscle with the intent of reducing a muscle spasm brought on by a cramp. The receptors most affected are _____.

    a. Joint kinesthetic
    b. Golgi tendon organ
    c. Muscle spindles
    d. Meissner's corpuscles

21. As slow, deep effleurage is applied to the left upper thigh, the practitioner notices and the client describes a twitching of the muscles in the back of the opposite leg. What type of reflex has been stimulated?

    a. Stretch reflex
    b. Tendon reflex
    c. Ipsilateral reflex
    d. Contralateral reflex

22. The portion of the autonomic nervous system that supports energy conservation is _____.

    a. Parasympathetic
    b. Peripheral
    c. Somatic
    d. Sympathetic

23. The thoracolumbar division of the autonomic nervous system contains ganglia located _____.

    a. Near the spine
    b. At the effector organs
    c. In the spinal column
    d. In the cranial and sacral areas

24. A client reports being prone to headaches from being in bright light. Bright light has been a problem only in the last few weeks. The client also reports an increase in workload. What might be the function of the autonomic nervous system that could be responsible for the sensitivity to light?

    a. Parasympathetic dilation of the pupil
    b. Sympathetic dilation of the pupil
    c. Parasympathetic contraction of the pupil
    d. Sympathetic contraction of the pupil

25. A client requests an outcome from the massage session that includes a good night's sleep and less fidgeting. The massage session then would need to be designed to accomplish what?

    a. Cranial sacral plexus inhibition
    b. Parasympathetic inhibition
    c. Sympathetic inhibition
    d. Sympathetic dominance

26. The release of epinephrine into the system is called _____.

    a. Parasympathetic dominance
    b. Adrenergic stimulation
    c. Sympathetic inhibition
    d. Parasympathetic facilitation

27. The primary neurotransmitter of the parasympathetic system is _____.

    a. Acetylcholine
    b. Epinephrine
    c. Norepinephrine
    d. Adrenaline

28. The sympathetic chain ganglia are located in an area similar to the back-shu points on which meridian?

    a. Spleen
    b. Kidney
    c. Liver
    d. Bladder

29. Acupuncture points often are located in the same area as _____.

    a. Motor points
    b. Synapse
    c. Root hair plexus
    d. Myotomes

30. Research seems to indicate that one of the most noticeable beneficial effects of acupuncture is that it produces what physiologic response?

    a. Parasympathetic inhibition
    b. Sympathetic inhibition
    c. Inhibition of endorphins
    d. Sympathetic facilitation

31. Which of the following physiologic effects do massage and acupuncture share?

    a. Increases sympathetic arousal
    b. Decreases levels of endorphins
    c. Blocks release of substance P
    d. Decreases parasympathetic arousal

32. A client appears particularly agitated during the initial history interview. What is the best voice pattern to use to calm the client and best ensure that the client understands you?

    a. A slow high pitch
    b. A fast deep pitch
    c. A slow deep pitch
    d. A fast deep pitch

33. The bones in the ear that respond to vibration of the tympanic membrane are called _____.

    a. Pinna
    b. Ossicles
    c. Cochlea
    d. Corti

34. The massage method that most affects the inner ear balance mechanisms is _____.

    a. Tapotement
    b. Compression
    c. Friction
    d. Rocking

35. When vision records a change in the environment, it causes a signal to be sent to which part of the brain?

    a. Frontal lobe
    b. Cerebellum
    c. Ventricles
    d. Sulcus

36. Righting reflexes combine information from vision and the vestibular mechanisms to maintain _____.

    a. Baroreceptors
    b. Equilibrium
    c. Sclera
    d. Vertigo

37. A client indicates in the history interview that he is prone to motion sickness. Which massage methods should be avoided?

    a. Active joint movement
    b. Stretching
    c. Rocking
    d. Compression

38. Which of the following senses exerts the strongest influence on the emotional limbic system?

    a. Smell
    b. Taste
    c. Hearing
    d. Sight

39. Which of the following is a structure of the nose?

    a. Ciliary body
    b. Canthus
    c. Turbinate
    d. Sclera

40. A client complains of radiating pain down the arm into the elbow and fingers. The client has not been evaluated by a physician, so a referral is indicated. Which diagnosis by the physician would be most helped by massage?

    a. Guillain-Barré syndrome
    b. Brachial plexus entrapment
    c. Cervical plexus compression
    d. Osteoporosis

41. A client reports having herpes zoster and is experiencing pain. Which of the following would be the best massage approach?

    a. A full-body, 1-hour massage with attention to universal precautions that uses tapotement, active joint movement, and fractioning methods
    b. A full-body massage lasting $1^1/_2$ hours that avoids the area of the rash and that actively engages the client in muscle energy lengthening and stretching
    c. A seated massage that lasts for 15 minutes
    d. A full-body, 1-hour massage that avoids the area of the rash with attention to universal precautions and a focus toward relaxation

42. A client seeks massage after a diagnosis of neuralgia in the left leg. Which of the following would be a realistic therapeutic massage outcome?

    a. Reduction of pain and regeneration
    b. Long-term symptom decrease
    c. Short-term pain management
    d. Short-term regeneration

43. A client is complaining of a recent inability to sleep and a feeling of agitation and reports concern over a change in management systems at work. The physician diagnosis was exogenous anxiety. Which of the following treatment plans is most appropriate?

    a. Mild exercise program, therapeutic massage, and a medication such as imipramine to control symptoms
    b. A hypoventilation syndrome management program including massage and chiropractic manipulation
    c. A mild exercise program, cognitive behavioral therapy, short-term use of diazepam, and relaxation massage
    d. Therapeutic massage, meditation, increase in caffeine consumption, and bed rest

44. A client is experiencing radiating pain in the abdomen and the buttocks. Which of the following is the most correct statement?

    a. The femoral nerve in the sacral plexus is impinged.
    b. The client has compression of the thoracodorsal nerve.
    c. The client's symptoms involve the lumbar plexus.
    d. The client's symptoms involve the brachial plexus.

45. Which of the following best responds to massage methods that move the joints?

    a. Free nerve endings
    b. Dermatomes
    c. Thermal receptors
    d. Proprioceptors

46. During assessment, the massage therapist notices that the client has dilated pupils. What would be the most logical cause of this condition?

    a. The client is experiencing sympathetic dominance.
    b. The client is experiencing parasympathetic dominance.
    c. The client has a somatic dysfunction.
    d. The accessory nerve is damaged.

47. A client is very sensitive to scent and can get anxious if the smell of something is not pleasing. Which of the following explains this reaction?

    a. Smell is controlled by the vagus nerve.
    b. Smell is an aspect of the limbic system.
    c. Smell affects the back-shu points.
    d. Smell is a vestibular process.

48. Which of the following are viral diseases of the nervous system?

    a. Herpes and vertigo
    b. Polio and neuralgia
    c. Entrapment and herpes
    d. Herpes and polio

Exercise

Using the foregoing questions as examples, now write at least three more questions—one of each type: factual recall and comprehension, application and concept identification, and clinical reasoning and synthesis. Make sure to develop plausible wrong answers, and be sure that the correct answer is clearly correct. Then write a rationale for each question. The more questions you write, the better you will understand the material.

Correct answers are on pages 54-57.

Answers and Discussion

1. **c**
   Factual recall
   Rationale: The question is a definition of somatic nerves.

2. **b**
   Factual recall
   Rationale: The question is a definition of nerves.

3. **c**
   Factual recall
   Rationale: The question uses terminology that would have to be defined to identify the correct answer.

4. **a**
   Factual recall
   Rationale: The question is representative of cranial nerve function. All of the functions of cranial nerves would be needed to answer the question correctly.

5. **a**
   Factual recall
   Rationale: The question is representative of peripheral nervous system anatomy. A strong knowledge of the terminology and function of this anatomy would be needed to answer the question correctly.

6. **a**
   Factual recall
   Rationale: The question is representative of peripheral nervous system anatomy. A strong knowledge of the terminology and function of this anatomy would be needed to answer the question correctly.

7. **c**
   Application and concept identification
   Rationale: Answering this question depends on an understanding of peripheral nervous system anatomy. Symptoms indicate that the lumbar plexus is involved.

8. **b**
   Application and concept identification
   Rationale: Answering this question depends on an understanding of peripheral nervous system anatomy. Symptoms indicate that the brachial plexus is involved.

9. **c**
   Factual recall
   Rationale: The question is representative of peripheral nervous system anatomy.

10. **a**
    Application and concept identification
    Rationale: Answering this question depends on an understanding of peripheral nervous system anatomy. Symptoms described in the question are from inappropriate pressure on the greater auricular nerve.

11. **d**
    Application and concept identification
    Rationale: Answering this question depends on an understanding of peripheral nervous system anatomy. Symptoms indicate that a range in dermatome distribution between L1 and L3 is likely. Answer d is the only answer that represents this area.

12. **b**
    Application and concept identification
    Rationale: Answering this question depends on an understanding of peripheral nervous system reflex functions. Also required is interpretation of the word elements. *Mono* means one, and *poly* means many. It takes many reflex actions to regain balance.

13. **c**
    Factual recall
    Rationale: The question is representative of peripheral nervous system function. A strong knowledge of the terminology would be needed to answer the question correctly. Blood pressure is monitored by visceroceptors that detect changes in the internal body environment.

14. **d**
    Factual recall
    Rationale: The question is representative of peripheral nervous system anatomy and physiology. A strong knowledge of the terminology and function of this anatomy would be needed to answer the question correctly. Most reflexes do not make their way past the brainstem, so the spinal cord is the correct answer.

15. **a**

    Clinical reasoning and synthesis
    Rationale: A decision based on factual data is
    required to answer the question correctly. The
    facts presented in the question indicate that the
    person has a learned training effect to golf.
    Coordination is disrupted, described as timing
    being off. Knowledge of the types of reflexes is
    necessary to choose the best answer. Golf is
    something learned, so the conditioned reflex is
    the best answer. Mono reflex does not exist. The
    tendon and stretch reflex are more involved in
    muscle tone.

16. **b**

    Application and concept identification
    Rationale: The question describes sensations
    that indicate that the client is not getting used to
    the draping material. The ability of the nervous
    system to adapt to sensation is what allows the
    body to tolerate ongoing sensation.

17. **d**

    Application and concept identification
    Rationale: The question is asking for a
    connection between massage methods that
    create deep compressive forces and the sensory
    receptor affected. This is important so that
    correct methods can be used to generate the
    type of sensation that specific receptors identify
    and to which they respond. Ruffini's end organs
    would respond to compressive force. The other
    mechanical sensory receptors listed respond
    more to light touch.

18. **a**

    Application and concept identification
    Rationale: The question is asking for a
    connection between massage methods that
    create deep compressive forces and the sensory
    receptor affected. This is important so that
    correct methods can be used to generate the
    type of sensation that specific receptors identify
    and to which they respond. Meissner's
    corpuscles adapt quickly.

19. **c**

    Factual recall
    Rationale: The question is representative of
    peripheral nervous system anatomy and
    physiology. A strong knowledge of the
    terminology and function of this anatomy would
    be needed to answer the question correctly. The
    question is the definition of a proprioceptor.

20. **c**

    Application and concept identification
    Rationale: The question is asking for a
    connection between massage methods that
    create compressive forces and the sensory
    receptor affected and location of that receptor.
    This is important so that correct methods can be
    used to generate the type of sensation that
    specific receptors identify and to which they
    respond. Muscle spindles are located primarily
    in the belly of the muscle and are active when a
    muscle cramps.

21. **d**

    Application and concept identification
    Rationale: The question is asking for a
    connection between massage methods and
    reflex responses. You must understand all the
    reflex patterns listed as possible answers.
    Because the question describes a pattern
    involving opposite sides of the body, the
    contralateral reflex is the correct answer.

22. **a**

    Factual recall
    Rationale: The question is representative of
    autonomic nervous system anatomy and
    physiology. A strong knowledge of the
    terminology and function of this anatomy would
    be needed to answer the question correctly. The
    question describes a function of the
    parasympathetic system.

23. **a**

    Factual recall
    Rationale: The question is representative of
    autonomic nervous system anatomy and
    physiology. A strong knowledge of the
    terminology and function of this anatomy would
    be needed to answer the question correctly. The
    question describes the location of sympathetic
    nerves and ganglia near the spine.

24. **b**

    Clinical reasoning and synthesis
    Rationale: The question presents a case that asks
    for a reason for light sensitivity combined with
    headache. You need to analyze the facts of the
    question. They are headache brought on by bright
    light, recent onset, and increased job stress. Next,
    you have to identify the various responses of the
    autonomic nervous system in relation to the facts.
    Increased workload is likely to stimulate
    sympathetic dominance. An effect of this is pupil
    dilation, which would increase light sensitivity.
    The incorrect answers do not describe correct
    function of the autonomic nervous system.

25. **c**
Application and concept identification
Rationale: The question is asking for a connection between massage methods and changes in the autonomic nervous system. You must understand all the reflex patterns listed as possible answers. Because the question describes a pattern of parasympathetic dominance, massage would have to be designed to inhibit sympathetic activation.

26. **b**
Factual recall
Rationale: The question is representative of autonomic nervous system physiology. A strong knowledge of the terminology and function of this physiology would be needed to answer the question correctly. The term *adrenergic* is used to describe sympathetic stimulation, and epinephrine is one of the neurotransmitters involved.

27. **a**
Factual recall
Rationale: The question is representative of autonomic nervous system physiology. A strong knowledge of the terminology and function of this physiology would be needed to answer the question correctly. The main neurotransmitter of the parasympathetic system is acetylcholine.

28. **d**
Application and concept identification
Rationale: The question is asking for a connection between the anatomy of the autonomic nervous system and the traditional meridian system.

29. **a**
Application and concept identification
Rationale: The question is asking for a connection between the anatomy of the peripheral nervous system and the traditional acupuncture system.

30. **b**
Application and concept identification
Rationale: The question is asking for a connection between the physiology of the autonomic nervous system and the traditional acupuncture system. When acupuncture is used, parasympathetic dominance usually is evident, so inhibition of the sympathetic functions also would be evident.

31. **c**
Application and concept identification
Rationale: The question is asking for a connection between massage effects, the physiology of the autonomic nervous system, and the traditional acupuncture system. Research indicates that massage and acupuncture inhibit substance P.

32. **c**
Application and concept identification
Rationale: The question is asking for a connection between the physiology of hearing and the use of voice tone. High-pitched, fast speaking indicates and can create sympathetic arousal. A slow deep pitch is more calming.

33. **b**
Factual recall
Rationale: Answering the question requires an understanding of the terminology in the question and possible answers. The terms in the answers are related to the ear, but only the term *ossicles* describes the bones.

34. **d**
Application and concept identification
Rationale: The question is asking for a connection between the vestibule mechanism and massage application. The rocking of the head in particular affects this system.

35. **a**
Factual recall
Rationale: Answering the question requires an understanding of the terminology in the question and possible answers and the function of these areas. The question asks for a specific visual interpretation, which is processed in the frontal lobes.

36. **b**
Factual recall
Rationale: Answering the question requires an understanding of the terminology in the question and possible answers and the functions of these areas. The only logical answer is answer b.

37. **c**
Application and concept identification
Rationale: The question is asking for a connection between the vestibule mechanism, a pathologic condition, and massage application. Rocking of the head in particular can result in motion sickness.

38. **a**
    Factual recall
    Rationale: Answering the question requires an understanding of the terminology in the question and possible answers and the functions of these areas. The only logical answer is answer a.

39. **c**
    Factual recall
    Rationale: The question asks for identification of terminology. Only the turbinate is located in the nose.

40. **b**
    Clinical reasoning and synthesis
    Rationale: The question is asking for identification of symptoms to support a referral. The facts of the question indicate brachial plexus involvement.

41. **d**
    Clinical reasoning and synthesis
    Rationale: The question is representative of a decision based on a pathologic condition. The question is asking for identification of symptoms to support an appropriate massage intervention. The facts of the question include a current outbreak of herpes zoster and pain. Each of the answers is a possible approach and would have to be analyzed to determine the best answer. The outcome would be increased tolerance to pain and reduced pain perception. These outcomes are best achieved with parasympathetic dominance and an increase in serotonin and endorphins. In addition, appropriate sanitation is a factor. The client also is immune compromised because an active infection is present. Only answer d addresses all these issues.

42. **c**
    Clinical reasoning and synthesis
    Rationale: The question is asking for the development of realistic outcomes for massage intervention. The possible answers have to be analyzed to identify which one is best in relation to the facts of the question. The only fact is a diagnosis of neuralgia, which would have to be researched. Neuralgia is a noninflammatory disorder of the nerve resulting in pain. Nerve pain is difficult to manage. The only logical answer is answer c.

43. **c**
    Clinical reasoning and synthesis
    Rationale: The question is representative of a decision based on a pathologic condition. The question is asking for identification of symptoms to support an appropriate massage intervention. The facts of the question include recent sleep disturbance, feeling of agitation, work stress, and a diagnosis of exogenous anxiety. Information about exogenous anxiety becomes part of the factual information and indicates that the client is reacting to changes in the environment. Each of the treatment plans offered needs to be analyzed to identify which one best addresses the needs of the client. In addition, information about standard treatment protocols including use of medication is necessary. For this type of reactive anxiety, short-term therapy and medication use are usually successful. Massage would need to support these interventions. The only logical treatment plan is given in answer c.

44. **c**
    Concept identification
    Rationale: The femoral nerve is not part of the sacral plexus, the thoracodorsal nerve innervates the latissimus dorsi muscle, and the brachial plexus supplies the arm. By elimination, the lumbar plexus would contain the nerve that would explain these symptoms.

45. **d**
    Factual recall
    Rationale: Only the proprioceptors are specific for detecting movement.

46. **a**
    Concept identification
    Rationale: Parasympathetic influence on the eye is to constrict the pupil. This is an autonomic function, and the accessory nerve is a cranial nerve that influences speaking and movement of the head.

47. **b**
    Concept identification
    Rationale: Smell can be emotional because of the connection to the emotional brain centers in the limbic system.

48. **d**
    Factual recall
    Rationale: Of the offered combinations, only answer d has both conditions that have a viral cause.

6
Endocrine System

Review Tips

The content concerning the endocrine system discusses the control mechanisms of the body. This material lends itself to the case study type of question because hormones influence how persons behave. As always, there are terms to memorize and to be able to use correctly or you will not be able to interpret the questions or identify the correct answer.

Review the content in your textbook that lists pathologic conditions relating to the body system and the related indications and contraindications for massage. Massage exams tend to target safe practice content. As a result, there is an emphasis on the appropriateness of massage for various pathologic conditions.

Questions

1. Which of the following ancient healing systems most correlates with the endocrine system?

   a. Meridian system
   b. Five elements
   c. Doshas
   d. Chakra system

2. Which of the following most accurately describes hormones?

   a. Secreted from exocrine glands
   b. Found in the synapse
   c. Transported in the blood
   d. Secretion regulated by positive feedback

3. A client is experiencing lingering anxiety from a minor auto accident 4 hours ago. What difference between the nervous system and the endocrine system would explain this condition?

   a. The nervous system is short acting and the endocrine system is long acting.
   b. The endocrine system is short acting and the nervous system is long acting.
   c. The nervous system transports hormones more consistently through blood and tissues.
   d. Neurotransmitters have a long duration of effect, and hormones are short acting.

4. A primary action of hormones is _____.

   a. Increasing or decreasing cellular processes
   b. Supporting positive feedback control of homeostasis
   c. Inhibiting synaptic uptake of neurotransmitters
   d. Suppressing tropic effects of cellular processes

5. Hypersecretion refers to _____.

   a. Normal decrease in endocrine secretion
   b. Abnormal decrease in endocrine secretion
   c. Normal increase in endocrine secretion
   d. Abnormal increase in endocrine secretion

6. Which of the following translates nerve impulses into hormone secretions by endocrine glands?

   a. The limbic system
   b. The pituitary gland
   c. The hypothalamus
   d. The adrenal glands

Correct answers are on pages 64-66.   **59**

7. An elderly client with a history of slow tissue healing and gradual weight loss begins to stabilize her weight and increase her ability to heal skin abrasions after receiving a weekly massage for 3 months. Which of the following offers the most concrete explanation for this outcome?

   a. Massage influences positive feedback mechanism to decrease adrenal output.
   b. Massage supports hypothalamic release of growth hormone-releasing hormone.
   c. Massage changes sleep patterns to increase dopamine influence.
   d. Massage beneficially influences tissue transport systems of neurotransmitters from endocrine tissues.

8. The pituitary gland is a primary source of _____.

   a. Tropic hormones
   b. Melatonin
   c. Adrenergic hormones
   d. Pitocin

9. Which of the following supports growth hormone function in the adult?

   a. High blood sugar
   b. Loving relationships
   c. Disrupted sleep
   d. Lack of exercise

10. Which of the following anterior pituitary hormones can be influenced positively by cold hydrotherapy applications?

    a. Melanocyte-stimulating hormone
    b. Follicle-stimulating hormone
    c. Thyroid-stimulating hormone
    d. Luteinizing hormone

11. A 38-year-old female client describes symptoms of constipation, increased edema, sensitivity to cold, muscle and joint pain, and hair loss. She indicates that there is an increase in stress in her life; she is tired and seems unable to cope as effectively as before. She had a general physical examination within the last 6 months, but no specific tests were done. Based on these symptoms, which condition might suggest a need for referral?

    a. Exophthalmos
    b. Hypothyroidism
    c. Hyperthyroidism
    d. Hypocalcemic tetany

12. A type II diabetic patient wishes to become a client for therapeutic massage. The physician is supportive. Which of the following statements is most accurate as a basic understanding of type II diabetes?

    a. A disruption of insulin production occurs in the islet cells of the pituitary gland.
    b. Insulin is a powerful diuretic, so increased edema is a warning sign of diabetic coma.
    c. Insulin is released when levels of blood sugar, amino acids, and fatty acids rise.
    d. Glucagon facilitates the ability of insulin to transport glucose across the cell membrane.

13. Which of the following hormones extends the response of the fight or flight produced by the sympathetic autonomic nervous system?

    a. Epinephrine
    b. Amylin
    c. Aldosterone
    d. Erythropoietin

14. The resistance phase of Selye's general adaptation response is most supported by which hormone?

    a. Progesterone
    b. Cortisol
    c. Noradrenaline
    d. Melatonin

15. Prolonged effects of lingering, unresolved stress can predispose a person to type II diabetes because _____.

    a. Cortisol supports a rise in blood levels of glucose, fatty acids, and amino acids
    b. Glucocorticoids reduce the activity of aldosterone, predisposing one to ketoacidosis
    c. Catecholamines inhibit sympathetic dominance pattern, resulting in excessive parasympathetic control over digestive processes
    d. Stress shuts down the production of adrenal cortex hormones, putting additional strain on the pancreas for glucose production

16. What two endocrine glands secrete androgens?

    a. Adrenal glands and pituitary
    b. Ovaries and thyroid
    c. Pineal and adrenal glands
    d. Testes and adrenal glands

17. A client who is a marathon runner developed an inflammatory condition of the knee. As part of the treatment process, the client received an injection of corticosteroid into the area of the knee. The client wishes to have a deep massage of the area to reduce the pain. Why is this not appropriate?

    a. The massage could decrease the inflammatory response and concentrate the medication at the injection site.
    b. Deep massage increases the potential for localized inflammation and would disturb the action of the corticosteroid injection.
    c. Deep massage would increase the tension of the muscles, causing instability, and inflammation would decrease.
    d. Corticosteroids reduce inflammation and increase tissue repair; because massage increases the tendency for tissue repair, excessive scarring could result.

18. A female client is experiencing some increase in coarse facial hair and acne. Which of the following hormones may be involved?

    a. Androgen
    b. Estrogen
    c. Progesterone
    d. Endorphin

19. Which of the following endocrine glands is most sensitive to light and dark cycles?

    a. Adrenal
    b. Parathyroid
    c. Pineal
    d. Thymus

20. Using the philosophy of the chakra system, a person practices compassion to self and others. Which endocrine gland is being supported?

    a. Adrenal
    b. Parathyroid
    c. Pineal
    d. Thymus

21. Which of the following is the most common tissue hormone?

    a. Prostaglandin
    b. Cholecystokinin
    c. Atrial natriuretic factor
    d. Insulin-like growth factor

22. In relationship to ancient chakra theory, if someone is concerned with not having enough money to pay bills, surviving a job change, and staying focused learning a new computer skill, which endocrine gland is likely to be affected?

    a. Pituitary
    b. Thyroid
    c. Adrenal
    d. Pineal

Correct answers are on pages 64-66.

23. A client has just experienced a job shift change from days to nights and is having difficulty adjusting to the sleep pattern. The client indicates feeling disconnected and out of sorts. Which endocrine gland initially might be affected, and which massage approach would be most beneficial?

    a. Pineal gland; a massage that focuses on sympathetic stimulations with active participation by the client

    b. Adrenal glands; a massage that generates localized inflammatory areas, such as is found with direct pressure and friction on trigger points

    c. Thymus gland; a massage that uses sufficient pressure but pain-free compression and rhythmic gliding methods to support parasympathetic dominance

    d. Pineal gland; a massage that uses sufficient pressure but pain-free compression and rhythmic gliding methods to support parasympathetic dominance

24. Which of the following best explains massage influence of the endocrine system?

    a. Stimulation of mechanoreceptors

    b. Decrease in lymphatic stagnation

    c. Influence on autonomic nervous system

    d. Direct release of hormones

25. An elderly client has been more alert and has gained a bit of weight since she has been receiving massage. Which of the following is the most logical explanation?

    a. Massage stimulates the hypothalamus.

    b. Excessive pituitary function is inhibited.

    c. The pancreas increases insulin output.

    d. Thyroid function increases melatonin production.

26. By supporting restorative sleep, on which of the following does massage have the most direct effect.

    a. Antidiuretic hormone

    b. Cortisol

    c. Luteinizing hormone

    d. Oxytocin

27. A client complains of the following: dry skin, joint pain, and edema. Which of the following endocrine functions should the client have checked by a physician?

    a. Glucagons

    b. Androgen

    c. Thymosin

    d. Thyroid

28. A client has a chronic inflammatory condition that is helped somewhat by aspirin. Which of the following is the most correct statement?

    a. Prostaglandins, which are tissue hormones, are involved.

    b. Progesterone, which is an androgen, needs to be inhibited.

    c. Pituitary hormones are overactive.

    d. The pancreas and gonads are hyperactive.

Exercise

Using the foregoing questions as examples, now write at least three more questions—one of each type: factual recall and comprehension, application and concept identification, and clinical reasoning and synthesis. Make sure to develop plausible wrong answers, and be sure that the correct answer is clearly correct. Then write a rationale for each question. The more questions you write, the better you will understand the material.

Answers and Discussion

1. **d**
   Application and concept identification
   Rationale: Ancient healing traditions were based on observation through the centuries. Although the technology was not available to validate theories by Western scientific methods, it is apparent that body anatomy and physiology were being observed. When one compares the chakra system to Western theories of anatomy and physiology, one understands the correlation with the endocrine system.

2. **c**
   Factual recall
   Rationale: The question is a portion of the definition of a hormone.

3. **a**
   Application and concept identification
   Rationale: The question is asking for a relationship between the two systems of control in the body. The nervous system responds quickly to emergency situations, and then the endocrine system sustains the effect over a longer period.

4. **a**
   Factual recall
   Rationale: The correct answer describes a function of a hormone. The three incorrect answers are flawed and do not state true information in relationship to the question.

5. **d**
   Factual recall
   Rationale: The question is representative of terminology used for endocrine system pathology. *Hyper* means too much.

6. **c**
   Factual recall
   Rationale: The question describes a function of the hypothalamus. You must know the function of the other structures listed to eliminate wrong answers and identify the correct answer.

7. **b**
   Clinical reasoning and synthesis
   Rationale: This question is representative of the type of case study found in relation to the content area—the endocrine system. Analysis of the question and possible answers leads to a correct decision. The facts presented by the question are elderly client, slow tissue healing, gradual weight loss, and improvement in all areas after 3 months of weekly massage. The question asks for the justification of this outcome. The possible answers also list facts—some correct and others incorrect, some appropriate in relation to the question and others not. Research has shown that touch stimulates the hypothalamus. A function of the hypothalamus is to stimulate the pituitary to produce and release growth hormone, which would account for the benefits seen.

8. **a**
   Factual recall
   Rationale: The question asks for an understanding of the terms listed. The pituitary is the main source of tropic hormones.

9. **b**
   Application and concept identification
   Rationale: The question is asking for a connection between growth hormone function and behavior that supports it in the body. Only the correct answer supports growth hormone function. The other three possible answers indicate stress, which suppresses growth hormone function.

10. **c**
    Application and concept identification
    Rationale: The question is asking for a connection between hydrotherapy applications and pituitary hormones. The three incorrect answers are anterior pituitary hormones that have not been shown to be influenced by cold applications.

11. **b**
    Clinical reasoning and synthesis
    Rationale: This question is representative of the type of case study found in relation to the content area—the endocrine system. Analysis of the question and possible answers would lead to a correct decision. The facts presented by the question are middle-aged woman, hypothyroid symptoms, increased stress and reduced ability to cope, and no blood work done during the physical. The four answers list terminology you would have to understand to identify the correct answer.

12. **c**

    Application and concept identification
    Rationale: The pancreatic pathology of type II
    diabetes is defined in the correct answer. The
    three incorrect answers provide misinformation.
    You would have to interpret all of the
    terminology to find the incorrect word usage
    and identify the correct answer.

13. **a**

    Factual recall
    Rationale: The question is asking for the
    identification of the correct adrenal hormone
    that stimulates sympathetic function of the
    autonomic nervous system. Epinephrine and
    aldosterone are adrenal hormones, but
    aldosterone is involved in water balance, so
    epinephrine is the correct answer.

14. **b**

    Application and concept identification
    Rationale: Selye's general adaptation response is
    described in many sources. This information is
    correlated with hormone function. Cortisol exerts
    a long-term effect on the body and therefore is
    more involved with resistance to stress.

15. **a**

    Application and concept identification
    Rationale: The question asks for a connection
    between long-term stress and the development
    of diabetes. The four possible answers provide
    explanations. You need to define each of the
    terms in the answers to identify the correct
    answer. Only answer a makes the correct
    correlation.

16. **d**

    Factual recall
    Rationale: You need to define the terms in the
    question to identify the correct answer.
    Androgens are gonadocorticoids and are
    produced by the gonads and the adrenal glands.

17. **b**

    Clinical reasoning and synthesis
    Rationale: The facts provided in the question are
    the client is a runner, has an inflamed knee,
    received a steroid injection at the site, and asks
    for deep massage to the area. The question
    indicates that this type of massage application is
    contraindicated, and the answer is to justify why
    this is so. Only answer b is a logical response.
    The other three answers present incorrect
    information. Massage of the site of a recent
    injection is contraindicated. Deep massage
    would tend to increase inflammation in the area.
    Corticosteroids decrease tissue repair processes.

18. **a**

    Application and concept identification
    Rationale: The question asks for a reason for the
    change in the condition of the client. An effect of
    androgen is increased facial hair and acne.

19. **c**

    Factual recall
    Rationale: The question is asking for an
    endocrine influence. The pineal gland is
    responsive to light and dark.

20. **d**

    Application and concept identification
    Rationale: The question is representative of how
    the ancient healing systems and Western thought
    are connected. You must understand the various
    chakra relationships to the endocrine glands to
    identify the correct answer. The thymus is
    correlated with the heart and spleen chakras.

21. **a**

    Factual recall
    Rationale: The four possible answers would need
    to be defined and identified to determine
    whether each is a tissue hormone and which is
    most common. Only prostaglandin is a tissue
    hormone.

22. **c**

    Application and concept identification
    Rationale: The question is representative of how
    the ancient healing systems and Western thought
    are connected. You must understand the various
    chakra relationships to the endocrine glands to
    identify the correct answer. The adrenal glands are
    correlated with the root chakra issues of survival.

23. **d**

    Clinical reasoning and synthesis
    Rationale: Three types of information are
    presented in the question and possible answers:
    the behavior change and result, what primary
    endocrine function is disrupted, and what
    massage intervention would support a return to
    homeostasis. All three areas must connect
    logically for a correct answer. Only the correct
    answer does this.

24. **c**

    Concept identification
    Rationale: The primary influence on the
    endocrine system by massage is a secondary
    effect when there is a shift in autonomic nervous
    system dominance. Lymphatic is more about
    fluids, and stimulation of mechanoreceptors has
    many different influences on the body, but
    mostly directed to the somatic nervous system.

25. **a**
    Concept identification
    Rationale: Touch stimulates the hypothalamus, which in turn regulates the endocrine responses. The other responses have not been shown to be a result of massage application or are flawed in terminology.

26. **b**
    Clinical reasoning and synthesis
    Rationale: Antidiuretic hormone influences water balance, and luteinizing hormone influences ovulation, progesterone, and testosterone. Oxytocin is influenced by touch and bonding and by parasympathetic dominance. Cortisol would be most influenced by sleep. The adrenal hormone is specific, and during deep restorative sleep, it would be least active.

27. **d**
    Concept identification
    Rationale: These are hypothyroid symptoms. The other answers are hormones, not endocrine function.

28. **a**
    Concept identification
    Rationale: The key is that prostaglandins are involved in inflammation and are influenced by aspirin. None of the other hormones is endocrine.

7
Skeletal System

Review Tips

The content on the skeletal system is almost exclusively memorization. The information will appear in questions that target joints, muscles, biomechanics, assessment, and various injuries and pathologic conditions. Use the study tools in this text and the flashcards. Questions that specifically target this content are factual recall or may be the case study type about injury or disease.

You must know the names of the bones and the names and location of the bony landmarks. A strong foundation in this content will make studying the joints and muscles much easier.

Questions

1. Which of the following is not a function of bone?

   a. Storing minerals
   b. Producing blood cells
   c. Generating heat
   d. Storing lipids

2. A type of bone that develops in a tendon or joint capsule is a(n) _____.

   a. Sesamoid bone
   b. Piezo-bone
   c. Articulation bone
   d. Compact bone

3. Which aspect of bone structure provides the elastic quality of bone?

   a. Inorganic mineral
   b. Organic material
   c. Trabeculas
   d. Endoskeleton

4. The main component of bone that has the piezoelectric quality is _____.

   a. Compact bone
   b. Cancellous bone
   c. Red marrow
   d. Collagen

5. The external connective tissue covering of bone is called the _____.

   a. Exoskeleton
   b. Endoskeleton
   c. Periosteum
   d. Endosteum

6. The continual changing of bone in response to functional demands is called _____.

   a. Remodeling
   b. Oppositional growth
   c. Haversian
   d. Articulation

7. Which type of bone contains trabeculas?

   a. Compact
   b. Cancellous
   c. Osteon
   d. Concentric

8. Which of the following bone types contains a diaphysis?

   a. Flat
   b. Irregular
   c. Long
   d. Sesamoid

9. A young male client is experiencing a growth spurt. He complains that the bones in his legs ache. What is responsible for this phenomenon?

   a. Increased testosterone promotes long bone growth.
   b. Increased estrogen promotes long bone growth.
   c. Decreased estrogen supports long bone growth.
   d. Decreased testosterone promotes long bone growth.

10. Which of the following is a depression on a bone?

    a. Condyle
    b. Fossa
    c. Line
    d. Tubercle

11. Which of the following bones is located in the appendicular portion of the skeleton?

    a. Ethmoid
    b. Clavicle
    c. Sternum
    d. Coccyx

12. Which suture joins the parietal bones and occipital bone?

    a. Squamous
    b. Coronal
    c. Lambdoidal
    d. Sagittal

13. Which of the following bones forms the structure of the nose?

    a. Vomer
    b. Zygomatic
    c. Sphenoid
    d. Fontanelle

14. What bone has a superior articular facet?

    a. Humerus
    b. Occipital
    c. Thoracic vertebra
    d. Carpal

15. Which of the following landmarks is located on the humerus?

    a. Glenoid fossa
    b. Xiphoid process
    c. Radial styloid
    d. Olecranon fossa

16. The coracoid process is located on which bone?

    a. Scapula
    b. Sternum
    c. Femur
    d. Talus

17. A client experienced an accident in which the trunk was thrust into extension. Which of the following structures might have been injured?

    a. Deltoid ligament
    b. Anterior longitudinal ligament
    c. Anterior superior iliac spine
    d. Linea aspera

18. Which of the following is part of the pelvis?

    a. Fovea
    b. Triquetrum
    c. Trochlear notch
    d. Acetabulum

19. When one is palpating over the spine, the structure most prominently felt is the _____.

    a. Centrum
    b. Spinous process
    c. Annulus fibrosis
    d. Pedicle

20. If an intervertebral disk rupture occurs, what is the possible outcome?

    a. Narrowed disk space because of leakage of the nucleus pulposus
    b. Narrowed intervertebral space because of rupture of the fontanelle
    c. Impingement of the nerve from pressure exerted by the sella turcica
    d. Increased space in the foramen impinging on the spinal cord

21. When one is palpating the posterior cervical area, the fibrous structure felt is the _____.

    a. Kyphosis ligament
    b. Odontoid process
    c. Nuchal ligament
    d. Demifacets

22. The costal angle is located on which bone?

    a. Sternum
    b. Clavicle
    c. Atlas
    d. Rib

23. The foot typically contains how many bones?

    a. 31
    b. 26
    c. 12
    d. 22

24. A client complains of pain in the lower back. Observation indicates an excessive lumbar curve. This is called _____.

    a. Scoliosis
    b. Kyphosis
    c. Lordosis
    d. Talipes

25. A female client, age 67, has a history of smoking. This could indicate caution for compressive force used during massage for which reason?

    a. Osteonecrosis
    b. Osteomyelitis
    c. Osteochondritis dissecans
    d. Osteoporosis

26. A client complains of pain in the tibia. The client completed a marathon 24 hours before the massage session. What contraindication to massage may account for the pain?

    a. Stress fracture
    b. Compound fracture
    c. Dislocation
    d. Whiplash

27. Which sequence of terms would all be bony landmarks?

    a. Trabeculas, lacunas, crest
    b. Epicondyle, sulcus, fissure
    c. Periosteum, osteon, trochanter
    d. Sesamoid, axial, meatus

28. Which sequence of terms are all axial skeleton bones?

    a. Coccyx, occipital, sternum
    b. Rib, sacrum, tibia
    c. Femur, clavicle, ulna
    d. Vertebrae, mandible, ilium

29. Which of the following are bony landmarks of the humerus?

    a. Radial tuberosity and styloid process
    b. Iliac fossa and coracoid process
    c. Olecranon fossa and lesser tubercle
    d. Intercondylar fossa and intertrochanteric line

30. Which of the following is located in the vertebral column?

    a. Manubrium
    b. Lamina
    c Vertebral border
    d. Scaphoid

Correct answers are on pages 72-74.

31. Which spinal deformity has the concavity in the
    lumbar and the convexity in the thorax?

    a. Scoliosis
    b. Scurvy
    c. Whiplash
    d. Lordosis

Exercise

Using the foregoing questions as examples, now write at least three more questions—one of each type: factual recall and comprehension, application and concept identification, and clinical reasoning and synthesis. Make sure to develop plausible wrong answers, and be sure that the correct answer is clearly correct. Then write a rationale for each question. The more questions you write, the better you will understand the material.

Answers and Discussion

1. **c**
Factual recall
Rationale: The question and possible answers identify bone function. Generating heat is a function of muscle, not bone.

2. **a**
Factual recall
Rationale: The question is the definition of a sesamoid bone.

3. **b**
Factual recall
Rationale: The question asks for the elastic component of bone provided by the organic material.

4. **d**
Factual recall
Rationale: The question asks for the piezo-material of bone, which is collagen.

5. **c**
Factual recall
Rationale: You need to define all the terms in the possible answers to answer the question. Periosteum is the external connective tissue covering of bone.

6. **a**
Factual recall
Rationale: You need to define all the terms in the possible answers to answer the question. The question asks for the name of a bone function described as change in the bone in response to demand. This is remodeling.

7. **b**
Factual recall
Rationale: You need to define all the terms in the question and possible answers to answer the question. Cancellous bone contains trabeculas.

8. **c**
Factual recall
Rationale: You need to define all the terms in the question and possible answers to answer the question. Long bones contain a diaphysis.

9. **a**
Application and concept identification
Rationale: The question is asking for the connection between hormone effect on bone and symptoms of aching. Answer a explains why this could be happening. The other three answers present incorrect information. Estrogen and testosterone produce long bone growth, but increasing estrogen levels, primarily in females, also stops the growth. Because a male is described in the question, answer a is the correct answer.

10. **b**
Factual recall
Rationale: The question is asking for the identification of a bony landmark. You would need to recognize all of the landmarks to answer this type of question correctly.

11. **b**
Factual recall
Rationale: The question is asking for a classification of a bone by regions of the axial and appendicular skeleton. You must know what bones fall into these classifications to answer the question.

12. **c**
Factual recall
Rationale: This question is representative of a multitude of questions that could be written on the anatomy of bones. To answer the question, you must identify correctly the location of the bones in the question and the suture that connects them.

13. **a**
Factual recall
Rationale: This question is representative of a multitude of questions that could be written on the anatomy of bones. To answer the question, you must identify correctly the location of the bones in the possible answers provided.

14. **c**
Factual recall
Rationale: This question is representative of a multitude of questions that could be written on the anatomy of bones. To answer the question, you must identify correctly which bone has the structure described in the question.

15. **d**
Factual recall
Rationale: This question is representative of a multitude of questions that could be written on the anatomy of bones. To answer the question, you must identify correctly which bony landmark is located on the humerus.

16. **a**
Factual recall
Rationale: This question is representative of a multitude of questions that could be written on the anatomy of bones. To answer the question, you must identify correctly which bone has a coracoid process. The scapula is the correct answer.

17. **b**
Application and concept identification
Rationale: This question is representative of many questions that could be written about movement and bone structure. This particular question asks for the connection between a structure connected with bone and an injury. If the trunk were put in exaggerated extension, the anterior longitudinal ligament could be overstretched.

18. **d**
Factual recall
Rationale: This question is representative of a multitude of questions that could be written on the anatomy of bones. To answer the question, you must identify correctly which bone or bony structure is part of the pelvis. You must identify the location of all of the structures provided in the possible answers to identify the acetabulum.

19. **b**
Factual recall
Rationale: This question is representative of a multitude of questions that could be written on the anatomy of bones. To answer the question, you must identify correctly which bone or bony structure is part of the spine that can be palpated easily. You must identify the location of all of the structures provided in the possible answers to identify the spinous process.

20. **a**
Application and concept identification
Rationale: The question is asking what happens if the disk ruptures. The correct answer needs to be logical and contain correct terminology usage. You would need to define all the terms to rule out wrong answers and to identify the correct answer, a.

21. **c**
Factual recall
Rationale: This question is representative of a multitude of questions that could be written on the anatomy of bones. To answer the question, you must identify correctly which bone or structure is part of the cervical spine that can be palpated easily. You must identify the location of all of the structures provided in the possible answers to identify the nuchal ligament. There is no structure called the kyphosis ligament. Incorrect use of terms is a common way to develop wrong answers.

22. **d**
Factual recall
Rationale: This question is representative of a multitude of questions that could be written on the anatomy of bones. To answer the question, you must identify correctly which bone has a costal angle. You must identify the location of all the structures provided in the possible answers to identify the ribs.

23. **b**
Factual recall
Rationale: This question is representative of a multitude of questions that could be written on the anatomy of bones.

24. **c**
Application and concept identification
Rationale: The question asks for the name of an excessive lumbar curve that may be responsible for low back pain. You would need to define all the terms to identify the correct answer, lordosis.

25. **d**
Clinical reasoning and synthesis
Rationale: The facts in the question would help you to identify the predisposition to the pathologic condition osteoporosis. The question also indicates that caution should be used during the massage because osteoporosis predisposes one to bone fracture.

26. **a**
Clinical reasoning and synthesis
Rationale: The facts in the question are pain in the tibia and endurance running the day before. The possible answers indicate reasons for the pain. You must define the various pathologic conditions of the skeletal system to rule out incorrect answers. The most logical answer is a stress fracture based on the history provided by the question.

27. **b**
    Factual recall
    Rationale: This is a terminology question.
28. **a**
    Factual recall
    Rationale: This is a terminology question.
29. **c**
    Factual recall
    Rationale: This a terminology question.
30. **b**
    Factual recall
    Rationale: This is a terminology question.
31. **d**
    Concept identification
    Rationale: Scoliosis has curves in both areas.
    Scurvy and whiplash are not spinal deformities.

8
Joints

Review Tips

The content concerning joints is more complex than studying for the skeletal system because you must know the parts of the joint and the function of the joints. The body has various types of joints. Joint structures also have specific pathologic conditions to understand. The main parts of a joint are bones, ligaments, cartilage, and in synovial joints, a joint capsule. Various types of movements occur at joints in response to muscle contraction.

Because there are so many factors involved in joint structure and function, it is easy to write many different types of questions that cover this content. The data are represented in all three question types.

Study strategies include flash cards, labeling activities, examples, and metaphors. Building simple models with clay, wood, hinges, and various types of craft materials or even structural toys such as Tinkertoys is also an excellent study strategy.

Questions

1. Joint function is a relationship between _____.

   a. Bones and landmarks
   b. Stability and mobility
   c. Articulations and diarthroses
   d. Synovial fluid and pathologic range of motion

2. The most complex joint design is likely to function in _____.

   a. Stability
   b. Viscoelasticity
   c. Mobility
   d. Synarthrosis

3. Principles and characteristics of joint design include all of the following except _____.

   a. The design of a joint depends on its function
   b. The breakdown of any joint structure will affect the entire joint function
   c. Generally, stability must be achieved before mobility
   d. Most joints serve only one function, stability or mobility

4. What type of cartilage is found in joints that function primarily for mobility?

   a. White fibrocartilage
   b. Hyaline cartilage
   c. Yellow fibrocartilage
   d. Synovial cartilage

5. An important component of connective tissue that supports pliability is _____.

   a. Water
   b. Synovial fluid
   c. Colloid
   d. Viscosity

6. The viscoelastic quality of connective tissue to modify in the direction of the force applied and then slowly return to the original state is called _____.

   a. Plastic range
   b. Fibrous
   c. Creep
   d. Avulsion

7. A client has been participating in a stretching program for more than a year. Initially the program was helpful, but during the last 3 months the program has become more aggressive and the client is complaining of joint pain. Which alteration in connective tissue may explain what has occurred?

   a. The client has experienced a rupture in the connective tissue structures and has developed lax ligaments.
   b. The client has exceeded the limits of the elastic range of the tissue, consistently deformed the tissue in the plastic range, and developed lax ligaments.
   c. An avulsion failure of connective tissue has occurred, creating a decrease in mobility.
   d. The tissue has become dehydrated, increasing creep tendency and contributing to stability provided by muscle contraction.

8. A client is complaining of a feeling of shortening and pulling in the area of the low back and sacroiliac joints. Assessment indicates decreased pliability in the connective tissue structures in this area. Which of the following massage applications is most appropriate to achieve an increase in short-term mobility without compromising stability or creating a remodeling process of the tissue?

   a. Application of massage methods that slowly introduce creep, increasing pliability at the plastic range of the tissue
   b. Application of therapeutic inflammation coupled with stretching to exceed the plastic range of the tissue
   c. Application of elongation stretching to breach the plastic range of the tissue, creating inflammation to restore an appropriate creep pattern
   d. Application of abrupt bending of the connective tissue to support the increase in ligament laxity, thereby increasing mobility

9. A client has been diagnosed with a hypermobile knee joint. Which of the following would be part of an appropriate treatment plan?

   a. Extend the elastic range of connective tissue structures by altering the plastic range.
   b. Elongate the plastic component of connective tissue in the direction of the shortening.
   c. Restore pliability.
   d. Manage muscle contraction around the joint using standard massage methods.

10. Which of the following joint types has the most limited mobility?

    a. Syndesmosis
    b. Amphiarthrosis
    c. Cartilaginous
    d. Diarthrosis

11. Which of the following is not a characteristic of a synovial joint?

    a. A joint capsule formed of fibrous tissue
    b. Bones are separated by fibrocartilage.
    c. Hyaline cartilage covers the joint surfaces.
    d. Synovial fluid forms a lubricating film over the joint surfaces.

12. Which of the following joint structures is highly innervated and a source of sensory data concerning movement and position of a joint?

    a. Stratum synovium
    b. Articular cartilage
    c. Stratum fibrosum
    d. Joint cavity

13. A client is experiencing muscle spasms and reduced mobility around a shoulder joint that has a history of dislocation. Which of the following applications of massage would be best in assisting this client?

    a. Increase the plastic range of the ligament structures and stretched tense muscles.
    b. Use friction on tendons and ligaments, and then incorporate a stretching program to increase flexibility.
    c. Reduce muscle spasms to the point that mobility is supported but stability is not compromised.
    d. Use massage methods and stretching to eliminate muscle spasms.

14. The accessory movements at a joint that describe how articulating surfaces move within the joint capsule and contribute to joint play are called _____.

    a. Closed packed position
    b. Arthrokinematics
    c. Osteokinematics
    d. Range of motion

15. Joints in which stability is reduced because of increased laxity of supportive ligaments also have an increase in _____.

    a. Joint play
    b. Hypomobility
    c. Muscle relaxation
    d. Plasma membrane

16. The closed packed position of a joint can be described as _____.

    a. The convex surface fitting minimally into the concave surface
    b. The position in which spin, roll, and slide most easily occur
    c. The position with the most joint play
    d. The convex surface fitting with maximal contact into the concave surface

17. A client sprained a joint in one finger. What is going to be the most comfortable position for the joint and why?

    a. The closed packed position because this is the most stable position of the joint
    b. The loose packed position so that movement can occur most easily
    c. The least packed position to accommodate swelling
    d. The closed packed position to accommodate increased synovial fluid

18. Which of the following describes a neurologic protective mechanism for normal joint function?

    a. Anatomic range of motion
    b. Physiologic range of motion
    c. Pathologic range of motion
    d. Osteokinematics

19. Which of the following joints has the least amount of bone structure creating the anatomic range of motion limits?

    a. Elbow
    b. Hip
    c. Ankle
    d. Knee

20. A client has a history of a broken wrist. The wrist was in a cast for an extended period because bone repair was slower than normal. The client now is experiencing a decrease in range of motion of the wrist. What might be the cause?

    a. Hypomobility because of contracture
    b. Hypomobility because of reduced muscle tension
    c. Hypermobility because of increased muscle tension
    d. Hypomobility because of increased anatomic range of motion

Correct answers are on pages 83-87.

21. During the massage session, passive joint movement is used for assessing the range of motion of the arm during circumduction. Which of the following best describes the action used during this process?

    a. Bending movement that decreased the angle of a joint
    b. Movement of arm medially toward the midline of the body
    c. Twisting and turning of a bone on its own axis
    d. Combined movements of flexion, extension, abduction, and adduction to create a cone shape

22. Before the massage session begins and during the initial physical assessment, active joint movement is used to assess the range of motion of the foot. Which term is most correct to use to describe a portion of this activity?

    a. Elevation
    b. Retraction
    c. Eversion
    d. Opposition

23. The term used to describe the movement of the scapula toward the spine is _____.

    a. Rotation
    b. Retraction
    c. Protraction
    d. Supination

24. During assessment you want the client to rotate the hip externally. What instructions would you give the client?

    a. Please move your leg so that you cross it over the other leg at the ankles.
    b. Please straighten your legs and turn the entire leg so that you point your toes toward each other.
    c. Please straighten your legs and turn the entire leg so that you point your toes away from each other.
    d. Please bring your knee toward your chest.

25. A ball-and-socket joint also is considered a _____.

    a. Pivot joint
    b. Biaxial joint
    c. Gliding joint
    d. Multiaxial joint

26. The name of the association between joints as they function in relationship to each other is called _____.

    a. Joint play
    b. Osteokinematics
    c. Kinematic chains
    d. Diarthrosis

27. The function of joints that often is going to result in a compensation pattern in one joint if there is a change in function in another joint is called the _____.

    a. Closed kinematic chain
    b. Open kinematic chain
    c. Loose packed kinematic chain
    d. Closed packed kinematic chain

28. The two articulating bones of the temporomandibular joint are the _____.

    a. Temporal and maxilla
    b. Mandible and maxilla
    c. Mandible and temporal
    d. Temporal and zygomatic

29. The glenohumeral joint has extensive mobility because _____.

    a. It has range-of-motion limits provided primarily by soft tissue
    b. Physiologic limits to range of motion provide for a loose fit between the humerus and the clavicle
    c. Of its biaxial joint structure, which allows movement in three planes
    d. Of the ball-and-socket joint structure, which allows movement only in two planes

30. Which is a movement allowed at the sternoclavicular joint?

    a. Flexion
    b. Rotation
    c. Inversion
    d. Extension

31. Should there be an injury to the sternoclavicular joint that limits its range of motion, what other structure will be affected?

    a. Radius
    b. Olecranon
    c. Scapula
    d. Deltoid ligament

32. The coracoclavicular ligament is part of what joint?

    a. Glenohumeral
    b. Temporomandibular
    c. Sternoclavicular
    d. Acromioclavicular

33. Which of the following joint is responsible for pronation and supination?

    a. Ulnar-humeral
    b. Radioulnar
    c. Radiohumeral
    d. Radiocarpal

34. A wrist movement is greatest in flexion and extension because _____.

    a. The joint capsule is loose in the superior and inferior directions
    b. The joint type is a hinge joint
    c. The joint capsule is loose laterally and medially
    d. The radiocarpal joint forms a direct contact between the ulna and the carpal bones

35. The joint where the fingers join the body of the hand is called the _____.

    a. Distal interphalangeal joint
    b. Proximal interphalangeal joint
    c. Metacarpophalangeal joint
    d. Intercarpal joint

36. The articulating bones of the sacroiliac joint are the _____.

    a. Sacrum and ischium
    b. Sacrum and iliac
    c. Sacrum and acetabulum
    d. Sacrum and pubis

37. Which of the following joints has no direct muscle action but is responsible for helping the vertebral column to remain relatively still during walking?

    a. Symphysis pubis
    b. Sacral lumbar
    c. Labrum
    d. Sacroiliac

38. The loose packed position of the hip joint is ____.

    a. Flexion, abduction, and lateral rotation
    b. Extension, adduction, and medial rotation
    c. Flexion, adduction, and lateral rotation
    d. Extension, abduction, and lateral rotation

39. If the leg is fixed and does not move and the pelvis moves forward into anteversion, what is the result?

    a. Increased kyphosis
    b. Increased lordosis
    c. Decreased lordosis
    d. Decreased scoliosis

40. The most stable position of the knee joint is ____.

    a. In slight flexion
    b. In full hyperextension
    c. In locked extension
    d. In locked flexion

41. A client was playing football when tackled. Pressure was put on the lateral side of the left knee. Which ligament would receive the most extension strain?

    a. Lateral collateral
    b. Medial collateral
    c. Posterior cruciate
    d. Posterior meniscofemoral

Correct answers are on pages 83-87.

42. Which fibrocartilaginous structure allows for more surface contact of the femur on the tibia?

    a. Cruciates
    b. Labrum
    c. Patella
    d. Menisci

43. The most stable position of the ankle joint is _____.

    a. Plantar flexion
    b. Plantar rotation
    c. Full dorsiflexion
    d. Rotated eversion

44. A client continues to sprain the ankles. You notice that the client wears boots with a 2-inch heel. How would this contribute to injury potential?

    a. The heel positions the ankle in dorsiflexion, making the ankle joint less stable.
    b. The heel positions the ankle in plantar flexion, making the ankle joint less stable.
    c. The weight is shifted to the ball of the foot, creating an open kinematic chain.
    d. The inferior tibiofibular joint is extended when the heel is raised and creates instability.

45. Which of the following joints allows rotation as a motion pattern?

    a. Atlantooccipital
    b. Atlantoaxial
    c. Intervertebral
    d. Costovertebral

46. Which movement of the vertebral joints is most stabilized by the anterior longitudinal ligament?

    a. Extension
    b. Flexion
    c. Rotation
    d. Lateral flexion

47. During the history interview, a client reports experiencing a disk herniation posterior in the low back. Which type of injury and what likely location would be indicated?

    a. Extension injury at the sacrolumbar junction
    b. Flexion injury at T12
    c. Flexion injury at the lumbosacral junction
    d. Extension injury at the thoracolumbar junction

48. Which two joints are most active during breathing?

    a. Intervertebral and costovertebral
    b. Vertebral arch and chondrosternal
    c. Costochondral and intervertebral
    d. Costovertebral and costochondral

49. What is the action of the ribs during inspiration?

    a. Ribs lowered
    b. Ribs raised
    c. Ribs protracted
    d. Ribs retracted

50. Which of the following pathologic conditions of the joints responds most positively to massage?

    a. Dislocation
    b. Rheumatoid arthritis
    c. Lateral epicondylitis
    d. Kyphosis

51. A client has received a diagnosis of degenerative joint disease. Conservative treatment measures are indicated. Which of the following treatment plans is most appropriate?

    a. Bed rest with over-the-counter antiinflammatory medication
    b. Cortisone injections and moderate exercise
    c. Ice, regular intense exercise, and connective tissue massage
    d. Ice, moderate exercise, general massage, and counterirritation ointments

52. A client has a sore shoulder from a work-related repetitive overuse injury. The client has held the shoulder in the least packed position with a sling and through muscle holding for more than 3 months. Now the client is experiencing reduced range of motion. Which of the following is most helped by massage?

    a. Protective muscle splinting that has developed shortened connective tissue patterns
    b. Nerve impingement
    c. Arthritis
    d. Adhesive capsulitis

53. Massage methods that move the body most influence which of the following?

    a. Synarthrosis joints
    b. Synchondrosis joints
    c. Synovial joints
    d. Interosseous ligaments

54. A client reports spraining a knee when hit on the lateral side, resulting in a convex position of the medial collateral ligament. Which of the following forces best describes the injury to the ligament?

    a. Shear
    b. Compression
    c. Tension
    d. Torsion

55. Which of the following joint movements are opposites?

    a. Retraction, protraction
    b. Plantar flexion, pronation
    c. Horizontal adduction, diagonal adduction
    d. Depression, downward rotation

56. If a joint has a normal movement of 0 degrees to 90 degrees of flexion and the range of motion of the joint is limited by 10%, what is the range of motion of the joint?

    a. 45 degrees of extension
    b. 80 degrees of flexion
    c. 80 degrees of abduction
    d. 100 degrees of flexion

57. The assessment form indicates that a client has an anterior tilt of the pelvis bilaterally. Which of the following would explain best what the massage therapist would see and feel during physical assessment?

    a. One hip is lower than the other.
    b. The client is twisted to the left.
    c. The client is flexed at the hips.
    d. The client is experiencing scapula retraction.

58. Which of the following would describe the movement of the ribs during inspiration?

    a. The ribs are rotated.
    b. The ribs are depressed.
    c. The ribs are fixed.
    d. The ribs are elevated.

Correct answers are on pages 83-87.

Exercise

Using the foregoing questions as examples, now write at least three more questions—one of each type: factual recall and comprehension, application and concept identification, and clinical reasoning and synthesis. Make sure to develop plausible wrong answers, and be sure that the correct answer is clearly correct. Then write a rationale for each question. The more questions you write, the better you will understand the material.

Answers and Discussion

1. **b**
Application and concept identification
Rationale: Function of joints is based on stability and mobility. Bones, landmarks, articulations, diarthroses, and synovial fluid do not describe function.

2. **c**
Factual recall
Rationale: The function of simple joint design is stability and that of complex joint design is mobility.

3. **d**
Factual recall
Rationale: The question is representative of the type that asks for identification of only the wrong answer. You need to read these types of questions carefully. In this question answer d is the correct choice because the other possible answers do describe characteristics of joint design. Many joints serve a dual function of stability and mobility.

4. **b**
Factual recall
Rationale: You need to define the terminology. Hyaline cartilage is found at the ends of bone in synovial joints.

5. **a**
Factual recall
Rationale: A major component of ground substance is water.

6. **c**
Factual recall
Rationale: You need to define the terms to understand the question and identify the correct answer. The question is the definition of creep.

7. **b**
Clinical reasoning and synthesis
Rationale: The facts presented in the question are a 1-year stretching program that was initially beneficial and increased intensity of the program in the last 3 months, resulting in joint pain. The question wants to know why this is the outcome based on changes in connective tissue structure. Each of the answers provides an explanation, but the three wrong answers present flawed data. Analysis is necessary to identify errors and find the correct answer. Only answer b presents correct information in relation to the facts of the question and indicates a logical explanation for the decrease in joint stability and development of joint pain.

8. **a**
Clinical reasoning and synthesis
Rationale: The case study format presents the following facts: sensation of shortening in the lumbosacral area, confirmed by assessment revealing decreased mobility of the tissue in the area. Next limits are put on the type of intervention allowed. The correct answer needs to stay within these limits yet address the problem. Knowledge of the physiologic effects of massage methods on connective tissue physiology is necessary to analyze correctly for the appropriate answer. The three incorrect answers are not logical and would present cautions with their use. Only answer a presents a treatment plan that is cautious yet effective.

9. **d**
Clinical reasoning and synthesis
Rationale: The facts presented by the question are limited to information about a hypermobile knee joint. Safe application of massage methods is always a priority. The three wrong answers would further increase the hypermobility; therefore answer d is the most logical approach because the protective and compensatory muscle contraction is not eliminated but instead is managed.

10. **a**
Factual recall
Rationale: Defining the terminology is necessary to answer the question.

11. **b**
Factual recall
Rationale: This is an example of identification of the incorrect statement as the answer of choice. Always read this type of question carefully. Synovial joints are freely movable, and fibrocartilage is found in synarthrodial joints.

12. **c**
Factual recall
Rationale: Defining the terms is necessary to answer the question.

13. **c**

    Clinical reasoning and synthesis
    Rationale: The facts presented by the question are information about multiple dislocations of a shoulder joint that now has reduced mobility and muscle spasms. Safe application of massage methods is always a priority. The three wrong answers would further increase the underlying hypermobility. Answer c is the most logical approach because the protective and compensatory muscle contraction is not eliminated but instead is managed.

14. **b**

    Factual recall
    Rationale: The question is the definition of arthrokinematics.

15. **a**

    Application and concept identification
    Rationale: The concepts presented in the question are stability and laxity, and in the answers they are joint play, hypomobility, and muscle relaxation. The term *plasma membrane* refers to cellular structure. The question wants to know what happens when lax ligaments reduce stability, and the answer is that joint play increases.

16. **d**

    Factual recall
    Rationale: The correct answer defines the closed packed position of a joint.

17. **c**

    Application and concept identification
    Rationale: The question asks why the least packed position is the most comfortable when a joint is injured.

18. **b**

    Factual recall
    Rationale: The question is the definition of physiologic range of motion.

19. **d**

    Factual recall
    Rationale: The question asks for information about joint structure. This question represents the type of question in which an understanding of how joints are designed is necessary to answer the question. The anatomic limits of motion of the knee are provided primarily by soft tissue, such as the joint capsule and ligaments, instead of bone, as found in the elbow and hip. The ankle is similar to the knee but is held more stable by the bone structure.

20. **a**

    Clinical reasoning and synthesis
    Rationale: The case study question structure requires an analysis of the data provided in the question and possible answers. The facts are a broken wrist, extended period of joint immobility while in a cast, and current limited range of motion of the wrist. The correct answer would explain why this has occurred. The condition described is hypomobility, so answer c can be eliminated. Muscles atrophy when immobile, so answer b can be eliminated. Answer d is an incorrect use of terminology. The only answer left is answer a, which would be the probable outcome.

21. **d**

    Application and concept identification
    Rationale: The question asks for the connection between a massage method (passive range of motion) and how the method would be implemented. Only answer d correctly describes circumduction.

22. **c**

    Factual recall
    Rationale: You need to define the terms in the possible answers to identify eversion as a movement of the foot.

23. **b**

    Factual recall
    Rationale: You need to define the terms in the possible answers to identify scapular retraction.

24. **c**

    Application and concept identification
    Rationale: The question is asking for how correct information is transmitted to a client so that a joint movement can be performed for assessment or intervention. The action described by the correct answer needs to result in the external rotation of the hip. Only answer c is correct.

25. **d**

    Factual recall
    Rationale: You need to define the terms to identify the correct answer.

26. **c**

    Factual recall
    Rationale: The question is the definition of kinematic chains.

27. **a**
Factual recall
Rationale: The question describes the outcome of functional change in closed kinematic chains. The terminology is used incorrectly in possible answers c and d. This is often a strategy for creating incorrect answers.

28. **c**
Factual recall
Rationale: This question is representative of many possible questions relating to joint anatomy. You must identify the two correct articulating bones of the joint to answer the question correctly.

29. **a**
Factual recall
Rationale: This question is representative of many possible questions relating to joint anatomy. You must identify the correct structural design of the joint to answer the question.

30. **b**
Factual recall
Rationale: This question is representative of many possible questions relating to joint function. You must identify the correct structural design of the joint to answer the question.

31. **c**
Application and concept identification
Rationale: The question is asking for the relationship between two joints, the sternoclavicular joint and the scapula.

32. **d**
Factual recall
Rationale: This question is representative of many possible questions relating to joint anatomy. You must identify the correct structural design of the joint to answer the question.

33. **b**
Factual recall
Rationale: This question is representative of many possible questions relating to joint function. You must identify the correct structural design and movement pattern of the joint to answer the question.

34. **a**
Factual recall
Rationale: This question is representative of many possible questions relating to joint anatomy. You must identify the correct structural design of the joint to answer the question. The question requires understanding of the terminology to identify the correct answer.

35. **c**
Factual recall
Rationale: This question is representative of many possible questions relating to joint anatomy. You must identify the correct articulating bones of the joint to answer the question. The question requires understanding of the terminology to identify the correct answer.

36. **b**
Factual recall
Rationale: This question is representative of many possible questions relating to joint anatomy. You must identify the correct articulating bones of the joint to answer the question. The question requires understanding of the terminology to identify the correct answer.

37. **d**
Factual recall
Rationale: This question is representative of many possible questions relating to joint function. You must identify the correct structural design of the joint to answer the question. The question requires understanding of the terminology to identify the correct answer.

38. **a**
Application and concept identification
Rationale: This question is representative of many possible questions relating to joint function. You must identify the correct movement of the joint into the loose packed position to answer the question. The question requires understanding of the terminology to identify the correct answer.

39. **b**
Application and concept identification
Rationale: This question is representative of many possible questions relating to joint movement patterns. You must identify the correct result in response to anteversion to answer the question. The question requires understanding of the terminology to identify the correct answer.

40. **c**
Application and concept identification
Rationale: This question is representative of many possible questions relating to joint function. You must identify the most stable position of the knee to answer the question. The question requires understanding of the terminology to identify the correct answer.

41. **b**
Application and concept identification
Rationale: This question is representative of many possible questions relating to joint anatomy in response to trauma. You must identify the correct outcome of the trauma to answer the question. In this instance the medial ligament would be pushed into extension, causing damage. The question requires understanding of the terminology to identify the correct answer.

42. **d**
Factual recall
Rationale: The question describes the function of the menisci.

43. **c**
Factual recall
Rationale: The most stable position is full dorsiflexion.

44. **b**
Application and concept identification
Rationale: The question asks for an explanation as to why the heel would increase the potential for sprained ankle. The heel puts the ankle into plantar flexion, which is a less stable position for the ankle, predisposing one to ankle sprains.

45. **b**
Factual recall
Rationale: Knowledge about the range of motion allowed at the listed joints is necessary to answer the question.

46. **a**
Application and concept identification
Rationale: The connection between the location of the anterior longitudinal ligament and its function in relation to the vertebral joints is required to answer the question. This ligament stabilizes against trunk extension.

47. **c**
Clinical reasoning and synthesis
Rationale: The facts presented in the question indicate that the disk bulged posteriorly, which would be the result of a flexion injury. The most common location in the lower back is at the lumbosacral junction.

48. **d**
Factual recall
Rationale: Knowledge about the range of motion allowed at the listed joints is necessary to answer the question.

49. **b**
Factual recall
Rationale: Recall of rib motion during breathing in is required to answer the question. The ribs are raised during inspiration.

50. **c**
Application and concept identification
Rationale: You need to define the pathologic conditions listed and then correlate the benefits of massage with possible outcomes. Dislocation is contraindicated. Rheumatoid arthritis has a limited response to massage and requires caution. Kyphosis is structural. Only answer c is correct.

51. **d**
Clinical reasoning and synthesis
Rationale: The question provides the following fact: the client has degenerative joint disease. The textbook provides additional information about this disorder. The question also places cautions on treatment, indicating use of conservative measures. The correct treatment plan would need to address the condition and the cautions. Bed rest is not indicated, nor is cortisone injection used for conservative treatment. Intense exercise and connective tissue massage are too aggressive. Answer d presents the best plan.

52. **a**
Clinical reasoning and synthesis
Rationale: The facts from the question are repetitive strain injury, long-term decreased mobility, and reduced range of motion. Of the possible reasons for the reduced range of motion, massage would best reverse muscle and connective tissue abnormality.

53. **c**
Concept identification
Rationale: Only synovial joints are freely movable. The rest of the terms indicate structures with limited movement.

54. **d**
Concept identification
Rationale: A convexity is characteristic of a bend force. The hit on the lateral side would cause a concavity. Shear force has concavities and convexities but does not fit the description of the injury.

55. **a**
Factual recall
Rationale: Plantar flexion occurs in the ankle, and pronation occurs in the wrist; c and d are similar actions.

56. **b**
    Clinical reasoning and synthesis
    Rationale: Zero degrees is the anatomic position.
    The question is measuring a limit in flexion, so
    eliminate answers a and c. Answer d would be
    an increase in range of motion, not a decrease.

57. **c**
    Clinical reasoning and synthesis
    Rationale: An anterior tilt means the ischial
    tuberosity is up and the iliac crest is moving
    forward. This would mean the hips need to flex.

58. **d**
    Concept identification
    Rationale: Inspiration is the inhale, and the ribs
    move up and out

CHAPTER

9

Muscles

Review Tips

The content concerning muscles is complex. You must know muscle structure, location, function, functional muscle groups (agonist, antagonist, synergist), innervations, and pathologic conditions. Muscle is largely connective tissue; therefore you must grasp the nature of connective tissue types and function.

You can drive yourself crazy if you are not realistic about studying muscles. Hopefully, the following information and suggestions can make this study less confusing.

Muscle names can provide clues about location, function, and shape.

Nerves often are named to reflect their location; that is, the ulnar nerve is located adjacent to the ulna bone, and the thoracodorsal nerve is located in the posterior thorax.

Function involves joints, so muscle function often is described with the terms flexion, extension, rotation, adduction, and abduction. Other movement terms used to described muscle functions are medial, lateral, depression, elevation, and tilt. Types of muscle function are concentric, which produces (accelerates) movement; eccentric, which controls (decelerates) movement; and isometric, which stabilizes.

Most exams do not ask specific questions about the exact attachment of muscles because textbooks do not agree. You must know bony landmarks to learn muscle attachments. Attachment terminology is changing. The shift is from origin and insertion to proximal and distal attachment. *Mosby's Essential Sciences for Therapeutic Massage* uses the most current terminology and explains that muscles attach from one location to another.

The proximal attachment (typically the old origin description) is described as "from" and the distal "attachment (old insertion terminology) is described as to."
• From-proximal-origin
• To-distal-insertion

Adding to the confusion is that different textbooks and atlases describe attachments in different ways. Exam questions on legally defensible exams need to be referenced to approved textbooks. When these resources do not agree, writing questions can be difficult. The most common solution is not to have many questions that involve content, which is a bit controversial and could be challenged. Therefore it is not necessary to memorize in precise detail the attachment of every single muscle. Concentrate on the function of muscles and the general location.

A great way to study muscles—location and function—is to build models. You can obtain skeletal models inexpensively at a store that carries educational supplies or can order them online. Then use a modeling compound (clay, playdough) to build the muscles. Coloring books are helpful. The author recommends the Muscolino text *Musculoskeletal Anatomy Coloring Book* (Mosby, 2004). The flash card set by Muscolino is also helpful (*Musculoskeletal Anatomy Flashcards,* Mosby, 2005).

Because muscles and massage so often are connected, it is common to find muscle system terminology in many of the questions on massage exams. This is especially common in the case study type of questions.

This content can appear in all three types of multiple-choice questions.

Questions

1. Muscle uses which of the following to produce mechanical energy to exert force?

    a. Myoglobin
    b. Adenosine triphosphate
    c. Perimysium
    d. Cholecystokinin

2. A client complains of fatigue and muscle soreness after attempting to push a car that was stuck. Which of the following best describes this action?

    a. No movement was produced, so static force was generated.
    b. Dynamic force was used because the car did not move.
    c. Static force produced movement and energy expenditure.
    d. Because the car did not move, little energy was expended.

3. During assessment, the massage professional realizes that a client has extremely mobile joints. Which muscle functions would seem to be impaired?

    a. Produce movement
    b. Generate heat
    c. Maintain posture
    d. Stabilize joints

4. When a joint flexes, the muscles producing the action will shorten. Which of the functional characteristics of muscles is being described?

    a. Excitability
    b. Contractility
    c. Extensibility
    d. Elasticity

5. The structural units of contraction in skeletal muscle fibers are _____.

    a. Myoglobin
    b. Myofibrils
    c. Sarcomeres
    d. Fascicles

6. The attachment of myosin to cross-bridges on actin requires _____.

    a. Calcium
    b. Maximal stimulus
    c. Endomysium
    d. Potassium

7. Delicate and precise movements such as found with the eye muscles are possible because_____.

    a. Multiple sensory neurons innervate the muscles
    b. Large motor units exist in the muscle
    c. The muscle fibers in a motor unit are clustered together
    d. A motor unit consists of a few muscle fibers

8. Anatomically there is a strong correlation between the location of motor points, acupuncture points, and _____.

    a. Motor end plates
    b. Tendons
    c. Trigger points
    d. Mitotic units

9. The nature of muscles to maintain a certain amount of tautness is called _____.

    a. Threshold stimulus
    b. Muscle tone
    c. Treppe
    d. All-or-none response

10. A client was a sprinter in high school track and was effective during short and quick runs. Now 10 years later the client is complaining of lacking the endurance to run 5 miles as part of a fitness program. The client is in good physical condition with no apparent reason for the difficulties. Which of the following offers the most plausible explanation for the client's condition?

    a. The person has an abundance of slow twitch fibers in relationship to fast twitch fibers.
    b. The person has an increased ability to manage oxygen debt.
    c. The person's legs have a genetic tendency toward a makeup of more white anaerobic fibers.
    d. The person has increased slow twitch fibers in the postural muscles.

11. A client is complaining of tender areas in the postural muscles along the spine. Assessment indicates a series of trigger points in these muscles. The massage professional must determine how much compressive force to apply to the trigger points and how long to hold the contraction. Which of the following will affect this decision?

    a. These muscles contain more slow twitch red fibers that are fatigue resistant.
    b. These muscles are prone to oxygen debt.
    c. These muscles have an abundance of fast twitch and intermediate fibers.
    d. These muscles require a maximal stimulus to respond to treatment.

12. Vascular structures in muscles are _____.

    a. Limited to the muscular aponeurosis
    b. Abundant and designed to accommodate stretch
    c. Found mainly in the epimysium
    d. Abundant within the ligament structures

13. The connective tissue aspect of muscles is _____.

    a. The active contractile unit
    b. The main heat-producing structure
    c. Responsive to adenosine triphosphate
    d. Inseparable and continuous with muscle fibers

14. Intermuscular septa are formed primarily from _____.

    a. Deep fascia
    b. Epimysium
    c. Perimysium
    d. Endomysium

15. A client complains of a sensation of thickness and stiffness in the myofascial structures of the body. Slow, sustained stretching provides the most benefit. What is the most plausible reason for this effect?

    a. The neuromuscular unit is deprived of calcium, allowing the actin and myosin to disengage.
    b. The viscous nature of connective tissue responds to this method by becoming more pliable.
    c. The colloid connective tissue ground substance decreases water binding with these methods.
    d. The compression against the capillaries increases blood flow.

16. Two clients describe accidents in which the muscles of their upper thigh were cut and now healed. Client A has a mobile scar with near normal function. Client B has tissue rigidity and reduced movement. What is the most plausible explanation?

    a. Client A limited exercise and kept the area tightly wrapped during the healing process.
    b. Client B had more satellite cell activity during healing, causing increased scar tissue.
    c. Client A exercised during healing to stimulate satellite cells.
    d. Client B experienced increased circulation and reduced adhesions.

17. The proximal attachment of a muscle is also known as the _____.

    a. Origin
    b. Insertion
    c. Direct attachment
    d. Indirect attachment

Correct answers are on pages 98-103.

18. A client is complaining of pain when straightening the elbow. Palpation of the triceps at the musculotendinous junction indicates more tenderness at the insertion when the muscle is activated. What is the most likely reason for this?

    a. The insertion is the fixed attachment and would be more tender during movement.
    b. The insertion is the proximal attachment and is straining at the intermuscular septa.
    c. The belly of the muscle located at the insertion is highly innervated.
    d. The insertion is the more movable attachment, so it would produce more tenderness upon motion.

19. If a strong and sustained contraction without extensive movement is required, which of the following muscle shapes provides the best design?

    a. Parallel
    b. Pennate
    c. Circular
    d. Convergent

20. A client is experiencing a limitation in range of motion of the hip into abduction. Assessment indicates shortening and tension in the adductor group of muscles. Which of the following is the most likely source of the limited range of motion?

    a. Agonists
    b. Synergists
    c. Antagonists
    d. Fixators

21. The ability to execute a coordinated and accurate pattern of movement requires cooperation among various muscle groups called _____.

    a. Myotatic units
    b. Stretch reflex
    c. Tendon reflex
    d. Inhibition

22. The polysynaptic reflex that coordinates muscle action on both sides of the body is the _____.

    a. Stretch reflex
    b. Flexor reflex
    c. Tendon reflex
    d. Fixator reflex

23. A client unexpectedly lifted a box that was much too heavy. Now the client is experiencing residual weakness in the biceps and brachialis muscles and tension in the triceps muscle group. Which of the following reflexes best explains this situation?

    a. Stretch reflex
    b. Tendon reflex
    c. Withdrawal reflex
    d. Crossed extensor reflex

24. Which of the following muscle types has the ability to contract in such a way as to produce peristalsis?

    a. Cardiac
    b. Circular
    c. Smooth
    d. Pennate

25. A client is complaining of a headache in the eye, ear, and scalp, especially above the ear. Assessment identifies a trigger point in which of the following muscles?

    a. Orbicularis oculi
    b. Buccinator
    c. Risorius
    d. Occipitofrontalis

26. Which of the following is a muscle of mastication?

    a. Platysma
    b. Lateral pterygoid
    c. Digastric
    d. Zygomaticus major

27. The muscles of the anterior triangle of the neck as defined by the sternocleidomastoid have a primary function of _____.

    a. Assisting in swallowing
    b. Cervical extension
    c. Stabilization of capital rotation
    d. Neck flexion

28. Compression by which of the following muscle groups against the brachial nerve plexus often refers pain to the pectoralis, to the rhomboid area, and into the arm and hand?

    a. Splenius capitis and cervicis
    b. Erector spinae group
    c. Scalene group
    d. Infrahyoid group

29. The abdominal and psoas muscles are the major antagonists for which of the following muscles?

    a. Splenius capitis
    b. Longissimus thoracis
    c. Intertransversarii thoracis
    d. Serratus posterior

30. A client complains of difficulty achieving a full and deep breath. Assessments indicate no problems with exhalation. There is a restriction with the lifting of the ribs during inhalation. Which muscle that lifts the ribs may be involved?

    a. Diaphragm
    b. Serratus posterior inferior
    c. Internal intercostals
    d. External intercostals

31. A client complains of low back pain that increases with coughing. Assessment indicates tenderness in the deep lumbar area with referred pain to the gluteal area, particularly around the sacroiliac joint. Which muscle is likely to be involved?

    a. Quadratus lumborum
    b. Iliacus
    c. Semispinalis
    d. Psoas minor

32. Which of the following muscles has its origin at the crest of the pubis and pubic symphysis and insertion at the cartilage of the fifth, sixth, and seventh ribs and at the xiphoid process?

    a. Pyramidalis
    b. External oblique
    c. Rectus abdominis
    d. Transversus abdominis

33. Which of the following muscles would be innervated by the perineal division of the pudendal nerve?

    a. Levator ani
    b. Cremaster
    c. Longus colli
    d. Levator labii inferioris

34. Which of the following muscles of scapular stabilization contains three distinct parts with distinct functions, allowing the muscle to be an antagonist to itself?

    a. Serratus anterior
    b. Trapezius
    c. Pectoralis minor
    d. Rhomboid major

35. Assessment indicates that a client has the left scapular area rounded forward and protracted. Which of the following muscles are likely to be tense and shortened?

    a. Trapezius and rhomboideus minor
    b. Levator scapulae and supraspinatus
    c. Pectoralis minor and serratus anterior
    d. Teres minor and infraspinatus

36. Assessment indicates that a client has bilateral medially rotated humerus. The subscapularis muscles are tight and short and contain trigger points. Which of the following muscles is likely to be inhibited?

    a. Anterior deltoid
    b. Pectoralis major
    c. Teres major
    d. Infraspinatus

37. A client is having difficulty raising the arm into a position to comb the hair. Which of the following muscles is likely to be tight and short?

    a. Coracobrachialis
    b. Biceps brachii
    c. Latissimus dorsi
    d. Teres minor

Correct answers are on pages 98-103.

38. Which muscle is attached as follows: distal half of the anterior surface of the humerus, medial and lateral intermuscular septa, and coronoid process and tuberosity of the ulna?

    a. Brachioradialis
    b. Pronator teres
    c. Supinator
    d. Brachialis

39. Which of the following muscles is synergistic to the triceps?

    a. Supinator
    b. Pronator quadratus
    c. Anconeus
    d. Pronator teres

40. A client has been working on a project that required gripping a hammer for an extended period. Now the client is complaining of weakness when attempting to extend the wrist. Which of the following is the most likely explanation?

    a. The flexor muscle group of the hand and wrist increased tone levels, resulting in inhibition of the extensor group of muscles in the forearm.
    b. The flexor digitorum superficialis and profundus are weak from fatigue, so the wrist extensors have been facilitated.
    c. The deep layer of the posterior wrist extensor group is antagonistic to the superficial layer of this same muscle group, resulting in weakness in the wrist extensors.
    d. The flexor carpi ulnaris and the extensor carpi ulnaris are in spasm, resulting in inhibition of the abductor pollicis longus.

41. Which of the following muscles is located in the thenar eminence?

    a. Opponens digiti minimi
    b. Opponens pollicis
    c. Lumbricales
    d. Dorsal interosseus

42. Which of the following muscles extends, laterally rotates the hip joint with lower fibers, assists in adduction of the hip with the femur fixed, and assists in extension of the trunk?

    a. Gluteus medius
    b. Gluteus minimus
    c. Gluteus maximus
    d. Tensor fasciae latae

43. When considering the layering of muscles from superficial to deep, which of the following is the deepest?

    a. Gluteus medius
    b. Gluteus minimus
    c. Gluteus maximus
    d. Piriformis

44. Observation and assessment of a client indicate that the left leg is externally (laterally) rotated. Which of the following muscles may be tense and shortened?

    a. Tensor fasciae latae
    b. Gemellus superior
    c. Gracilis
    d. Pectineus

45. Which of the following pairs of muscles are synergistic with each other?

    a. Biceps femoris and gluteus maximus
    b. Adductor brevis and gluteus medius
    c. Semimembranosus and obturator externus
    d. Piriformis and semitendinosus

46. If the legs are fixed, which of the following is a flexor of the hip and also assists in flexion of the torso to the thigh?

    a. Vastus lateralis
    b. Vastus medialis
    c. Sartorius
    d. Semitendinosus

47. A client complains of difficulty extending the knee. Which group of muscles is likely to be tense and short?

    a. Adductor group

    b. Quadriceps femoris group

    c. Anterior leg group

    d. Hamstring group

48. When beginning flexion, a client feels a "catch" sensation in the back of the knee. The doctor does not find any problem with the joint and indicates that it is a muscular problem. Which muscle is likely to be involved?

    a. Peroneus brevis

    b. Tibialis posterior

    c. Popliteus

    d. Peroneus longus

49. Which muscles are most responsible for dorsiflexion?

    a. Anterior leg muscles

    b. Posterior leg muscles

    c. Lateral arm muscles

    d. Medial arm muscles

50. A dancer is finding it difficult to sustain movement requiring him to be on his toes. Which muscle may be inhibited?

    a. Plantar interossei

    b. Soleus

    c. Extensor digitorum

    d. Peroneus tertius

51. Which of the following muscles plantar flexes the ankle and assists with knee flexion?

    a. Tibialis posterior

    b. Tibialis anterior

    c. Peroneus longus

    d. Plantaris

52. If the gastrocnemius is tight and short, which of the following muscles is likely to be inhibited?

    a. Soleus

    b. Tibialis anterior

    c. Flexor hallucis longus

    d. Flexor digitorum longus

53. Which of the following muscles has its attachment on the larger or great toe?

    a. Flexor digitorum brevis

    b. Quadratus plantae

    c. Flexor hallucis brevis

    d. Abductor digiti minimi

54. A client's job requires her to perform the same repetitive lift and hand squeeze task. She has been doing this job for 8 months. In the beginning, her arms were sore and a bit swollen but that went away. In the past 3 months the pain and tension in the arms have returned and have begun to increase. Which of the following best describes the client's current condition?

    a. Chain reaction in myotatic units has occurred.

    b. Pain increases tension or spasm, which increases pain.

    c. Joint restriction and fascial shortening decrease mobility.

    d. Generalized fatigue has developed from an interrupted sleep pattern.

55. Which of the following medications likely would be prescribed for tendinitis?

    a. Antibiotic

    b. Muscle relaxant

    c. Anticoagulant

    d. Antiinflammatory

Correct answers are on pages 98-103.

56. A client is taking an over-the-counter analgesic. What concern would the massage professional have while providing massage?

    a. Feedback mechanisms for pain will be altered.
    b. Blood pressure may fall dangerously low.
    c. The infection may be spread.
    d. Inflammation may be increased.

57. Which of the following conditions is most likely to benefit directly from a nonspecific general massage session?

    a. Contusion
    b. Anterior compartment syndrome
    c. Muscle tension headache
    d. Spasticity

58. Which of the following conditions presents regional contraindications for massage as long as physician approval has been obtained?

    a. Post-polio syndrome
    b. Myositis ossificans
    c. Muscular dystrophy
    d. Myasthenia gravis

59. A client with fibromyalgia has been referred from the physician for massage. A treatment plan has been requested for approval before treatment begins. Which of the following would be the best approach?

    a. General massage with active assisted joint movement and stretching
    b. General massage with friction methods to active tender points
    c. Localized massage to the feet and ischemic compression to active trigger points
    d. General massage to support restorative sleep and symptomatic pain management

60. If the concentric function of a muscle is extension and lateral flexion, then which of the following is the eccentric function of that same muscle?

    a. Stabilizes the adjacent joint
    b. Elevation and rotation of the area
    c. Restrains flexion and controls extension
    d. Assists extension and lateral flexion

61. If the major function of a muscle is to stabilize, then which of the following muscle functions is involved?

    a. Isometric
    b. Concentric
    c. Eccentric
    d. Kinetic

62. If the concentric function of a muscle is to extend and laterally rotate the thigh at the hip joint, which of the following would be synergist and antagonist muscles?

    a. Hamstrings and iliopsoas
    b. Quadratus femoris and fibularis
    c. Popliteus and plantaris
    d. Quadratus lumborum and transverse abdominis oblique

63. What relationship do the tibialis anterior and the extensor digitorum longus have?

    a. They are located in the thigh.
    b. Both muscles are synergists to each other.
    c. The muscles are concentric eccentric antagonists.
    d. Both muscles function at the knee.

64. If the attachment of a muscle is located closer to the torso and would be listed as from in attachment description, which of the following would be correct?

    a. Distal insertion
    b. Distal origin
    c. Proximal origin
    d. *To* insertion

Exercise

Using the foregoing questions as examples, now write at least three more questions—one of each type: factual recall and comprehension, application and concept identification, and clinical reasoning and synthesis. Make sure to develop plausible wrong answers, and be sure that the correct answer is clearly correct. Then write a rationale for each question. The more questions you write, the better you will understand the material.

Answers and Discussion

1. **b**
Factual recall
Rationale: You would need to define all the possible answers to identify adenosine triphosphate as the correct answer.

2. **a**
Application and concept identification
Rationale: The question asks for the connection between an action (pushing a car), the result (fatigue and muscle soreness), and the best description for the action. Generating static force expends energy with no result in movement.

3. **d**
Application and concept identification
Rationale: Assessment identifies hypermobile joints. The correct answer explains the role of muscles in joint stability.

4. **b**
Factual recall
Rationale: You need to define the terms listed as possible answers to answer the question.

5. **c**
Factual recall
Rationale: You need to define the terms listed as possible answers to answer the question.

6. **a**
Factual recall
Rationale: You need to define the terms listed as possible answers to answer the question.

7. **d**
Factual recall
Rationale: The questions and possible answers describe a physiologic process in terms of muscle contractile ability and control based on the number of muscle fibers per motor unit. The fewer the fibers, the more precise the movement.

8. **c**
Factual recall
Rationale: You need to define the terms in the question and possible answers to answer the question.

9. **b**
Factual recall
Rationale: You need to define the terms in the question and possible answers to answer the question. The question is a definition of tone.

10. **c**
Application and concept identification
Rationale: The question identifies the genetic tendency for fast twitch and slow twitch fiber types in muscles. The wrong answers are not logical in relation to the facts in the question or misuse terminology in relation to other terms in the sentence. This is a common strategy for creating wrong answers.

11. **a**
Application and concept identification
Rationale: Postural muscles are fatigue resistant and usually are made of a higher percentage of slow twitch red fibers. To affect these muscles, a sustained force at threshold stimulus needs to be applied.

12. **b**
Factual recall
Rationale: You need to define the terms in the question and possible answers to answer the question. The structure of capillaries is long and winding to accommodate the changes in muscle shape.

13. **d**
Factual recall
Rationale: The connective tissue is continuous with muscle fibers. The three incorrect answers describe functions of muscles.

14. **a**
Factual recall
Rationale: You need to define the terms in the question and possible answers to answer the question.

15. **b**
Application and concept identification
Rationale: The question asks for the rationale for the massage method described. Slow stretching affects the viscous aspect of the connective tissue more than the neurologic or chemical action of muscle fibers. Slow stretching has minimal effect on blood flow. Answer c is incorrect because slow stretching would increase, not decrease, water binding.

16. **c**
Clinical reasoning and synthesis
Rationale: The facts in the question describe two different healing outcomes to a similar injury. Client A has near normal function, whereas client B has dysfunction. You need to decide why this occurred based on correct information. You need to analyze the answers in relation to the question and general factual data about tissue healing. Only answer c meets these criteria. Limiting exercise and wrapping the area would result in less mobility, and client A had near-normal function. Satellite cell activity results in replacement during healing, not increased scar development. Increased circulation and decreased adhesions result in mobility, not rigidity.

17. **a**
Factual recall
Rationale: You need to define the terms in the question and possible answers to answer the question.

18. **d**
Application and concept identification
Rationale: The question asks for an understanding of movement, muscle attachments, and terminology. You need to define all the terminology to understand the question and possible answers. You need to identify the correct answer based on muscle anatomy and physiology. The wrong answers use all the right words in the wrong context. This is common strategy for writing wrong answers. Only answer d correctly describes the reason for the increased tenderness on palpation.

19. **b**
Factual recall
Rationale: You need to define the terms listed as possible answers to answer the question. The question defines a function of pennate muscle shape.

20. **c**
Application and concept identification
Rationale: The question describes a myotatic unit. The answers listed are the components of myotatic units, and you need to define these terms. The agonist for abduction requires that the antagonist (the adductor) relax to allow for the movement. If this is not happening, then the antagonist is the likely cause.

21. **a**
Factual recall
Rationale: You need to define the terms listed as possible answers to answer the question. The question provides a definition of myotatic units.

22. **b**
Factual recall
Rationale: You need to define the terms listed as possible answers to answer the question. The question provides a definition of the flexor reflex.

23. **b**
Application and concept identification
Rationale: The action described in the question stimulated the protective action of the tendon reflex. The question asks for a correlation of the reflex physiology to an actual situation. An understanding of agonist and antagonist interaction and the response patterns of all the reflexes listed in the possible answers is necessary to identify the correct answer.

24. **c**
Factual recall
Rationale: You need to define the terms listed as possible answers to answer the question. The question provides a function of smooth muscle.

25. **d**
Factual recall
Rationale: This question is representative of hundreds of questions that can be written about muscle anatomy and physiology. To answer these types of questions there needs to be a factual basis about attachments, innervation, function, myotatic unit, common trigger points, and referred pain patterns of the individual muscles. This question asks for referred pain pattern.

26. **b**
Factual recall
Rationale: This question is representative of hundreds of questions that can be written about muscle anatomy and physiology. To answer these types of questions there needs to be a factual basis about attachments, innervation, function, myotatic unit, common trigger points, and referred pain patterns of the individual muscles. This question asks for function.

27. **a**
Factual recall
Rationale: This question is representative of hundreds of questions that can be written about muscle anatomy and physiology. To answer these types of questions there needs to be a factual basis about attachments, innervation, function, myotatic unit, common trigger points, and referred pain patterns of the individual muscles. This question asks for function of a group based on location.

28. **c**
Factual recall
Rationale: This question is representative of hundreds of questions that can be written about muscle anatomy and physiology. To answer these types of questions there needs to be a factual basis about attachments, innervation, function, myotatic unit, common trigger points, and referred pain patterns of the individual muscles. This question asks for referred pain pattern.

29. **b**
Factual recall
Rationale: This question is representative of hundreds of questions that can be written about muscle anatomy and physiology. To answer these types of questions there needs to be a factual basis about attachments, innervation, function, myotatic unit, common trigger points and referred pain patterns of the individual muscles. This question asks for myotatic unit interaction.

30. **d**
Factual recall
Rationale: This question is representative of hundreds of questions that can be written about muscle anatomy and physiology. To answer these types of questions there needs to be a factual basis about attachments, innervation, function, myotatic unit, common trigger points, and referred pain patterns of the individual muscles. This question asks for function.

31. **a**
Factual recall
Rationale: This question is representative of hundreds of questions that can be written about muscle anatomy and physiology. To answer these types of questions there needs to be a factual basis about attachments, innervation, function, myotatic unit, common trigger points, and referred pain patterns of the individual muscles. This question asks for referred pain pattern.

32. **c**
Factual recall
Rationale: This question is representative of hundreds of questions that can be written about muscle anatomy and physiology. To answer these types of questions there needs to be a factual basis about attachments, innervation, function, myotatic unit, common trigger points, and referred pain patterns of the individual muscles. This question asks for origin and insertion.

33. **a**
Factual recall
Rationale: This question is representative of hundreds of questions that can be written about muscle anatomy and physiology. To answer these types of questions there needs to be a factual basis about attachments, innervation, function, myotatic unit, common trigger points, and referred pain patterns of the individual muscles. This question asks about nerve supply.

34. **b**
Factual recall
Rationale: This question is representative of hundreds of questions that can be written about muscle anatomy and physiology. To answer these types of questions there needs to be a factual basis about attachments, innervation, function, myotatic unit, common trigger points, and referred pain patterns of the individual muscles. This question asks about function.

35. **c**
Factual recall
Rationale: This question is representative of hundreds of questions that can be written about muscle anatomy and physiology. To answer these types of questions there needs to be a factual basis about attachments, innervation, function, myotatic unit, common trigger points, and referred pain patterns of the individual muscles. This question asks about function.

36. **d**
Factual recall
Rationale: This question is representative of hundreds of questions that can be written about muscle anatomy and physiology. To answer these types of questions there needs to be a factual basis about attachments, innervation, function, myotatic unit, common trigger points, and referred pain patterns of the individual muscles. The question asks for the myotatic unit, particularly the antagonist to the subscapularis.

37. **c**
Factual recall
Rationale: This question is representative of hundreds of questions that can be written about muscle anatomy and physiology. To answer these types of questions there needs to be a factual basis about attachments, innervation, function, myotatic unit, common trigger points, and referred pain patterns of the individual muscles. This question asks for impaired function of an antagonist pattern.

38. **d**
Factual recall
Rationale: This question is representative of hundreds of questions that can be written about muscle anatomy and physiology. To answer these types of questions there needs to be a factual basis about attachments, innervation, function, myotatic unit, common trigger points, and referred pain patterns of the individual muscles. This question describes a muscle location.

39. **c**
Factual recall
Rationale: This question is representative of hundreds of questions that can be written about muscle anatomy and physiology. To answer these types of questions there needs to be a factual basis about attachments, innervation, function, myotatic unit, common trigger points, and referred pain patterns of the individual muscles. This question asks for the myotatic unit.

40. **a**
Clinical reasoning and synthesis
Rationale: The facts presented in the question are extended contraction of the muscles used to grip (the flexor group of the forearm and the intrinsic muscles of the palm) and inhibition of the wrist extensors. The possible answers provide a reason for this condition. You need to analyze each to determine the correct use of terminology and logical information based on the facts of the question.

41. **b**
Factual recall
Rationale: This question is representative of hundreds of questions that can be written about muscle anatomy and physiology. To answer these types of questions there needs to be a factual basis about attachments, innervation, function, myotatic unit, common trigger points, and referred pain patterns of the individual muscles. This question asks for location.

42. **c**
Factual recall
Rationale: This question is representative of hundreds of questions that can be written about muscle anatomy and physiology. To answer these types of questions there needs to be a factual basis about attachments, innervation, function, myotatic unit, common trigger points, and referred pain patterns of the individual muscles. This question describes function.

43. **d**
Factual recall
Rationale: This question is representative of hundreds of questions that can be written about muscle anatomy and physiology. To answer these types of questions there needs to be a factual basis about attachments, innervation, function, myotatic unit, common trigger points, and referred pain patterns of the individual muscles. This question asks for location.

44. **b**
Factual recall
Rationale: This question is representative of hundreds of questions that can be written about muscle anatomy and physiology. To answer these types of questions there needs to be a factual basis about attachments, innervation, function, myotatic unit, common trigger points, and referred pain patterns of the individual muscles. This question asks for function.

45. **a**
Factual recall
Rationale: This question is representative of hundreds of questions that can be written about muscle anatomy and physiology. To answer these types of questions there needs to be a factual basis about attachments, innervation, function, myotatic unit, common trigger points, and referred pain patterns of the individual muscles. This question asks for the myotatic unit.

46. **c**
Factual recall
Rationale: This question is representative of hundreds of questions that can be written about muscle anatomy and physiology. To answer these types of questions there needs to be a factual basis about attachments, innervation, function, myotatic unit, common trigger points, and referred pain patterns of the individual muscles. This question asks for function.

47. **d**
Factual recall
Rationale: This question is representative of hundreds of questions that can be written about muscle anatomy and physiology. To answer these types of questions there needs to be a factual basis about attachments, innervation, function, myotatic unit, common trigger points, and referred pain patterns of the individual muscles. This question asks for the myotatic unit.

48. **c**
Factual recall
Rationale: This question is representative of hundreds of questions that can be written about muscle anatomy and physiology. To answer these types of questions there needs to be a factual basis about attachments, innervation, function, myotatic unit, common trigger points, and referred pain patterns of the individual muscles. This question asks for function and location.

49. **a**
Factual recall
Rationale: This question is representative of hundreds of questions that can be written about muscle anatomy and physiology. To answer these types of questions there needs to be a factual basis about attachments, innervation, function, myotatic unit, common trigger points, and referred pain patterns of the individual muscles. This question asks for function.

50. **b**
Factual recall
Rationale: This question is representative of hundreds of questions that can be written about muscle anatomy and physiology. To answer these types of questions there needs to be a factual basis about attachments, innervation, function, myotatic unit, common trigger points, and referred pain patterns of the individual muscles. This question asks for function.

51. **d**
Factual recall
Rationale: This question is representative of hundreds of questions that can be written about muscle anatomy and physiology. To answer these types of questions there needs to be a factual basis about attachments, innervation, function, myotatic unit, common trigger points, and referred pain patterns of the individual muscles. This question asks for function.

52. **b**
Factual recall
Rationale: This question is representative of hundreds of questions that can be written about muscle anatomy and physiology. To answer these types of questions there needs to be a factual basis about attachments, innervation, function, myotatic unit, common trigger points, and referred pain patterns of the individual muscles. This question asks for the myotatic unit.

53. **c**
Factual recall
Rationale: This question is representative of hundreds of questions that can be written about muscle anatomy and physiology. To answer these types of questions there needs to be a factual basis about attachments, innervation, function, myotatic unit, common trigger points, and referred pain patterns of the individual muscles. This question asks for location.

54. **b**
Application and concept identification
Rationale: The question is describing the pain-spasm-pain cycle.

55. **d**
Factual recall
Rationale: This question is representative of many questions that can be written about muscle pathology. To answer these types of questions there needs to be a factual basis about attachments, innervation, function, myotatic unit, common trigger points, and referred pain patterns of the individual muscles along with medications, common pathologic conditions, and methods of treatment. This question asks for identification of antiinflammatory medication.

56. **a**
Factual recall
Rationale: This question is representative of the many questions that can be written about muscle pathology. To answer these types of questions there needs to be a factual basis about attachments, innervation, function, myotatic unit, common trigger points, and referred pain patterns of the individual muscles along with medications, common pathologic consditions, and methods of treatment. This question asks for the cautions for applying massage.
An analgesic is a painkiller.

57. **c**

Application and concept identification
Rationale: The question requires an understanding of the pathologic conditions listed correlated with the benefits of a general massage. The three wrong answers present contraindications or complex conditions requiring specific intervention. Muscle tension headache commonly responds well to general massage, which generates a parasympathetic effect.

58. **b**

Factual recall
Rationale: This question is representative of hundreds of questions that can be written about muscle pathology. This question asks for the cautions for applying massage. The three wrong answers indicate general contraindications. Only myositis ossificans has a regional contraindication.

59. **d**

Clinical reasoning and synthesis
Rationale: The facts are related to the condition of fibromyalgia. The decision is what is the best massage approach to use. Fibromyalgia is muscle pain syndrome, which responds best to general massage to support sleep and relieve pain symptoms. Any type of massage that creates inflammation or excessively strains the system is contraindicated.

60. **c**

Concept identification
Rationale: Typically the eccentric function of any muscle is to restrain and decelerate the opposite action.

61. **a**

Factual recall
Rationale: Stabilization is produced in this contraction, but not movement.

62. **a**

Concept identification
Rationale: A synergist assists a movement, and an antagonist produces the opposite movement. For answers c and d the muscles are in the wrong location, as is fibularis.

63. **b**

Concept identification
Rationale: The muscles are located in the leg, not the thigh; do not cross the knee; and share function at the ankle.

64. **b**

Concept identification
Rationale: Because of reverse actions of muscles where the stabilizing and moving attachments can change based on action, the terms origin and insertion are being phased out in favor of proximal and distal. Proximal attachments would be *from,* and the distal attachment would be *to.*

10
Biomechanics Basics

Review Tips

The content concerning biomechanics basics combines all the previous information into understanding how the body maintains posture and produces movement. This area has new terminology to understand. The content provides the foundation for assessment procedures. Assessment is necessary to determine indications and contraindications for massage.

This material often is represented in the concept identification and the case study/clinical reasoning synthesis question style. The terminology often is found in factual recall and comprehension questions.

An effective study strategy is to explain a concept in words different from those in the text or to give an example of what the text is talking about or to develop a metaphor about the content. As for the previous sections, look up any terminology you do not understand and make sure you know why the wrong answers are wrong.

Questions

1. What type of contraction occurs when the muscle lengthens while under tension, changes in tension occur to control the descent of resistance, and joint angle increases?

   a. Isometric eccentric
   b. Isotonic concentric
   c. Isometric concentric
   d. Isotonic eccentric

2. The amount of force on a specific area is called _____.

   a. Pressure
   b. Inertia
   c. Acceleration
   d. Center of gravity

3. A person who is maintaining an upright posture while reaching for an object is displaying _____.

   a. Static balance
   b. Dynamic balance
   c. Static equilibrium
   d. Inertia

4. Which of the following statements would describe the least amount of balance?

   a. Greater weight centered over a large base of support
   b. The center of gravity outside the base of support
   c. A low center of gravity with rotation around the axis
   d. An enlarged base of support in response to oncoming force

---

Correct answers are on pages 112-115.   **105**

5. The most efficient movement of the body into forward motion begins with the _____.

   a. Legs
   b. Arms
   c. Head
   d. Hips

6. Which of the following most often would be considered the fulcrum?

   a. Quadriceps muscles
   b. Radius
   c. Deltoid ligament
   d. Glenohumeral joint

7. When one is carrying a massage table from the car to the office, what is the responsibility of the muscles?

   a. Create a lever to distribute the load
   b. Exert effort to move the load
   c. Provide a fulcrum for the lever
   d. Maintain static balance

8. Because the body movements of the limb most often require rapid movement and insertions of the muscles close to the joint, which lever type most often is found?

   a. First-class lever
   b. Second-class lever
   c. Third-class lever
   d. Combined lever

9. During normal gait in the adult, the lumbar rotation is countered by a cervical spine rotation in the opposite direction for what reason?

   a. To keep the eyes on a level plane and the head oriented forward with the trunk
   b. To maintain the same-side counterbalance action of the arms and legs
   c. To coordinate the lever action of the elbows with the knees
   d. To activate the second-class lever system of the lift of the heel when moving onto the toes

10. An individual was running up stairs carrying a heavy briefcase in the left hand. Later that day the person felt increased tension in the left biceps muscle. Two days later, during a regular massage session, the client describes weakness and heaviness in one leg when walking up stairs or a hill. If normal gait reflexes are functioning, where would assessment likely find an inhibited muscle pattern?

    a. Right arm extensors
    b. Left hip flexors
    c. Right hip flexors
    d. Left hip extensors

11. During normal gait, when one foot is in contact with the floor, it is called the _____.

    a. Stance phase
    b. Double stance
    c. Swing phase
    d. Double swing

12. Which of the following aspects of the gait cycle would result in the most concentric contraction of the plantar flexors?

    a. Heel strike
    b. Midstance
    c. Toe-off preswing
    d. Midswing

13. When one is moving correctly from a seated to a standing position, the head moves forward and the hips bend, which moves the torso forward, then _____.

    a. The arms are contracted and push the body upright into a standing position
    b. The legs lift the body from the semisquat position into a standing position
    c. The leg muscles tense to provide stability while the back muscles straighten the torso
    d. The arms support the torso on the thighs so that the psoas and gluteal muscles can lift the body into a standing position

14. After tripping down a stair, but not falling, a client describes a sudden onset of pain during twisting and reaching movements. Which type of biomechanical dysfunction is most likely to be occurring?

    a. Neuromuscular
    b. Myofascial
    c. Joint related
    d. Capsular pattern

15. A reversible limitation of range of movement that occurs as a result of change in connective tissue following long-term muscle spasms is called _____.

    a. Nonoptimal motor function
    b. Capsular pattern
    c. Regional postural muscular imbalance
    d. Functional block

16. A client reports information during the history-taking process, which is confirmed with physical assessment, indicating that postural muscles are moderately short with mild connective tissue changes. Antagonist muscle patterns show some inhibition. What degree of imbalance is being observed?

    a. First degree
    b. Second degree
    c. Third degree
    d. Fourth degree

17. A client has been referred by the physician for massage. The diagnosis is functional stress with second-degree distortion of motor function. Which of the following symptoms would the client likely be experiencing?

    a. Minor recruitment of synergist muscles but not postural change
    b. Weakness of antagonist patterns and specific nonoptimal movement
    c. Fatigue with daily activities, mild pain, and localized functional blocks
    d. Instability of vertebral motion segments with painful muscle tension and connective tissue shortening

18. A client experienced an auto accident 4 years ago that resulted in a bulging disk at L4. The injury has since healed with minimal difficulties. During assessment, palpation indicates a moderate decrease in pliability of the lumbar dorsal fascia and mild shortening in the lumbar muscles. Forward flexion and rotation of the lumbar area are impaired mildly. Massage was focused to reduce the muscle shortening in the lumbar area and increase connective tissue pliability. Immediately after the massage the client reported increased mobility but within 15 minutes began to complain of lower back pain. What is the most likely explanation for this occurrence?

    a. A shift of the condition from second-degree functional stress to first-degree functional tension
    b. Increase in stability around the past injury
    c. Decrease in mobility in the area around the past injury
    d. Destabilization of resourceful compensation in lumbar area around past injury

19. When a joint is moved so that the joint angle is decreased, what is occurring?

    a. Prime movers and synergist concentrically contract. The antagonist eccentrically functions while lengthening to allow the movement.
    b. Prime movers concentrically contract with the antagonist so that synergists lengthen to allow movement.
    c. Movement occurs as the antagonist contracts and prime movers eccentrically control the movement.
    d. Resistance is applied to the fixators, providing the movement activating the prime movers.

20. A massage professional positions the client's body to assess the strength of the hip flexors. Which is the correct position for the hand applying resistance?

    a. Near the hip
    b. At the ankle
    c. At the distal end of the femur
    d. On the tibia

21. During joint movement and muscle strength assessment, it is important to isolate the movement to the jointed area being assessed. This is called _____.

    a. Force
    b. Resistance
    c. Balance
    d. Stabilization

22. Wrist flexion has a normal range of 0 to 80 degrees. A client is assessed with a range of motion of 100 degrees. This jointed area would be considered _____.

    a. Balanced
    b. Hypermobile
    c. Hypomobile
    d. Inhibited

23. A client complains of joint pain in the knee, and assessment indicates hypermobility with pain on passive movement. Which of the following would be the most appropriate treatment plan?

    a. General massage to the body with specific muscle energy work and lengthening of the extensors and flexors of the knee
    b. General massage with regional contraindications to the knee area and referral for more appropriate diagnosis of possible capsular dysfunction
    c. Referral for diagnosis before any massage
    d. General massage with attention to friction methods at the joint capsule

24. A client is experiencing an upper chest breathing pattern. Which of the following muscle(s) may test as short and too strong from this type of breathing?

    a. Diaphragm
    b. Suprahyoid muscles
    c. Scalene muscles
    d. Infraspinatus

25. The typical range of motion in extension for the lumbar spine is _____.

    a. 25 degrees
    b. 5 degrees
    c. 40 degrees
    d. 60 degrees

26. A client complains of pain and tension in the lower back more to the left side. Physical assessment indicates that the pelvis is elevated on the left compared with the right. The client also indicates difficulty raising the left arm over the head. Which of the following muscles may be involved?

    a. Psoas
    b. Rectus abdominis
    c. Latissimus dorsi
    d. Semispinalis

27. A client is having difficulty moving the head into cervical extension beyond 10 degrees. Which of the following cervical flexor muscles may be restricting mobility?

    a. Longissimus capitis
    b. Sternocleidomastoid
    c. Splenius capitis
    d. Iliocostalis cervicis

28. A client is unable to rotate the cervical area to turn the head past 20 degrees to the left. Muscle testing should indicate what?

    a. Even strength on both sides
    b. Increased tension in the right cervical rotators
    c. Weakness in the right cervical rotators
    d. Increased strength in the cervical flexors

29. Which of the following muscles is able indirectly to affect the sternoclavicular joint?

    a. Deltoid
    b. Triceps
    c. Pectoralis minor
    d. Pectoralis major

30. If the scapula remains fixed and immobile, what would result at the glenohumeral joint?

    a. Range of motion would be limited.
    b. Internal and external rotation would be enhanced.
    c. Flexion would be unaffected.
    d. Horizontal abduction would be the only limitation.

31. The glenohumeral joint is a good example to describe which of the following correct biomechanical principles?

    a. When mobility increases, stability also increases.
    b. When stability is less, mobility also decreases.
    c. The more mobility, the less stability.
    d. Mobility is supported before stability.

32. The primary function of the shoulder girdle muscles that have attachments at the axial skeleton, the scapula, and the clavicle is _____.

    a. Extension of the shoulder joint
    b. Stability of the scapula
    c. Mobility of the humerus
    d. Mobility of the glenohumeral joint

33. A client is experiencing pain with any activity involving external or lateral rotation of the right shoulder. Range of motion is limited to 40 degrees. This condition has been coming on gradually. Muscle testing indicates weakness when resistance is applied to move the shoulder from external rotation to internal rotation. There is shortening in the muscles of internal rotation. Which of the following would be the most logical treatment plan?

    a. Muscle energy methods to support lengthening of the infraspinatus and methods to increase tone in the subscapularis
    b. Deep massage to the rhomboid muscles and stretching of the lumbar fascia
    c. Traction of the scapulothoracic junction
    d. Massage to reduce tension in the pectoralis major and latissimus dorsi with tapotement to increase tone in the infraspinatus and teres major

34. A client has elbow flexion of 90 degrees. This is considered _____.

    a. Normal
    b. Hypermobility
    c. Hypomobility
    d. Instability

35. A client is unable to turn the palm up past 45 degrees. Which of the following movements is hypomobile?

    a. Supination
    b. Pronation
    c. Flexion
    d. Extension

36. How is the area positioned and where is resistance applied to perform a muscle test for the normal function of the wrist flexors?

    a. The elbow is flexed, and resistance is applied against the forearm.
    b. The wrist is flexed, and resistance is applied against the palm of the hand.
    c. The wrist is extended, and resistance is applied against the palm of the hand.
    d. The wrist is flexed, and resistance is applied against the dorsal side of the hand.

37. When the left hip moves into flexion, what is the biomechanically correct movement of the pelvic girdle and the lumbar spine?

    a. Anterior rotation for the pelvic girdle and extension for the lumbar spine
    b. Posterior rotation for the pelvic girdle and flexion for the lumbar spine
    c. Left lateral rotation for the pelvic girdle and right lateral flexion for the lumbar spine
    d. Left transverse rotation for the pelvic girdle and external rotation for the lumbar spine

38. Concentric contraction occurs in which muscles when the thigh is flexed toward the trunk?

    a. Hamstrings
    b. Gluteus maximus
    c. Iliopsoas
    d. Vastus lateralis

Correct answers are on pages 112-115.

39. A client lying prone is unable to lift the thigh off the table when attempting hip extension. Which muscle is not able to contract effectively?

    a. Sartorius
    b. Adductor magnus
    c. Rectus femoris
    d. Semimembranosus

40. A client is lying supine, and observation indicates that the left leg is rotated internally. What should muscle testing reveal?

    a. Muscles that externally rotate the hip are short, and muscles that internally rotate the hip are inhibited.
    b. Muscles that externally rotate the hip are inhibited, and muscles that internally rotate the hip are overly strong.
    c. Gluteus medius should test weak.
    d. Adductor longus should test weak.

41. A massage practitioner wishes to assess the ability of the knee to move into slight internal and external rotation. How should the knee be positioned?

    a. Full extension
    b. 5 degrees of hyperextension
    c. 30 degrees of flexion
    d. 10 degrees of flexion

42. The knee is placed in 100 degrees of extension, and the client is asked to hold this position. Resistance is applied to the concentrically contracting muscles. Pain and weakness are felt. What is a logical explanation for this?

    a. The hamstring muscle group is weak.
    b. The Q angle is being altered in a lateral direction by the contraction of the vastus medialis.
    c. The popliteus muscle has been unable to unlock the screw-home mechanism.
    d. The quadriceps muscle group is unable effectively to hold a contraction against resistance.

43. A client experienced a second-degree ankle sprain when the foot was forced into inversion. Which of the following muscles would have experienced an extension injury?

    a. Fibularis longus
    b. Soleus
    c. Flexor digitorum longus
    d. Interossei

44. The sequence of muscle contraction determined by the nervous system to produce optimal movement is called a _____.

    a. Stabilization action
    b. Gait action
    c. Firing pattern
    d. Lower crossed syndrome

45. If during assessment the rhomboid muscles, posterior deltoid, and infraspinatus muscle test inhibited, which of the following most logically is indicated?

    a. Lower crossed syndrome
    b. Myofascial-related dysfunction
    c. Gait assessment
    d. Upper crossed syndrome

46. Which of the following is likely to result in joint-related dysfunction?

    a. Constant loading of a joint
    b. Generalized edema
    c. Closed kinematic chain
    d. Optimal firing pattern

47. An example of a core stabilization inner unit muscle would be?

    a. Latissimus dorsi
    b. Adductor longus
    c. Quadriceps
    d. Transversus abdominis

48. Which of the following muscle joint complexes would have 80 degrees of internal rotation?

    a. Knee
    b. Shoulder
    c. Cervical area
    d. Trunk

Exercise

Using the foregoing questions as examples, now write at least three more questions—one of each type: factual recall and comprehension, application and concept identification, and clinical reasoning and synthesis. Make sure to develop plausible wrong answers, and be sure that the correct answer is clearly correct. Then write a rationale for each question. The more questions you write, the better you will understand the material.

Correct answers are on pages 112-115.

Answers and Discussion

1. **d**
   Factual recall
   Rationale: As in all questions, you need to define the terminology to interpret the question and possible answers correctly. The question is the definition of an isotonic eccentric contraction.

2. **a**
   Factual recall
   Rationale: After you define the possible answers, you see that the question is a definition of pressure.

3. **b**
   Factual recall
   Rationale: After you define the possible answers, you see that the question describes dynamic balance.

4. **b**
   Factual recall
   Rationale: After you analyze the possible answers in relation to balance principles and compare them to the question, which asks for a condition that increases instability, you see that only answer b is logical.

5. **c**
   Factual recall
   Rationale: The weight of the head carries the body forward.

6. **d**
   Application and concept identification
   Rationale: A fulcrum is a fixed point around which a lever rotates. Only the joint can be a fulcrum; bones are levers and muscles provide force.

7. **b**
   Application and concept identification
   Rationale: The question describes an action and asks for muscle function. Muscles exert a force to generate effort to overcome resistance.

8. **c**
   Factual recall
   Rationale: The lever types need to be defined. There is no combined lever type. A third-class lever provides the greatest speed.

9. **a**
   Application and concept identification
   Rationale: Visual input during gait requires that the eyes remain forward and be kept level.

10. **b**
    Clinical reasoning and synthesis
    Rationale: The question requires an analysis of normal gait patterns against the disrupted gait described in the question. The arms counterbalance the legs, with the right arm counterbalancing the left leg and vice versa. This would mean that when the shoulder flexors contract on the right, the thigh flexors on the left also are contracting. If the tension in the biceps muscle on the left has increased, it would inhibit the thigh flexors on the left and the thigh flexors on the right would increase in tone.

11. **a**
    Factual recall
    Rationale: You need to understand the entire gait cycle to answer the question. The answers name certain aspects of gait. When the foot is on the floor, it is the stance phase. There is no double swing during gait.

12. **c**
    Factual recall
    Rationale: This question requires interpretation of the terminology and understanding of muscle involvement creating the steps in the gait cycle listed as answers. Plantar flexors move the foot onto the toes; therefore toe-off preswing is the correct answer.

13. **b**
    Factual recall
    Rationale: The question is asking for the sequential steps in moving from a seated to a standing position.

14. **a**
    Application and concept identification
    Rationale: To answer the question, you need to define the four types of dysfunction, and then relate to the facts presented. Because of the recent onset in response to a slight trauma, answer a is the most logical.

15. **d**
    Factual recall
    Rationale: The question is the definition of functional block.

16. **b**
    Factual recall
    Rationale: The question is describing a second-degree pattern.

17. **c**
Factual recall
Rationale: The question is asking for symptoms related to the diagnosis.

18. **d**
Clinical reasoning and synthesis
Rationale: The case study provides history, assessment data, methods used, and outcomes. You need to analyze the answers in relation to the facts in the question. Because the condition changed from reduced range of motion without pain to increased range of motion but onset of pain, a shift from a second-degree to a first-degree dysfunction would not be logical. With mobility increasing, stability would decrease around the area. Answer d describes a change in compensation patterns and is the most logical reason for the pain.

19. **a**
Factual recall
Rationale: You need to define all the terms and interpret the question and the possible answers. This question is an example of terminology usage. The wrong answers are misusing the language.

20. **c**
Application and concept identification
Rationale: This question is representative of many different questions that can be written about biomechanical assessment and intervention. Resistance is applied to the distal end of the lever.

21. **d**
Factual recall
Rationale: The question defines stabilization.

22. **b**
Factual recall
Rationale: Range of motion beyond normal is considered hypermobility.

23. **b**
Clinical reasoning and synthesis
Rationale: Facts presented in the question are knee joint pain with hypermobility and pain with passive movement. Facts provided by the textbook include the knee is moving beyond 150 degrees of flexion and 135 degrees of extension. Pain on passive movement is often a joint dysfunction or nerve entrapment. The question asks for the best massage intervention based on this condition. The outcome is assumed to be a reversal of the condition. Answer a would increase the hypermobility. Answer b provides massage but refers the client for specific work on the knee because joint or nerve involvement is indicated by the assessment. This is the best answer. Answer c is too conservative, and answer d is too aggressive.

24. **c**
Application and concept identification
Rationale: The question is asking for a condition of a muscle group in response to a repetitive strain to the scalene muscles caused by the inappropriate breathing pattern.

25. **a**
Factual recall
Rationale: This question is representative of the many questions that can be written about range of motion. You need to remember the degrees of movement for each joint to answer this type of question.

26. **c**
Application and concept identification
Rationale: The question asks for muscle involvement based on symptoms and assessment. To answer this type of question, you must understand muscle anatomy and physiology along with myotatic units presented in Chapter 9. Then you need to integrate the muscle information into biomechanical function. The information from the question indicates the latissimus dorsi.

27. **b**
Factual recall
Rationale: This question is representative of the many questions that can be written about range of motion. You need to remember the degrees of movement for each joint and the muscles that produce the movement identified to answer this type of question. In this question only sternocleidomastoid is a cervical flexor.

28. **b**
Factual recall
Rationale: This question is representative of the many questions that can be written about range of motion. You need to remember the degrees of movement for each joint and the muscles that produce the movement identified to answer this type of question. In this question restricted mobility on the left should indicate shortened and contracted muscles on the right.

29. **d**
Factual recall
Rationale: This question requires knowledge of the particular joint and the muscle that is directly or indirectly working on the joint. Information about all the muscles listed as possible answers is necessary to eliminate wrong answers. Only the pectoralis major exerts influence on the sternoclavicular joint.

30. **a**
Application and concept identification
Rationale: The entire shoulder complex moves as a unit.

31. **c**
Application and concept identification
Rationale: A joint function is provided to identify a biomechanical principle. Information about the glenohumeral joint design is necessary to answer the question. Because this joint is one with the most mobility, answer c is the most logical.

32. **b**
Factual recall
Rationale: The question is asking for the function of a group of muscles in terms of biomechanics.

33. **d**
Clinical reasoning and synthesis
Rationale: The facts presented by the question are right shoulder pain on external rotation with a slow onset. Range of motion is 40 degrees and normal is 90 degrees. Infraspinatus, posterior deltoid, and teres minor are inhibited by the subscapularis, pectoralis major, latissimus dorsi, teres major, and anterior deltoid. The correct answer would need to bring a reversal of the condition in a safe and conservative manner. You have to interpret the terminology in each answer. Only answer d addresses the muscle listed as causal and applies proper methods to normalize the condition.

34. **c**
Factual recall
Rationale: Normal elbow flexion is 150 degrees, so the joint is hypomobile.

35. **a**
Application and concept identification
Rationale: The action limited is supination.

36. **b**
Factual recall
Rationale: This question is representative of proper positioning to isolate and test muscles.

37. **a**
Factual recall
Rationale: The hip, pelvic girdle, and lumbar spine are in a closed kinematic chain.

38. **c**
Factual recall
Rationale: The question describes a function of the iliopsoas.

39. **d**
Factual recall
Rationale: The question asks for what muscle is testing weak for hip extension. Semimembranosus is the only listed muscle involved in hip extension.

40. **b**
Application and concept identification
Rationale: The question is asking for a relationship between observed internal rotation and the outcome of muscle testing. Answer a reverses the information. The two muscles in answers c and d are not involved in the movement described.

41. **c**
Factual recall
Rationale: The loose packed position of the knee is at about 30 degrees of flexion, allowing for the movement of internal and external rotation.

42. **d**
Application and concept identification
Rationale: The concentrically contracting group of muscles in the knee being held in extension is the quadriceps.

43. **a**
Application and concept identification
Rationale: The fibularis longus is the only muscle that would be overstretched by this action.

44. **c**
Factual recall
Rationale: This is the definition of a firing pattern.

45. **d**
    Factual recall
    Rationale: The muscles listed are not in the lower body, nor are they actively involved in gait. Myofascial dysfunction typically is not assessed with muscle testing.

46. **a**
    Concept identification
    Rationale: Edema usually would not cause joint dysfunction, and loading of a joint more likely would cause the damage. Closed kinematic chain and optimal firing pattern are names of function not dysfunction.

47. **d**
    Concept identification
    Rationale: Core muscles stabilize the trunk, so eliminate answers b and c. Inner unit muscles attach intrinsically, which eliminates answer a. Therefore d is the answer.

48. **b**
    Factual recall
    Rationale: All the other areas have less rotational movement.

11

Integumentary, Cardiovascular, Lymphatic, and Immune Systems

Review Tips

Knowledge of the integumentary, cardiovascular, lymphatic, and immune systems usually is tested with factual recall and comprehension questions. Also the pathologic conditions for each of these systems is targeted in exam questions. A common aspect of question development is to connect the anatomy and physiology of each body system to a specific application of massage. The classic example of this is massage targeted to influence the cardiovascular and lymphatic function.

As previously explained, you must know the definition of the terms and must be able to use the terms correctly. More complex questions use the terminology in the question and possible answers, and unless you can decipher the language, you will not know what the question or the provided answers mean. There is no easy way study terminology. Using flashcards, reading glossaries, and doing labeling exercises reinforce the definitions of the various terms. Use the study tools in this guide, and make sure that when you read your textbooks, you know what the words mean. Also make sure that you understand the meaning of general language used to write the questions. If you are not sure of the meaning of a word, look it up in the dictionary.

Questions

1. Which of the following functions of the integumentary system is supported by maintaining sanitary procedures?

   a. Protecting against water loss
   b. Detecting sensory stimuli
   c. Preventing entry of bacteria and viruses
   d. Excreting sweat and salts

2. The outer layer of the skin is called the_____.

   a. Epidermis
   b. Dermis
   c. Superficial fascia
   d. Keratin

3. The pigment of our skin is produced by _____.

   a. Dermis
   b. Stratum corneum
   c. Adipose
   d. Melanocytes

4. Erector pili muscles are attached to_____.

   a. Nails
   b. Hair
   c. Fat cells
   d. Lunula

5. Sebum is produced by _____.

   a. Sweat glands
   b. Mammary glands
   c. Sebaceous glands
   d. Root plexus

6. Sweat produced by which of the following glands has the strongest odor?

   a. Eccrine
   b. Apocrine
   c. Ceruminous
   d. Sebaceous

7. A massage practitioner notices that a client's skin has a yellowish gold color. This would be a indication of _____.

   a. Cyanosis
   b. Anemia
   c. Fever
   d. Jaundice

8. Which of the following is a contagious skin disease?

   a. Impetigo
   b. Alopecia
   c. Scleroderma
   d. Vitiligo

9. Which of the following benign skin growths has the most potential for becoming malignant?

   a. Angioma
   b. Mole
   c. Lipoma
   d. Seborrheic keratosis

10. A massage professional identifies a few small lumps in the axillary area of a female client. What might be a pathologic concern?

    a. Basal cell carcinoma
    b. Candidiasis
    c. Psoriasis
    d. Fibrocystic disease

11. The heart muscle is called the _____.

    a. Pericardium
    b. Myocardium
    c. Epicardium
    d. Endocardium

12. Which of the following heart valves controls the flow of blood from the ventricles into the aorta?

    a. Atrioventricular
    b. Mitral
    c. Tricuspid
    d. Semilunar

13. Which of the following vessels carries blood to the lungs?

    a. Aorta
    b. Superior vena cava
    c. Pulmonary trunk
    d. Inferior vena cava

14. A client has a history of heart attack and has reduced blood flow to the heart. Which of the following vessels is most involved?

    a. Coronary
    b. Left external carotid
    c. Celiac
    d. Renal

15. What is the first heart chamber to receive blood from the superior and inferior venae cavae?

    a. Right ventricle
    b. Right atrium
    c. Left ventricle
    d. Left atrium

16. Which portion of the cardiac cycle performs relaxation of the ventricles during filling?

    a. Sinoatrial node
    b. Systole
    c. Atrioventricular bundle
    d. Diastole

17. A client complains of pooling of blood in the lower extremities. Which of the following circumstances would be a likely cause?

    a. Increased walking
    b. Lying with the feet above the heart
    c. Standing still for extended periods
    d. Regular deep breathing

18. During a general massage, the massage practitioner notices that the dorsalis pedis pulse is weaker on the left. Where is the practitioner palpating?

    a. Upper arm
    b. Wrist
    c. Knee
    d. Ankle

19. Which of the following would be an indication for referral?

    a. A radial pulse of 85 beats per minute
    b. A femoral pulse of 55 beats per minute
    c. A carotid pulse of 70 beats per minute
    d. A dorsalis pedis pulse of 52 beats per minute

20. A client reports commonly having a blood pressure of 90/50 mm Hg. What would this condition be called?

    a. Tachycardia
    b. Hypertension
    c. Hypotension
    d. Bradycardia

21. After a 1-hour massage focused on relaxation, a client becomes dizzy when sitting up. What is the likely cause?

    a. Stimulation of baroreceptors
    b. Increase of sympathetic stimulation
    c. Pulse rate of 65 beats per minute
    d. Decrease in parasympathetic tone

22. Applying deep pressure during massage to the neck near the sternocleidomastoid muscles could compress which artery?

    a. Basilar
    b. External carotid
    c. Axillary
    d. Mesenteric

23. Deep extended pressure behind the knee is contraindicated because of potential damage to which artery?

    a. Celiac
    b. Femoral
    c. Popliteal
    d. Posterior tibial

24. Which of the following veins is located in the arm?

    a. Basilic
    b. Jugular
    c. Renal
    d. Iliac

25. A client has had surgery for varicose veins in the legs. Which vein was removed?

    a. Azygus
    b. Brachiocephalic
    c. Hepatic
    d. Saphenous

26. Which of the following contributes to hematopoiesis?

    a. Erythrocyte
    b. Monocyte
    c. Stem cell
    d. Thrombocyte

27. Which of the following is a temporary deficiency or diminished supply of blood to a tissue?

    a. Aneurysm
    b. Embolus
    c. Blockage of a vessel
    d. Ischemia

Correct answers are on pages 123-125.

28. A pulmonary embolism may begin as _____.

    a. Deep vein thrombosis
    b. Hemophilia
    c. Angina pectoris
    d. Arrhythmia

29. Clear interstitial tissue fluid is called _____.

    a. Lymphocytes
    b. Lymph
    c. Plasma
    d. Fibrin

30. Both lymphatic ducts empty lymph fluid into the _____.

    a. Mediastinal nodes
    b. Subclavian veins
    c. Mesenteric artery
    d. Cisterna chyli

31. Massage that provides a pumping compression to the foot encourages lymphatic flow because _____.

    a. The palmar plexus is stimulated
    b. The parotid nodes are drained
    c. The plantar plexus is stimulated
    d. The mammary plexus is stimulated

32. Which of the following acts to store lymphocytes and blood?

    a. Thymus
    b. Peyer's patches
    c. Bone marrow
    d. Spleen

33. Which of the following is considered contagious?

    a. Hodgkin's disease
    b. Mononucleosis
    c. Leukemia
    d. Lymphoma

34. A person had the measles as a child and is no longer susceptible. This is called _____.

    a. Nonspecific immunity
    b. Immune deficiency
    c. Specific immunity
    d. Phagocytosis

35. Antigens are destroyed or suppressed by _____.

    a. The thymus
    b. Antibodies
    c. Nonspecific immunity
    d. Lymph nodes

36. The immune function of mucus results because _____.

    a. It is sticky
    b. It creates inflammation
    c. Of phagocytosis
    d. It washes pathogens from the body

37. Allergy is a condition of _____.

    a. Immune system suppression
    b. Lack of T-cell activity
    c. Overactive immune response
    d. Immune deficiency

38. A client has been experiencing ongoing work and family stress and cannot seem to recover from an upper respiratory infection. What is the most logical cause?

    a. Ongoing stress increases natural killer cells.
    b. Ongoing stress supports the development of autoimmune disease.
    c. Ongoing stress suppresses T-cell activity.
    d. Decrease in cortisol suppresses the immune system.

39. What is the contribution of the urinary system to immune function?

    a. Protective acid balance
    b. Mechanical barrier
    c. Development of lymphocytes
    d. Nutrient delivery to cells

40. Which of the following is considered sterilization for aseptic pathogen control?

    a. Iodine
    b. Chlorine
    c. Alcohol
    d. Extreme heat

41. The most likely transmission route for human immunodeficiency virus and hepatitis is _____.

    a. Handshaking
    b. Body fluids
    c. Environmental contact
    d. Droplets in the air

42. A client is immune suppressed. The physician has provided approval for massage. What would be the best massage treatment plan?

    a. General massage with specific use of stimulation techniques to encourage sympathetic dominance
    b. General massage with a focus on aggressive lymphatic drainage
    c. General massage with active stretching to encourage parasympathetic dominance
    d. General massage to support nonspecific homeostatic regulation and restorative sleep

43. Which of the following are aspects of the venous pump?

    a. Capillaries and arteries
    b. Breathing and muscle contraction
    c. Entrainment and pulses
    d. Bradycardia and arrhythmia

44. Which of the following is a result of congestive heart failure?

    a. Edema
    b. Cerebral arthrosclerosis
    c. Aortic aneurysm
    d. Anemia

45. A ventricular thrombus is located where?

    a. Leg
    b. Brain
    c. Heart
    d. Kidney

46. Which aspect of lymphatic circulation is most affected by skin stretching?

    a. Lymphatic plexuses
    b. Superficial lymphatic circulation
    c. Deep lymphatic circulation
    d. Movement of lymph though nodes

47. Which of the following is an autoimmune disorder?

    a. Callus
    b. Stress fracture
    c. Gangilion
    d. Rheumatoid arthritis

Correct answers are on pages 123-125.

Exercise

Using the foregoing questions as examples, now write at least three more questions—one of each type: factual recall and comprehension, application and concept identification, and clinical reasoning and synthesis. Make sure to develop plausible wrong answers, and be sure that the correct answer is clearly correct. Then write a rationale for each question. The more questions you write, the better you will understand the material.

Answers and Discussion

1. **c**
Application and concept identification
Rationale: Sanitary practices support the protective barrier of the skin.

2. **a**
Factual recall
Rationale: You need to define the terms to identify the correct answer. Aterward you can identify the epidermis as the outer layer of the skin.

3. **d**
Factual recall
Rationale: You need to define the terms to identify the correct answer.

4. **b**
Factual recall
Rationale: The location of the erector pili muscles is at the hair root.

5. **c**
Factual recall
Rationale: You need to define all the terms to answer the question.

6. **b**
Factual recall
Rationale: You need to define the terms and understand the different types of sweat to answer the question.

7. **d**
Application and concept identification
Rationale: Color changes in the skin can be an indication of a pathologic condition. A yellow cast may indicate jaundice.

8. **a**
Factual recall
Rationale: It is important to be able to recognize the various pathologic conditions of the skin. Contagious skin diseases are especially important to recognize. You should define all of the listed pathologic conditions of the skin, and then impetigo emerges as the correct answer.

9. **b**
Factual recall
Rationale: It is important to be able to recognize the various pathologic conditions of the skin. Those with the potential to malignant skin diseases are especially important to recognize. You should define all of the listed pathologic conditions of the skin, and then a mole emerges as the correct answer.

10. **d**
Factual recall
Rationale: It is important to be able to recognize the various pathologic conditions of the integumentary system. You should define all of the listed pathologic conditions, and then fibrocystic disease emerges as the correct answer.

11. **b**
Factual recall
Rationale: You need to define the terms to identify the correct answer.

12. **d**
Factual recall
Rationale: The question provides information to differentiate among the heart valves listed as possible answers.

13. **c**
Factual recall
Rationale: You need to determine the location and function of all the vessels listed as possible answers to answer the question.

14. **a**
Application and concept identification
Rationale: The question provides information about the location of the vessels by stating that the client had a heart attack and reduced blood flow to the heart. The coronary arteries supply blood to the heart.

15. **b**
Factual recall
Rationale: Answering the question requires knowledge of blood flow through the heart.

16. **d**
Factual recall
Rationale: Answering the question requires knowledge about the cardiac cycle and the structures and functions listed as possible answers. Systole and diastole are part of the cardiac cycle, with diastole being the portion when the ventricles relax.

17. **c**
Application and concept identification
Rationale: The client has a reduced return of blood in the veins, and the correct answer explains why. The three wrong answers would increase blood flow in the veins. Only standing still for long periods would reduce blood flow.

18. **d**
    Factual recall
    Rationale: The question is representative of the many types of questions that can be developed about the arteries. This question asks for the location of a particular pulse point.

19. **a**
    Application and concept identification
    Rationale: A normal pulse is between 50 and 70 beats per minute. Although 85 beats per minute is below what is considered tachycardia, it is faster than what is usually normal.

20. **c**
    Factual recall
    Rationale: A normal blood pressure is somewhere around 120/80 mm Hg. The blood pressure described in the question is low, indicating hypotension.

21. **a**
    Application and concept identification
    Rationale: Care needs to be taken so that clients do not have low blood pressure after a massage. The three wrong answers would indicate an increase in blood pressure, and pressure on the baroreceptors can lower it.

22. **b**
    Factual recall
    Rationale: The question asks for the name of the artery located in the neck near a particular muscle that would interfere with blood flow. The arteries named in the wrong answers are not located in the neck.

23. **c**
    Factual recall
    Rationale: The question asks for the name of the artery located in the knee that is susceptible to compressive force. The arteries named in the wrong answers are not located behind the knee.

24. **a**
    Factual recall
    Rationale: The question is representative of many questions that can be developed about the location of blood vessels. This question asks for the identification of the basilic vein.

25. **d**
    Factual recall
    Rationale: The question is representative of many questions that can be developed about the location of blood vessels and pathologic conditions connected to them. This question asks for the identification of the saphenous vein.

26. **c**
    Factual recall
    Rationale: You need to define all the terms to answer the question. Stem cells are involved in blood cell development.

27. **d**
    Factual recall
    Rationale: As in all of these types of questions, you have to define the terms to answer the question.

28. **a**
    Factual recall
    Rationale: This question relates to pathologic conditions of the cardiovascular system. You need to define all the terms to identify the correct answer and eliminate incorrect answers. In this question an embolism often begins as a thrombus.

29. **b**
    Factual recall
    Rationale: As in all of these types of questions, you need to define the terms to answer the question.

30. **b**
    Factual recall
    Rationale: As in all of these types of questions, you need to define the terms to answer the question. Knowledge about the anatomy of the lymphatic system and the path of lymph flow also is required.

31. **c**
    Application and concept identification
    Rationale: An understanding is needed of the lymphatic plexus on the bottom of the foot and that compression to the area results in stimulation of lymphatic fluid movement.

32. **d**
    Factual recall
    Rationale: The question describes a function of the spleen.

33. **b**
    Factual recall
    Rationale: The question is asking about pathologic conditions of the lymphatic system. You need to define all of the diseases listed and to identify the one that is contagious.

34. **c**
    Factual recall
    Rationale: The question is an example of specific immunity.

35. **b**
Factual recall
Rationale: The question describes a function of antibodies.

36. **a**
Factual recall
Rationale: The correct answer describes the nonspecific immune defense of mucus.

37. **c**
Factual recall
Rationale: The correct answer is a definition of allergy.

38. **c**
Application and concept identification
Rationale: The question is asking for a correlation with immune suppression and stress levels. Only answer c is correct because stress tends to suppress the entire immune function through an increase in cortisol levels.

39. **a**
Factual recall
Rationale: This function of the urinary system acts to support nonspecific immunity.

40. **d**
Factual recall
Rationale: Sanitary measures support the immune system by isolating and destroying pathogens. Extreme heat kills most pathogens.

41. **b**
Factual recall
Rationale: These two diseases are transmitted in body fluids.

42. **d**
Clinical reasoning and synthesis
Rationale: The facts in the question indicate that the immune system is unable to fight pathogens. Precautions need to be taken to protect the client. No methods should be used to increase the stress response or strain the adaptive capacity of the client. Only the last answer meets these criteria.

43. **b**
Concept identification
Rationale: Capillaries, arteries, and pulses are not involved directly in the venous pump. Answer d indicates pathologic conditions of the heart.

44. **a**
Factual recall
Rationale: This is a terminology-based question.

45. **c**
Factual recall
Rationale: Medical terminology should be of help in identifying the correct answer because a ventricle is part of the heart.

46. **b**
Concept identification
Rationale: Plexuses and nodes respond most to compression and deep lymphatic circulation by muscle action and respiration.

47. **d**
Factual recall
Rationale: Answers a, b, and c usually occur from overuse or trauma.

CHAPTER

12
Respiratory, Digestive, Urinary, and Reproductive Systems

Review Tips

Knowledge of the respiratory, digestive, urinary, and reproductive systems usually is tested with factual recall and comprehension questions. The pathologic conditions for each of these systems is targeted in exam questions. Another aspect of question development is to connect the anatomy and physiology of each body system to specific applications of massage. The classic example of this is massage targeted to influence the respiratory and digestive systems. Massage during pregnancy requires an understanding of the gestation and birthing process, so this content will appear in exam questions.

As previously explained, you must know the definitions of the terms and must be able to use the terms correctly. More complex questions use the terminology in the question and possible answers, and unless you can decipher the language, you will not know what the question or the provided answers mean. Use the study tools in this guide, and make sure that when you read your textbooks, you know what the words mean. Also make sure that you understand the meaning of general language used in the questions. If you are not sure of the meaning of a word, look it up in the dictionary.

Questions

1. Which of the following is a mechanical action of inhalation and exhalation that draws oxygen into the lungs and releases carbon dioxide into the atmosphere?

   a. Breathing
   b. External respiration
   c. Internal respiration
   d. Egestion

2. The nasal cavity is separated into a right and left portion by _____.

   a. Nares
   b. Sinuses
   c. Ethmoid
   d. Septum

3. A client complains of a congested nose and low back stiffness. What is the logical connection between the two?

    a. The respiratory mucus is too thin and allows bacteria to enter the body, causing a kidney infection.

    b. The swell bodies in the nose are not able to function properly, so the normal movement during sleep is disrupted.

    c. The olfactory nerves are increasing parasympathetic arousal, causing an increase in muscle tension.

    d. Nasal congestion is blocking the sinus cavities and inner ear, changing muscle tone in the lower extremities.

4. The air sacs in the lungs are called_____.

    a. Epiglottis
    b. Bronchioles
    c. Lobes
    d. Alveoli

5. A client is displaying behavior consistent with sympathetic autonomic nervous system dominance. What would be the state of the bronchioles?

    a. Bronchodilation
    b. Bronchoconstriction
    c. Pneumothorax
    d. Hyperventilation

6. Why would a person with a spinal cord injury at C6 be able to breathe without a ventilator?

    a. The intercostal nerves exit at C5.
    b. The phrenic nerve originates at C3.
    c. The mediastinum is intact.
    d. The pleural cavity is innervated at C1.

7. The external intercostal muscles create a vacuum in the thorax in which way?

    a. The upper ribs expand.
    b. The ribs are pulled together.
    c. The lower ribs are lifted up and out.
    d. The diaphragm muscle arches upward.

8. During assessment a client is observed with mild tachypnea, tension in the muscles of the neck and shoulder, and nervousness. Which of the following is most true?

    a. Nitrogen levels have risen and oxygen levels have decreased, creating a decrease in tidal volume.

    b. Oxyhemoglobin is saturated with carbon dioxide, and the muscles display tetany.

    c. An increase in carbon dioxide in the blood is triggering sympathetic activation.

    d. Oxygen levels have increased and carbon dioxide levels have dropped, predisposing to breathing pattern disorder.

9. A client with a diagnosis of asthma is referred for massage. What would be the most likely benefits of massage?

    a. Activation of the sympathetic nervous system that would support bronchoconstriction

    b. Reduction in anxiety and increased mobility of the ribs

    c. Stimulation of the client's ability to inhale but inhibition of excessive exhalation

    d. Increase in tone of respiratory muscles, supporting effective exhalation

10. Which of the following is contagious?

    a. Tuberculosis
    b. Hay fever
    c. Emphysema
    d. Cystic fibrosis

11. Massage methods that modulate the breathing rhythm also _____.

    a. Predispose a person to pulmonary embolism
    b. Interfere with treatment for sleep apnea
    c. Interact with the autonomic nervous system
    d. Interfere with most meditation methods

12. What supports addictive behavior related to food consumption?

    a. Need for nutrients
    b. Pleasure sensations
    c. Energy requirement
    d. Peristalsis activation

13. The abdominal cavity is lined with a mucous membrane called the _____.

    a. Peritoneum
    b. Gastrointestinal tract
    c. Omentum
    d. Mesentery

14. The enzyme amylase found in saliva is part of the digestive process for _____.

    a. Proteins
    b. Fats
    c. Lipids
    d. Carbohydrates

15. The folds in the stomach that expand when food is ingested are called _____.

    a. Bolus
    b. Rugae
    c. Chyme
    d. Pylorus

16. Which portion of the small intestine contains ducts from the liver, gallbladder, and pancreas?

    a. Ileum
    b. Jejunum
    c. Duodenum
    d. Mesentery

17. Which of the following acts as a digestive organ and also detoxifies the blood?

    a. Pancreas
    b. Stomach
    c. Liver
    d. Gallbladder

18. A major function of the large intestine is to _____.

    a. Absorb water
    b. Concentrate bile
    c. Remove and store glycogen
    d. Convert amino acids

19. Which of the following structures of the colon also contains lymphatic tissue?

    a. Cecum
    b. Appendix
    c. Ascending colon
    d. Sigmoid colon

20. A regular client reports various digestive upsets including dry mouth and constipation. The physician who wants a treatment plan and justification has cleared the client for massage. Which of the following would be the best plan to submit to the physician?

    a. Stimulating massage coupled with teaching self-help breathing supporting an increase in oxygen and a decrease in carbon dioxide to support ongoing autonomic nervous system sympathetic dominance
    b. General massage combined with deep massage to the colon to suppress peristalsis and break down concentrated fecal matter
    c. General massage focused to generate relaxation with diaphragmatic breathing and rhythmic stroking to the colon to stimulate peristalsis
    d. General massage to create parasympathetic dominance and lymphatic drainage, with visceral massage to the liver to increase detoxification and support upper chest breathing

21. The food source that breaks down into amino acids is _____.

    a. Protein
    b. Carbohydrate
    c. Fat
    d. Vitamins

22. A client has severely limited all dietary fat. Which of the following might occur?

    a. Inability to digest protein
    b. Difficulty with hormone production
    c. Interference with the absorption of water-soluble vitamins
    d. Decreased conversion of galactose

Correct answers are on pages 134-136.

23. Which of the following pathologic conditions of the digestive system affects the liver?

    a. Cystic fibrosis
    b. Diverticular disease
    c. Cirrhosis
    d. Gastritis

24. Of the following, which is contagious?

    a. Appendicitis
    b. Hepatitis
    c. Reflux esophagitis
    d. Irritable bowel syndrome

25. Which of the following pathologic conditions is considered a medical emergency and requires immediate referral?

    a. Gastroenteritis
    b. Peptic ulcer disease
    c. Inflammatory bowel disease
    d. Strangulated hernia

26. Appropriate massage for the colon _____.

    a. Begins at the ascending colon, ends at the rectum, and moves toward the cecum
    b. Begins at the sigmoid colon and ends at the cecum, with directional flow toward the rectum
    c. Begins at the rectum and ends at the cecum, with a directional flow toward the cecum
    d. Begins at the splenic flexure and ends at the hepatic flexure, with directional flow toward the sigmoid colon

27. Micturition is _____.

    a. Parasympathetic action to void urine
    b. Sympathetic action to increase retention of feces
    c. Movement of blood through the nephrons
    d. Restoration of blood acid-base balance

28. When stretch receptors signal that the bladder needs to empty, what muscle contracts?

    a. Pectineus
    b. Coccygeus
    c. Pyramidalis
    d. Detrusor

29. Cystitis is _____.

    a. Inflammation of the medulla of the kidney
    b. Infection of the glomerulus
    c. Bladder infection
    d. Obstruction of the urethra

30. Why might massage be contraindicated for those with renal insufficiency?

    a. Massage causes increase in blood pressure
    b. Massage increases blood volume through the kidneys
    c. Massage spreads bacteria through the urinary system
    d. Massage increases the difficulty with incontinence

31. Erectile tissue is able to become firmer because _____.

    a. This tissue engorges with blood
    b. Muscles contract, stiffening the tissue
    c. The tissue absorbs water from the lymph
    d. Smooth muscles encircle the tissue, acting as a sphincter

32. Thirty minutes into a relaxation massage a male client has an erection. What is the most logical reason for this response?

    a. The client has been "sexualizing" the massage.
    b. Erection is a parasympathetic response.
    c. Stimulation of the skin shifts blood flow.
    d. Activation of sympathetic reflexes triggers the response.

33. Which of the following secretes a lubricating fluid in the female external genitalia?

    a. Fundus
    b. Bartholin gland
    c. Clitoris
    d. Symphysis pubis

34. During sexual development in the female, which occurs last?

    a. Hypothalamus matures.
    b. Estradiol is produced.
    c. Adrenal cortex hormone signals pubic hair growth.
    d. Ovulation

35. The alkaline nature of semen is to _____.

    a. Stimulate orgasm.
    b. Counteract the acid nature of vaginal fluid.
    c. Thin the protective coating of the ovum.
    d. Lubricate the ejaculatory duct.

36. If a female client is in the second trimester of a pregnancy, which of the following would most apply?

    a. Massage will be most comfortable if it is given with the client prone.
    b. Massage will be most comfortable if client is positioned on the side.
    c. Massage of the feet is contraindicated.
    d. Massage should focus most on lymphatic drainage.

37. During massage, a lactating client experiences the let-down response. What would be the most likely cause?

    a. Massage stimulates the release of oxytocin.
    b. Massage stimulates the production of testosterone.
    c. Massage decreases colostrum.
    d. Massage decreases libido.

38. Which of the following sexually transmitted diseases has a bacterial origin?

    a. Genital warts
    b. Herpes genitalis
    c. Gonorrhea
    d. Hepatitis B

39. A 56-year-old male client complains of difficulty voiding urine. What would be the most likely diagnosis from his physician?

    a. Endometriosis
    b. Trichomonas vaginitis
    c. Bartholin cyst
    d. Benign prostatic hypertrophy

40. A client is experiencing weakness and exhaustion; impaired concentration, memory, and performance; disturbed sleep; and emotional sweating. A complete physical has ruled out any existing pathologic condition. Stress is indicated as a probable cause. Which of the following treatment plans would best reverse the stress response?

    a. Massage to promote lymphatic drainage and stimulate arterial circulation
    b. Massage to support proper breathing function and reverse hyperventilation syndrome
    c. Massage to reduce scar tissue and prevent adhesions
    d. Massage to stimulate increase in heart rate and blood pressure

41. A couple has experienced difficulties conceiving a third child. The doctors can find no reason for the difficulties. The man is a regular client. He asks if massage could be of help. The answer is yes. Which of the following justification statements is most logical?

    a. Massage can assist in the success of sexual intercourse by encouraging adrenaline secretion.
    b. Massage can increase the rate of ovulation by stimulating the hypothalamus to secrete follicle-stimulating hormone.
    c. Massage can encourage more efficient homeostatic mechanisms in the body, promoting general health, including fertility.
    d. Massage can increase the levels of testosterone, prolactin, and progesterone, promoting ovulation.

Correct answers are on pages 134-136.

42. A massage therapist feels restless on days off and finds it more difficult to sleep. What is the most logical reason for this phenomenon?

    a. Providing massage usually promotes a parasympathetic response in the client and the practitioner; on days when no massage is performed, the practitioner does not stimulate relaxation responses as effectively.

    b. Providing massage is fatiguing; on days off the massage practitioner has more energy.

    c. Providing massage interferes with natural entrainment responses, and on days off the practitioner is more in tune with biorhythms.

    d. Providing massage increases adrenaline and other stimulating hormones and neurotransmitters; when this occurs, hyperventilation syndrome is common, resulting in restlessness and sleep disturbances.

43. The amount of energy expended by the body at any given time is called _____.

    a. Citric acid cycle
    b. Total metabolic rate
    c. Basal metabolic rate
    d. Digestion

44. Most body water is located in _____.

    a. Interstitial fluid
    b. Lymph
    c. Intracellular fluid
    d. Plasma

45. Force exerted by water is called _____.

    a. Hydrostatic pressure
    b. Dehydration
    c. Osmosis
    d. Electrolyte balance

46. During the first trimester there is an increase in progesterone. Which of the following results can therapeutic massage directly and mechanically influence?

    a. Increased urination
    b. Constipation
    c. Nausea
    d. Lymphatic stagnation

47. Which of the following is a medical emergency?

    a. Lactation
    b. Vaginitis
    c. Ectopic pregnancy
    d. Prelabor

Exercise

Using the foregoing questions as examples, now write at least three more questions—one of each type: factual recall and comprehension, application and concept identification, and clinical reasoning and synthesis. Make sure to develop plausible wrong answers, and be sure that the correct answer is clearly correct. Then write a rationale for each question. The more questions you write, the better you will understand the material.

Correct answers are on pages 134-136.

Answers and Discussion

1. **a**
Factual recall
Rationale: Defining the terminology is necessary to answer the question. The question is the definition of breathing.

2. **d**
Factual recall
Rationale: The question describes the location of the septum. Make sure to know the location of all the structures listed.

3. **b**
Application and concept identification
Rationale: You must analyze each of the answers for correct information and in relationship to the question. Only answer b meets both criteria.

4. **d**
Factual recall
Rationale: The question defines alveoli. Always define the terminology and identify the location of the structures for questions of this type.

5. **a**
Factual recall
Rationale: The question describes a physiologic state and asks for how a structure would respond. You need to define and understand all the terminology in relation to the sympathetic state.

6. **b**
Factual recall
Rationale: The question is asking about anatomy in relationship to function. Because the phrenic nerve allows the diaphragm to function and the injury is below this area, breathing without assistance is possible.

7. **c**
Factual recall
Rationale: The question is about muscle function resulting in rib movement up and out, which creates the vacuum drawing air into the lungs.

8. **d**
Application and concept identification
Rationale: This question and the possible answers first require that the terminology be defined and the meaning of the question and answers be interpreted. This is a common question type. Then the answers need to be analyzed to identify the correct answer. Tachypnea is fast breathing, which would increase oxygen levels, drop carbon dioxide levels, and trigger sympathetic dominance. This is a cause of hyperventilation syndrome.

9. **b**
Clinical reasoning and synthesis
Rationale: The facts are located in the question and in the textbook. You need to understand the symptoms and treatment of asthma. This is true of any pathologic condition before attempting to decide what benefit massage has to offer and to identify contraindications and need for referral. You must analyze the possibilities offered in the possible answers for safe and effective application. The problem is bronchoconstriction, so answer a is incorrect. Answer b is correct. Answers c and d would increase the problem.

10. **a**
Factual recall
Rationale: You need to define all the listed pathologic conditions and identify the one that is contagious.

11. **c**
Application and concept identification
Rationale: The question is asking for the physiologic interaction with massage, autonomic nervous system, and breathing. The three wrong answers present information contrary to the identified effects of massage.

12. **b**
Factual recall
Rationale: Addictive behavior is related to stimulation of pleasure sensations.

13. **a**
Factual recall
Rationale: Defining the terminology and identifying the location of the structures are necessary to answer the question. The question describes the peritoneum.

14. **d**
Factual recall
Rationale: You need to identify digestive enzymes in relation to the food groups they work on to choose the correct answer.

15. **b**
Factual recall
Rationale: Defining the terminology and identifying the location of the structures are necessary to answer the question. The question describes the rugae.

16. **c**
    Factual recall
    Rationale: Defining the terminology and identifying the location of the structures are necessary to answer the question. The question describes the duodenum.

17. **c**
    Factual recall
    Rationale: Defining the terminology and identifying the function of the structures are necessary to answer the question. The question describes the liver.

18. **a**
    Factual recall
    Rationale: Defining the terminology and function of the large intestine is necessary to answer the question.

19. **b**
    Factual recall
    Rationale: Defining the terminology and identifying the location and function of the structures are necessary to answer the question. The question describes the appendix.

20. **c**
    Clinical reasoning and synthesis
    Rationale: The answer is the correct justification for why massage would achieve the outcome of managing the symptoms listed. You must analyze each of the presented treatment plans for effectiveness and safety. You need to define all terms and interpret the statements before choosing the correct answer. Sympathetic dominance tends to aggravate digestive problems. Answer b is not a safe practice. Answer c is correct. Answer d includes supporting upper chest breathing, indicating sympathetic dominance, so the content in the answer is flawed.

21. **a**
    Factual recall
    Rationale: Defining the terminology is necessary to answer the question. The question describes protein.

22. **b**
    Application and concept identification
    Rationale: The question is asking for the connection between fats and hormone production.

23. **c**
    Factual recall
    Rationale: Defining the pathologic conditions is necessary to answer the question. The question describes cirrhosis.

24. **b**
    Factual recall
    Rationale: Defining the pathologic conditions is necessary to answer the question. The question describes hepatitis.

25. **d**
    Factual recall
    Rationale: Defining the pathologic conditions is necessary to answer the question. The question describes strangulated hernia.

26. **b**
    Application and concept identification
    Rationale: Stimulation of movement of fecal material through the large intestine may be assisted by massage that simulates the peristaltic action of the large intestine and flows along the same anatomic route.

27. **a**
    Factual recall
    Rationale: You need to define the terms to identify the correct answer.

28. **d**
    Factual recall
    Rationale: The question is asking for a muscle function. You need to identify all listed muscles for location and function to answer the question correctly.

29. **c**
    Factual recall
    Rationale: The question is asking for a definition of a pathologic condition. To identify the correct answer, you need to learn the common diseases of the urinary system. Medical terminology interpretation is helpful. *Cyst-* means bladder.

30. **b**
    Application and concept identification
    Rationale: The question asks for an effect of massage that may be contraindicated if a particular pathologic condition is present. Renal insufficiency would make it difficult for the kidneys to handle increased blood volume.

31. **a**
    Factual recall
    Rationale: The correct answer explains the physiology of erectile tissue.

32. **b**
    Application and concept identification
    Rationale: The correct answer explains the physiology of the male erection in response to parasympathetic dominance.

33. **b**
Factual recall
Rationale: You need to define all the terms to answer the question.

34. **d**
Factual recall
Rationale: Ovulation is the last to occur as the female sexually matures.

35. **b**
Factual recall
Rationale: The question asks for the reason for the pH of semen.

36. **b**
Application and concept identification
Rationale: An understanding of the stages of pregnancy, positioning of the client, and indications and contraindications for massage is required to answer the question.

37. **a**
Application and concept identification
Rationale: You need to define the terms and understand the relationship of oxytocin to massage and lactation.

38. **c**
Factual recall
Rationale: You need to define all the pathologic conditions listed to identify gonorrhea as the correct answer.

39. **d**
Factual recall
Rationale: You need to define all the pathologic conditions listed to identify benign prostatic hypertrophy as the correct answer.

40. **b**
Clinical reasoning and synthesis
Rationale: Based on the symptoms described in the question, the most logical cause is disrupted breathing function, which creates sympathetic dominance. The treatment described in answer b would address this situation best.

41. **c**
Clinical reasoning and synthesis
Rationale: The correct answer would provide correct justification for how massage may help some types of infertility conditions that are related to stress. You need to analyze each answer for correct information in relationship to the outcome. Adrenaline does not promote decreased stress response. Massage has not been shown to affect follicle-stimulating hormone. Answer c is the correct answer. Massage has not been shown to affect the hormones listed, and these same hormones may inhibit ovulation.

42. **a**
Clinical reasoning and synthesis
Rationale: This question asks for a decision based on accumulated knowledge from textbooks in relation to massage practice and physiologic effects. The facts in the question indicate sympathetic autonomic nervous system activation. The correct answer would explain why this is so. Answer a is the most logical. Massage done correctly should not be excessively fatiguing. Massage promotes entrainment. Answer d is not logical.

43. **b**
Factual recall
Rationale: This is a terminology question. You need to define the words and compare them to the question. The citric acid cycle is how food becomes energy. Digestion breaks food down, and basal metabolic rate concerns energy usage while one is awake.

44. **c**
Factual recall
Rationale: The combined fluid inside the cells accounts for most of the body fluid.

45. **a**
Factual recall
Rationale: This is a definition question.

46. **b**
Concept identification
Rationale: The key words are "directly and mechanically influence," which is possible with constipation.

47. **c**
Factual recall
Rationale: Prelabor is normal, as is lactation. Vaginitis is an infection that needs to be treated, but ectopic pregnancy could cause the fallopian tube to burst.

SECTION

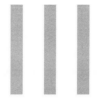

13

Foundations of Therapeutic Applications of Touch

Review Tips

The information in this content area is used to determine a foundation for professional behavior. Test questions written on the foundations of therapeutic applications of touch include vocabulary, professional behavior, and historical influence on current trends in the professional evolution of therapeutic massage. This content often is found in case study type of questions, especially in combination with ethical behavior and communication skills.

The vocabulary targets terms used to describe interactions of persons in social and professional settings.

When studying the vocabulary, pay particular attention to words used in each of the example questions. Use textbooks and the glossary in this book to look up terms that are unclear.

Most certification exams do not have questions about historical dates; therefore do not spend time memorizing dates. Questions about historical figures may appear on some exams, but typically not many. Target most study time to understanding the professional aspects of therapeutic touch.

Questions

1. Professionalism is defined as _____.

   a. An occupation that helps people
   b. A service provided for others
   c. An intricate system that is structured and systematic
   d. Adherence to professional status, methods, standards, and character

2. A middle-aged client is reluctant to work with a 22-year-old massage therapist. This is an example of _____.

   a. Gender issues
   b. Genetic predisposition
   c. Age issues
   d. Body sensitivity

3. An individual response to professional therapeutic touch _____.

   a. Is consistent with cultural influences
   b. Cannot be predetermined
   c. Is gender specific
   d. Depends on outcomes

4. Culture is defined by _____.

   a. Race as defined by color and where you live
   b. Arts, beliefs, customs, institutions, and all products of human work and thought created by a specific group of people at a particular time
   c. What you study, the profession you choose, the family you grew up in, and whom you marry
   d. The work place including the people, environment, physical location, and financial management

5. Which of the following is a form of touch technique?

   a. Socially stereotyped touch
   b. Mechanical touch
   c. Inadvertent touch
   d. Ritualized touch

6. The word massage is derived from all the following languages except _____.

   a. English
   b. French
   c. Arabic
   d. Greek

7. The practice of acupuncture involves _____.

   a. The stimulation of specific points along the body, usually by the insertion of tiny, solid needles
   b. The stimulation of specific points along the body, usually by the pressing of the thumb into the point
   c. The stimulation of broad points along the body, usually by accomplishing a series of ever-deepening compressive strokes
   d. Using counterirritation, such as scraping, cutting, or burning of skin, to relieve pain

8. Polarity therapy was created by _____.

   a. Dr. James B. Mennell
   b. Randolph Stone
   c. Wilhelm Reich
   d. Dr. Janet Travell

9. Henrick Ling was a noted _____.

   a. Physician who developed massage techniques for joint stiffness and wound healing
   b. Swedish writer who wrote De Medicina, a series of eight books covering the body of knowledge of the day
   c. Teacher who is credited with developing Swedish massage
   d. Physician credited with bringing massage to the scientific community

10. The National Certification Examination for Therapeutic Massage and Bodywork was first devised in _____.

    a. 1980
    b. 1992
    c. 1974
    d. 1998

11. One of the prominent reasons that Ling's work had a difficult time being accepted was because _____.

    a. He worked only with healthy people
    b. He used poetic and mystic language in his writings
    c. He based it on newly discovered knowledge of the circulation of the blood and lymph
    d. The primary focus was on gymnastics

12. What is the massage trend that developed in 1991 that supported acceptance for the benefits of massage?

    a. Increase in valid research
    b. Deregulation of massage education
    c. Decrease in influential women in the profession
    d. Resistance to integrating massage into traditional health care settings

Exercise

Using the foregoing questions as examples, now write at least three more questions—one of each type: factual recall and comprehension, application and concept identification, and clinical reasoning and synthesis. Make sure to develop plausible wrong answers, and be sure that the correct answer is clearly correct. Then write a rationale for each question. The more questions you write, the better you will understand the material.

Answers and Discussion

1. **d**
   Factual recall
   Rationale: The correct answer is the definition of professionalism.

2. **c**
   Factual recall
   Rationale: The question provides an example of age issues and the interpretation of professional touch. You need to understand the entire issue of touch perceptions to answer the question.

3. **b**
   Application and concept identification
   Rationale: The question addresses the issue of how touch interaction can be experienced by an individual.

4. **b**
   Factual recall
   Rationale: The correct answer is the definition of culture.

5. **b**
   Factual recall
   Rationale: You need to define the various forms of touch to identify touch technique and mechanical touch.

6. **a**
   Factual recall
   Rationale: The history of massage has a basis in the terminology and historical origins.

7. **a**
   Factual recall
   Rationale: The correct answer is a definition of acupuncture.

8. **b**
   Factual recall
   Rationale: You should remember major historical figures who have contributed to the body of knowledge of massage and bodywork. Although Randolph Stone is the correct answer to the question, the others also made significant contributions.

9. **c**
   Factual recall
   Rationale: You should remember major historical figures who have contributed to the body of knowledge of massage and bodywork.

10. **b**
    Factual recall
    Rationale: You should remember major historical events that have influenced massage and bodywork.

11. **b**
    Factual recall
    Rationale: You should remember major historical events that have influenced massage and bodywork.

12. **a**
    Factual recall
    Rationale: You should remember major historical events that have influenced massage and bodywork. Research currently is a major influence on the profession.

CHAPTER

14
Professionalism and Legal Issues

Review Tips

Professionalism and legal issues are considered important on most exams because they influence ethical professional behavior. One of the purposes of exams is to determine whether persons will behave in an appropriate manner so that the clients are not harmed. The reason for legislation is to protect the public, and questions on this content attempt to determine safe and professional practice.

A specific vocabulary is used to describe this content and concepts. Use the vocabulary in the questions as a guide for study. Use textbooks and the glossary in this book to look up terms that are unclear.

This content often is tested in the case study/ example type of format. A clinical reasoning process is necessary to determine the correct answer. As previously explained, the facts are presented in the question and the possibilities are in the four potential answers. Analyze each potential answer against the facts in the question to determine the correct response.

Questions

1. The knowledge base and practice parameters of a profession are called _____.

    a. Scope of practice
    b. Informed consent
    c. Dual role
    d. Therapeutic relationship

2. A massage professional becomes angry with a client who complains about personal problems during the massage. The massage practitioner is displaying _____.

    a. Transference
    b. Therapeutic relationship
    c. Ethical behavior
    d. Countertransference

3. A massage professional does not regularly drape all clients in a modest and professional manner. Which of the following best describes this conduct?

    a. The massage professional practices a dual role.
    b. The massage professional has breached a standard of practice.
    c. The massage professional is involved in misuse of the scope of practice.
    d. The massage professional needs additional training in draping.

4. A massage professional works with three main populations: athletes, those with chronic pain, and clients requiring stress management. The therapist uses a variety of methods. Which of the following best describes the massage application style being used?

    a. Structural and postural approaches
    b. Applied kinesiology
    c. Integrated approaches
    d. Myofascial methods

5. A massage professional has been working with a particular client for 12 months. Recently the client has been experiencing increasing difficulties with the family communications. The biggest problem is stress and tension between son and father. Discussions during massage are centered around solving this problem. Which of the following best describes this situation?

   a. Massage professional is having difficulty maintaining informed consent.
   b. Scope of practice violations, particularly with psychology, are occurring.
   c. The client should be referred for acupuncture or chiropractic.
   d. The client is engaged in countertransference.

6. A client, a professional dancer, is basically healthy but is seeking massage to manage minor injury and support recovery. Which scope of practice description best describes these outcomes?

   a. Wellness/normal function
   b. Health care services
   c. Dysfunction and athletic performance
   d. Illness/trauma

7. A massage professional with entry-level training has been seeing a client recently diagnosed with diabetes. The massage professional is becoming more uncomfortable providing massage as the client displays more symptoms. What is occurring?

   a. The massage professional is in a dual role now that the client is ill.
   b. The client is more demanding of the professional.
   c. The massage professional has failed to abide by the definition of massage.
   d. The massage professional is functioning outside the personal scope of practice.

8. A massage professional is careful to provide an informed consent process for each client and updates informed consent regularly. Which of the following ethical principles is being followed?

   a. Confidentiality
   b. Justice
   c. Proportionality
   d. Client autonomy and self-determination

9. Taking a client's history and providing a physical assessment to develop a massage care plan is called a _____.

   a. Needs assessment
   b. Brochure and policy statement
   c. Release of information
   d. Chart

10. A massage professional has worked hard to develop a policy statement and has included types of service offered, information on training and experience, appointment policies, client and practitioner expectations, sexual appropriateness, and recourse policy. What did the professional forget to include?

    a. Number of appointments to meet therapeutic goals
    b. Fee structure
    c. Objective progress measurements
    d. Methods of clinical reasoning

11. Which of the following is a violation of confidentiality?

    a. Maintaining client records in a secure location
    b. Asking the client questions about work environment
    c. Approaching and speaking to a client in a restaurant
    d. Speaking to a client's chiropractor with appropriate releases

12. Which of the following would be an appropriate disclosure to a client?

    a. The fact that the massage professional has a cold
    b. Business financial concerns
    c. Discussion about a mutual acquaintance
    d. Marital difficulties

13. A massage professional has been asked to work with a support group for persons with cerebral palsy. The therapist is well trained and has 7 years of experience but is uncomfortable with persons with disabilities, especially if communication is problematic. Which of the following is grounds for refusal on the part of the massage professional?

    a. Lack of skills
    b. Lack of peer support
    c. Inability to serve without bias
    d. Only wishes to work with females

14. A massage professional with 15 years of experience but minimal continuing education is in charge of a massage clinic. A recent massage graduate has obtained a position at the clinic. The new graduate notices that his current skills, particularly in charting and critical thinking, are more sophisticated than those of his supervisor but is hesitant to discuss the issue. What is the best description for this situation?

    a. Power differential
    b. Dual role
    c. Maintenance of professional environment
    d. Reciprocity

15. Which of the following is the best example of transference?

    a. A massage professional is biased toward a client because of political beliefs.
    b. A massage professional is receiving small gifts from a client expressing affection.
    c. A massage professional asks a client to attend a meeting about a nutritional product with him.
    d. A client is angry with the massage professional for being late for the last three appointments.

16. Which of the following would be the best explanation for a client who is confused over an incident of becoming mildly sexually aware during the last massage?

    a. The massage practitioner was sexualizing the massage.
    b. The client was sexualizing the massage.
    c. The client was experiencing parasympathetic sensations.
    d. The massage practitioner was massaging erotic zones.

17. A massage practitioner made a practice of careful and modest draping during the massage, used low lighting and soft music to help clients relax, always locked the door to maintain privacy, provided informed consent, and maintained charting. Where is the greatest potential for ethical concerns?

    a. Locked door
    b. Low lighting
    c. Soft music
    d. Confidential charting

18. A massage professional is troubled over a client's responses during the last four massage sessions. There is nothing specific about the client's behavior, but something has changed in the client's response to the massage. What could be helpful to the massage professional?

    a. Credentialing review with certification
    b. Managing intimacy issues
    c. Changing body language
    d. Decision making with peer support

19. A client seems to interrupt often when the massage practitioner is attempting to gather information about the client's condition before the massage. The client often provides inaccurate information when asked questions. Where might the client need assistance in the communication process?

    a. Formulating I-messages
    b. Listening
    c. Open-ended question
    d. Word choice

20. A client informs a massage professional that another massage practitioner in the practice is soliciting clients to move to a new private practice the therapist is starting. The massage professional knows that everyone in the massage practice signed a contract agreeing not to behave in this manner. After carefully consideration of the situation and discussion with a peer in a similar situation in another state, what is the next step in dealing with this type of unethical behavior of a peer?

    a. Formal reporting
    b. Contacting a lawyer
    c. Talking with those involved
    d. Speaking to fellow workers

Correct answers are on pages 148-149.

21. Local legislation controlling the location of a business is _____.

    a. Licensing
    b. Building codes
    c. DBA
    d. Zoning

22. What is the struggle between at least interdependent parties?

    a. Communication skills
    b. Reflective listening
    c. Conflict
    d. Brainstorming

23. A massage therapist is angry with a co-worker about the scheduling of the massage room. They are more busy than their co-worker and want to schedule more time on Saturdays. What type of conflict is this?

    a. Relationship conflict
    b. Data conflict
    c. Interest conflict
    d. Value conflict

24. A massage therapist is frustrated with his supervisor over being told he has to chart each massage using new forms. When he voiced his concerns, the supervisor told him there was no point in arguing and if he did not like it, he could leave. Which of the following described the conflict resolution method the supervisor used?

    a. Power/dominance
    b. Denial
    c. Collaboration
    d. Negotiation

25. Which of the following describes HIPPA?

    a. Credentials
    b. Clinical reasoning
    c. Reciprocity
    d. Privacy standards

Exercise

Using the foregoing questions as examples, now write at least three more questions—one of each type: factual and recall and comprehension, application and concept identification, and clinical reasoning and synthesis. Make sure to develop plausible wrong answers, and be sure that the correct answer is clearly correct. Then write a rationale for each question. The more questions you write, the better you will understand the material.

Correct answers are on pages 148-149.

Answers and Discussion

1. **a**
   Factual recall
   Rationale: The question is the definition of scope of practice. As with all of these types of questions, you need to define all the terms to understand and answer the question.

2. **d**
   Application and concept identification
   Rationale: The question gives an example of countertransference. As with all of these types of questions, you need to define all the terms to understand and answer the question. You need to compare the behavior of the massage professional described in the question with the definition.

3. **b**
   Application and concept identification
   Rationale: The question provides an example of breach of a standard of practice. You need to define the terms.

4. **c**
   Application and concept identification
   Rationale: The question addresses various approaches to massage and bodywork. A description of the population and indication of application of a variety of methods indicate that this professional uses an integrated approach.

5. **b**
   Application and concept identification
   Rationale: The question provides an example of a breach in scope of practice. To identify the correct answer, you need to define and understand all the terms in relation to the behavior.

6. **c**
   Factual recall
   Rationale: The question provides an example of the scope of practice for working with those with complex situations but who are not ill.

7. **d**
   Application and concept identification
   Rationale: The question gives an example, and the correct answer would explain a logical reason why the practitioner is uncomfortable. This is not a dual role, transference, or even a technical breach of scope of practice for massage, but the personal scope of practice is affected because the massage professional did not receive enough training to address this complex disease condition.

8. **d**
   Factual recall
   Rationale: You need to define the ethical principles to identify the correct answer.

9. **a**
   Factual recall
   Rationale: The question is the definition of a needs assessment.

10. **b**
    Factual recall
    Rationale: The question lists all the components of a policy statement except fee structure. The wrong answers are part of a treatment plan or a clinical reasoning process.

11. **c**
    Application and concept identification
    Rationale: The correct answer would indicate that confidentiality has been breached. The three wrong answers are examples of maintaining confidentiality.

12. **a**
    Application and concept identification
    Rationale: First, define the term *disclosure,* and then you can identify the correct example. Only information that would directly affect the massage interaction is to be disclosed. The three wrong answers are examples of inappropriate conversation with a client.

13. **c**
    Application and concept identification
    Rationale: The question asks for a rationale for the right of refusal. The only answer that is logical based on the facts in the question is answer c.

14. **a**
    Application and concept identification
    Rationale: The question gives an example of the power differential but in a different context than the examples in the textbook. The other terms, once defined, would not be logical in relation to the facts of the question.

15. **b**
    Application and concept identification
    Rationale: First, define *transference* and then compare it with the examples provided in the possible answers. Answer a is countertransference, answer b is correct, answer c is dual role, and answer d is justifiable anger, not transference.

16. **c**
    Application and concept identification
    Rationale: The most logical answer is answer c. The facts of the question indicate that the client is confused over the sensations and indicate no intentional acts by either party.

17. **a**
Factual recall
Rationale: Locking the door could be considered entrapment.

18. **d**
Application and concept identification
Rationale: The question provides an example of a situation in which peer support is helpful in ethical decision making. The three wrong answers would indicate that the professional has decided what the problem is, but the question indicates otherwise. Peer support and ethical decision making are helpful in identifying the area of concern and developing plans to rectify the situation.

19. **b**
Factual recall
Rationale: The question gives examples of listening difficulties.

20. **c**
Factual recall
Rationale: The question is asking for the steps in dealing with peer behavior.

21. **d**
Factual recall
Rationale: This question is representative of how information about credentialing and legal operation can be tested. You need to define the terms to answer the question.

22. **c**
Factual recall
Rationale: This is the definition of conflict.

23. **c**
Concept identification
Rationale: The nature of the conflict is "not enough to go around." This is an interest conflict.

24. **a**
Factual recall
Rationale: The supervisor has the authority to use power regardless if it is the best method or not.

25. **d**
Factual recall
Rationale: The Health Insurance Portability and Accountability Act encompasses three primary areas and involves privacy standards, patient rights, and administrative requirements.

15
Medical Terminology for Professional Record Keeping

Review Tips

Medical terminology for professional record keeping lends itself to definition-type factual recall questions. The most effective study strategy for this type of content is memorization. Use flashcards and similar study aids to prepare for testing on this content.

Various types of record keeping procedures are acceptable. The massage community tends to follow the SOAP style. Intake procedures are relatively standardized—history taking, assessment, needs assessment, and treatment plan development.

Questions

1. Record keeping for clients involves _____.

   a. Charting each session of the ongoing process
   b. Having the client fill out a general information packet
   c. Written record of intake procedures, informed consent, needs assessments, recording of each session, and release of information
   d. Filing each piece of information received from physicians and insurance companies or payments received from clients

2. Charting can be defined as _____.

   a. A record of each payment made by the client
   b. A record of the time spent with each client
   c. A written record of the intake procedure
   d. The ongoing process of recording each session

3. Massage treatment goals must be quantified, meaning _____.

   a. That they are achievable
   b. That they are measured in terms of objective criteria
   c. How they will be done
   d. What they will cost

4. The purpose of building a database is to _____.

   a. Gather information on which to build the professional interaction, establish client goals, and develop a plan for achieving them
   b. Develop a comprehensive knowledge base of medical terms to be able to reason clinically and chart effectively
   c. Develop procedures for writing records and the ways to use various forms
   d. Set achievable goals and outline a general plan

5. A database consists of _____.

   a. Charts on the actual session
   b. All the information available that contributes to therapeutic interaction
   c. The client's description of the problem
   d. Goals that are quantified and qualified and are functionally oriented

---

Correct answers are on page 155.   **151**

6. The purpose of assessment is to _____.

    a. Provide methods to correct deviations from the norm
    b. Identify effective functioning to eliminate massage to that area
    c. Do a visual and functional assessment but not a palpation assessment
    d. Identify effective functioning and deviations from the norm

7. Which of the following is a quantified outcome goal?

    a. Client will be able to increase range of motion of the lateral flexion of the cervical area by 15 degrees.
    b. Client will be able to resume normal work activities.
    c. Client will be reassessed in 12 sessions.
    d. Client will recover ability to play golf.

8. To analyze the data gathered during the assessment, one must _____.

    a. Increase mechanical application of skills for application of the treatment plan
    b. Generate quantifiable goals and methods to achieve client goals
    c. Consider the information based on examination, investigation, and analysis in relation to outcomes
    d. Compare information to generalized norms and protocols for treatment

9. The treatment plan _____.

    a. Is an exact protocol developed by client and practitioner
    b. Is a fluid guideline developed by client and practitioner
    c. Must be complete at the end of the first session and not revised
    d. Must be complete before the massage begins, because information gathered during the massage is not relevant

10. Problem-oriented medical records including SOAP require that _____.

    a. The qualified goals and the outcome of the massage be noted on the record
    b. The facts, possibilities, logical consequences of cause and effect, and impact on persons be noted on the record
    c. The results of palpation assessment but not the client history be recorded
    d. Only the interventions be noted on the record

11. Which of the following would be recorded in the objective data section of a SOAP note?

    a. Client states she has interrupted sleep.
    b. Client is currently taking melatonin.
    c. Observation and palpation indicate upper chest breathing.
    d. Client wishes to have weekly appointments.

12. The most important area in terms of determining future intervention procedures based on results is _____.

    a. S: subjective—what the client states
    b. O: objective—what was observed from assessment and examination
    c. A: analysis—what worked/did not work
    d. P: plan—what client wants to work on and what needs to be done during the next session

13. The P (plan) part of SOAP should include _____.

    a. Client medication history
    b. Client self-care
    c. Key symptoms
    d. Relation of outcomes to goals

14. The purpose of using a clinical reasoning model is _____.

    a. To be able to think through an intervention process and justify the effectiveness of a therapeutic interaction
    b. To provide a primary means of effectively supporting diagnosis to other health care professionals
    c. To integrate all the modalities and techniques into a user-friendly charting process for all to understand
    d. To provide a framework for the client charting protocols and data collection

15. A client presents a physician referral that states that only general massage with light pressure is to be used because of a recent angioplasty. The suffix in angioplasty means _____.

    a. Tumor
    b. Enlargement
    c. Surgical repair
    d. Disease

16. Reading the history, the massage professional sees that the client lists having myalgia. Which of the following defines myalgia?

    a. Muscle condition
    b. Spine pain
    c. Muscle pain
    d. Muscle paralysis

17. While reviewing a file on a client referred from another massage therapist, the massage professional finds information in the SOAP charting that indicates that applications of effleurage to the legs resulted in vasodilation. Which body system was affected directly?

    a. Cardiovascular
    b. Urinary
    c. Immune
    d. Digestive

18. What needs to be done to develop a valid analysis of massage benefits in a SOAP chart?

    a. Completion of a treatment plan
    b. Preassessment and postassessment procedures
    c. Prior development of a problem-oriented medical record
    d. Dates of reassessment

19. A massage professional lists reducing neuritis as a long-term client goal in the treatment plan. Which of the following describes the outcome?

    a. Provide relief from intestinal spasm
    b. Provide a decrease in joint mobility
    c. Produce an increase in nerve conduction
    d. Provide a decrease in nerve inflammation

20. Where would a massage professional record this statement on a SOAP note: "Palpation identified mild scoliosis"?

    a. S
    b. O
    c. A
    d. P

Correct answers are on page 155.

Exercise

Using the foregoing questions as examples, now write at least three more questions—one of each type: factual recall and comprehension, application and concept identification, and clinical reasoning and synthesis. Make sure to develop plausible wrong answers, and be sure that the correct answer is clearly correct. Then write a rationale for each question. The more questions you write, the better you will understand the material.

Answers and Discussion

1. **c**
Factual recall
Rationale: The answer describes record-keeping responsibilities.

2. **d**
Factual recall
Rationale: The correct answer is the definition of charting.

3. **b**
Factual recall
Rationale: The correct answer is the definition of a quantifiable goal.

4. **a**
Factual recall
Rationale: The correct answer describes the use of a database.

5. **b**
Factual recall
Rationale: The correct answer describes the components of a database.

6. **d**
Factual recall
Rationale: The correct answer describes the reason for assessment.

7. **a**
Application and concept identification
Rationale: First, you must define a quantified outcome goal and then analyze the possible answers for which one fits the criteria. Two of the wrong answers are examples of qualified goals.

8. **c**
Factual recall
Rationale: The correct answer describes the proper reason for data analysis.

9. **b**
Factual recall
Rationale: The correct answer is a definition of a treatment plan. The incorrect answers present inaccurate information.

10. **b**
Factual recall
Rationale: The correct answer describes the contents of proper charting.

11. **c**
Application and concept identification
Rationale: A type of objective data is information collected from assessment, as described in the correct answer. Answers a and b are subjective data, and answer d is information for the treatment plan.

12. **c**
Application and concept identification
Rationale: The decision-making process is being described in the question, and this happens during the analysis.

13. **b**
Factual recall
Rationale: The answer describes data recorded as part of the plan.

14. **a**
Application and concept identification
Rationale: The wrong answers are reasons for record keeping. Clinical reasoning is a process of thinking.

15. **c**
Factual recall
Rationale: This is a common approach to question development about medical terminology.

16. **c**
Factual recall
Rationale: This is a common approach to question development about medical terminology.

17. **a**
Factual recall
Rationale: This is a common approach to question development about medical terminology.

18. **b**
Application and concept identification
Rationale: The question asks for components of analysis. Required is a preassessment and postassessment to determine results.

19. **d**
Application and concept identification
Rationale: Knowledge of medical terminology is required to interpret the question. Neuritis is nerve inflammation.

20. **b**
Factual recall
Rationale: This is a common approach to question development about SOAP charting.

16

Scientific Art of Therapeutic Massage

Review Tips

The scientific art of therapeutic massage describes the research that validates the benefits of massage. The methods of scientific inquiry are described, and this is supported by an appendix in *Mosby's Fundamentals of Therapeutic Massage*. Research is important to the massage profession, but this content is difficult to write text questions on because the information changes often in response to research findings. Test questions need to have clearly right and wrong answers, and if the knowledge base shifts, then the questions may be flawed.

The more consistent content is the terminology and the generally accepted effects of massage.

The questions in this chapter rely heavily on correct use of terminology. When using the questions for study, make sure to define all terms in the questions and possible answers. Use the textbooks and references and the glossary in this book to look up any terms you do not understand.

This content also lends itself to the case study type of question, and the correct answer is identified by using the clinical reasoning process. As previously explained, the facts are presented in the question and the possibilities are in the four potential answers. Analyze each potential answer against the facts in the question to determine the correct response.

Questions

1. Science is defined as _____.

   a. Knowing something without going through a conscious process of thinking
   b. The ability to pay attention to a specific area and maintain an unconscious focus and intent
   c. The intellectual process of using all mental and physical resources available to better understand, explain, and predict normal and unusual natural phenomena
   d. Craft, skill, and technique that enable a person to monitor and adjust involuntary or subconscious responses

2. Centering is _____.

   a. A craft, skill, technique, and talent
   b. The ability to pay attention and maintain specific focus
   c. Knowing something without going through a conscious process of thinking
   d. The objective researching of a concept to see whether it is valid

3. The purpose of valid research in massage is to _____.

   a. Generate more questions about massage
   b. Objectively research the physiologic process
   c. Subjectively research the massage process
   d. Justify massage as an art

4. The techniques of therapeutic massage provide manual external sensory stimulation. Which of the following would be a good example?

   a. Entrainment
   b. Rubbing
   c. Centering
   d. Breathing

5. Most agree that the effects of massage can be explained by two categories: _____.

   a. Reflexive and mechanical methods
   b. Centering and intuition
   c. Art and experimentation
   d. Art and intuition

6. Which methods directly affect (stimulate) the nervous system?

   a. Mechanical methods
   b. Circulatory methods
   c. Reflexive methods
   d. Connective tissue methods

7. We now know that biochemicals are responsible for most problems in behavior, mood, and perception of stress and pain. Which of the following is an example of this type of problem?

   a. Anxiety
   b. Obstructive sleep apnea
   c. Eczema
   d. Farsightedness

8. Massage can increase a person's fine motor movements such as handwriting. Which neurotransmitter is influenced?

   a. Serotonin
   b. Oxytocin
   c. Dopamine
   d. Growth hormone

9. Massage has been demonstrated to reduce some individual's craving for food and/or reduce hunger. Which neurotransmitter is responsible?

   a. Epinephrine
   b. Serotonin
   c. Dopamine
   d. Norepinephrine

10. If I wanted my employees to be more attentive, I would do massage for _____.

    a. 5 minutes
    b. 45 minutes
    c. 15 minutes
    d. 60 minutes

11. Connectedness and intimacy in massage are most likely the results of an increased level of _____.

    a. Cortisol
    b. Endorphins
    c. Serotonin
    d. Oxytocin

12. Massage has been shown to reduce levels of _____, which decreases sympathetic arousal.

    a. Cortisol
    b. Oxytocin
    c. Growth hormone
    d. Enkephalins

13. A client states a goal of wanting to relax and complains of having headaches, gastrointestinal problems, and high blood pressure. The client is likely to be experiencing _____.

    a. An excessive parasympathetic output
    b. An excessive sympathetic output
    c. An entrainment process normalization
    d. Sleep deprivation

14. Hans Selye described body responses to stress in three stages. The middle stage is called _____.

    a. Alarm reaction
    b. Exhaustion reaction
    c. Resistance reaction
    d. Entrainment reaction

15. What is the general term used to describe the initial activation of the sympathetic nervous system?

    a. Alarm
    b. Stress
    c. Entrapment
    d. Entrainment

16. A person experiencing fluid retention, muscle weakness, vertigo, hypersensitivity, fatigue, weight gain, and breakdown in connective tissue most likely has _____.

    a. Test anxiety
    b. Long-term high blood levels of cortisol
    c. First-stage/alarm reaction
    d. Conservation withdrawal

17. What type of massage has been demonstrated to be most helpful for a client who has reached the exhaustive reaction phase of the general adaptive response to stress and has been there for more than 6 months?

    a. Several appointments over 1 month using 15 minutes of tapotement and shaking
    b. A massage using pulling and pressing with light pressure for weekly sessions for 3 months
    c. A massage that primarily focuses on long, slow strokes; broad-based compression; and rocking for weekly appointments for 6 months
    d. A staccato, fast deep pressure during weekly massage for 6 months

18. Parasympathetic patterns are _____.

    a. Restorative—adrenaline is secreted, mobility is decreased, and the bronchioles are constricted
    b. Physical activity is curtailed, digestion and elimination are increased, and the bronchioles are constricted
    c. Physical activity is increased, pupils are dilated, saliva secretion is stopped, and stomach secretion is increased
    d. Restorative—heartbeat speeds up, bladder delays emptying, and saliva secretion increases

19. If a conservation withdrawal pattern is apparent, it can be the result of _____.

    a. Intense negative experiences
    b. Synchronization to a rhythm
    c. A reflex response
    d. Reduction of air impingement

20. In the human body, what initiates entrainment?

    a. Digestive glands
    b. Autonomic nerves
    c. Brain
    d. Biologic oscillators

21. A client becomes very relaxed in response to the music and the rhythm of the strokes used during the massage session. What has occurred?

    a. Mechanical effects
    b. Circulation decrease
    c. Entrainment
    d. Client education

22. An altered state of consciousness can be achieved by massage. For its most therapeutic effect, the massage must be how long?

    a. 5 minutes
    b. 10 minutes
    c. 90 minutes
    d. 45 minutes

23. State-dependent memory can be triggered by massage because _____.

    a. The massage triggers, through movement or pressure, a stored pattern and stored release of chemical codes of emotions
    b. The massage presentation of stimuli teaches the body to manage more efficiently with sympathetic stress responses
    c. The massage itself influences the course of the memory, even if the massage is not specific to that memory
    d. Massage influences biologic oscillators such as the heart and thalamus, which sets rhythm patterns opposite the memory pattern

24. There are three main types of proprioceptors: muscle spindles, tendon organs, and _____.

    a. Cervical/lumbar plexus
    b. Spinal nerves
    c. Joint kinesthetic receptors
    d. Sphincter muscles

25. A client gets a cramp in the hamstring when stretching too quickly. Which reflex prompted the action?

    a. Stretch reflex
    b. Hooke's reflex
    c. Flexor reflex
    d. Extensor reflex

Correct answers are on pages 163-165.

26. The most common bodywork technique that involves the tendon reflex is _____.

    a. Muscle toning
    b. Post-isometric relaxation
    c. Acupuncture
    d. Counterirritation

27. What reflex is involved in maintaining balance?

    a. Flexor reflex
    b. Withdrawal reflex
    c. Tendon reflex
    d. Crossed extensor reflex

28. The Arndt-Schulz law states that weak stimuli activate physiologic processes; very strong stimuli inhibit them. What are the implications for massage?

    a. Massage is a strong sensory stimulation.
    b. Techniques have to be intense to produce responses.
    c. It is difficult to figure out whether a pain originates from a joint or surrounding tissue.
    d. To encourage a specific response, use gentler methods; to shut off the response, use deeper methods.

29. The law of facilitation states that when an impulse has passed through a certain set of neurons to the exclusion of others one time, it will tend to take the same course on a future occasion, and each time it travels this path, the resistance will be smaller. What are the implications for massage?

    a. If a sensory receptor is activated, it will respond in a certain way.
    b. Methods must override a sensation to produce a response.
    c. The body likes sameness; after a pattern has been established, less stimulation is required to activate the response.
    d. For a massage method to change a sensory perception, the intensity of the method must match and then exceed the existing sensation.

30. Some methods of massage affect the ground substance by increasing pliability. These methods include skin rolling, gliding strokes, and _____.

    a. Abrupt compression
    b. Tapotement
    c. Petrissage
    d. Shaking

31. The best way to increase arterial circulation during massage is _____.

    a. A 50-minute massage using effleurage but not heavy pressure
    b. A 45-minute compressive massage against the arteries proximal to the heart and moving in a distal direction
    c. A 50-minute massage using short pumping effleurage and gliding toward the heart
    d. A 30-minute massage emphasizing gliding strokes to passive/active joint movement distal to proximal

32. Gate-control theory is _____.

    a. Reduction of perception of a sensation of a sensory receptor by adaptation
    b. Control of homeostasis by alteration of tissue or function
    c. A method of teaching the body to deal with stress
    d. The hypothesis that painful stimuli can be prevented from reaching higher levels of the central nervous system by stimulating lower sensory nerves

33. The gallbladder 30 acupuncture point location correlates with which of the following motor points?

    a. Triceps
    b. Gastrocnemius
    c. Gluteus maximus
    d. Brachioradialis

34. The triple heater meridian location corresponds with which nerve?

    a. Ulnar nerve
    b. Tibial nerve
    c. Sciatic nerve
    d. Lateral plantar nerve

35. Traditional chakra locations correspond to _____.

    a. Oxytocin
    b. Arndt-Schulz law
    c. Trigger points
    d. Autonomic nerve plexuses

36. When a research experiment is performed more than once to make sure that the results were not biased, it is called _____.

    a. Double blind
    b. Control
    c. Hypothesis
    d. Replication

37. What is the first aspect of research?

    a. The conclusions
    b. The question
    c. The hypothesis
    d. The experiment

38. What is it called when the researcher is exploring existing information about a research question?

    a. Discovery
    b. Discussion
    c. Scientific method
    d. Framework

39. What is the broad explanation that synthesizes many different, unrelated facts and findings to explain a process or phenomenon?

    a. The experiment
    b. The introduction
    c. The variable
    d. The theory

40. Which of the following has the variable present?

    a. The control group
    b. The experimental group
    c. The replication group
    d. The discussion group

41. The experiment is what?

    a. Testing the conclusions
    b. Discovering the variables
    c. Testing the hypothesis
    d. The compared results

42. A researcher is conducting an experiment in which massage is introduced to determine whether endorphin levels change. What is the massage?

    a. The hypothesis
    b. The controlled variable
    c. The independent variable
    d. The dependent variable

43. In a typical research paper, where is the actual experiment described?

    a. Introduction
    b. Results
    c. Conclusions
    d. Methods

44. When a researcher's opinions influence the outcome of the research, what has happened?

    a. The research is valid.
    b. The research is biased.
    c. The research has an abstract.
    d. The experiment is replicated.

Correct answers are on pages 163-165.

Exercise

Using the foregoing questions as examples, now write at least three more questions-one of each type: factual recall and comprehension, application and concept identification, and clinical reasoning and synthesis. Make sure to develop plausible wrong answers, and be sure that the correct answer is clearly correct. Then write a rationale for each question. The more questions you write, the better you will understand the material.

Answers and Discussion

1. **c**
   Factual recall
   Rationale: The correct answer is a definition of science.

2. **b**
   Factual recall
   Rationale: The correct answer is a definition of centering.

3. **b**
   Factual recall
   Rationale: Research objectively validates massage.

4. **b**
   Factual recall
   Rationale: Only rubbing provides manual stimulation.

5. **a**
   Factual recall
   Rationale: This question is testing terminology knowledge.

6. **c**
   Factual recall
   Rationale: You need to define all the terms to answer the question.

7. **a**
   Factual recall
   Rationale: The question states a fact and then asks for the correct disorder. Anxiety is a mood disorder.

8. **c**
   Factual recall
   Rationale: The question is an example of how massage affects physiology. Information about neurotransmitter function also is required. Dopamine coordinates fine motor movement, and research shows that dopamine availability increases with massage.

9. **b**
   Factual recall
   Rationale: The question is an example of how massage affects physiology. Information about neurotransmitter function also is required. Serotonin is involved with satiety, and its availability increases with massage.

10. **c**
    Factual recall
    Rationale: The question is an example of how massage affects physiology. Information about neurotransmitter function also is required. Norepinephrine availability increases during the first 15 minutes of massage.

11. **d**
    Factual recall
    Rationale: The question is an example of how massage affects physiology. Information about neurotransmitter function also is required. Oxytocin availability increases with massage and is implicated in bonding.

12. **a**
    Factual recall
    Rationale: The question is an example of how massage affects physiology. Information about neurotransmitter function also is required. Cortisol decreases with a 30-minute or longer massage, which increases parasympathetic dominance.

13. **b**
    Application and concept identification
    Rationale: The question asks for a correlation between relaxation, the sympathetic symptoms displayed, and a massage outcome.

14. **c**
    Factual recall
    Rationale: Knowledge of the stages of the stress response is being tested. Entrainment is not part of the stress response.

15. **a**
    Factual recall
    Rationale: Terminology is being assessed by the question and possible answers. You need to define all terms to answer the question.

16. **b**
    Application and concept identification
    Rationale: Answers a and c indicate an adrenaline response. The symptoms provided in the question indicate resistance response and the result of long-term exposure to cortisol. Answer d is a parasympathetic response pattern.

17. **c**
    Clinical reasoning and synthesis
    Rationale: The facts provided in the question are long-term stress and a breakdown in adaptive capacity (exhaustion). Textbook facts would provide additional information about long-term cortisol effects, indications, and contraindications. Because the body is overstressed, care needs to be taken that the massage does not add excessive stress to the system. The wrong answers strain the system or do not provide for a long enough intervention.

18. **b**
Factual recall
Rationale: The correct answer describes parasympathetic functions. Answer d uses terminology incorrectly.

19. **a**
Factual recall
Rationale: This is the emergency response of the parasympathetic system.

20. **d**
Factual recall
Rationale: You need to define the terms to understand the connection between entrainment and the rhythms produced by biologic oscillators.

21. **c**
Application and concept identification
Rationale: The question asks for the reason for a physiologic response to massage and music in relation to the rhythm, which indicates an entrainment effect.

22. **d**
Factual recall
Rationale: It takes 45 minutes for the autonomic nervous system to make a state change.

23. **a**
Application and concept identification
Rationale: State-dependent memory is a conditioned response pattern that can be triggered by massage.

24. **c**
Factual recall
Rationale: This is a terminology question. You need to define all terms to identify the correct answer.

25. **a**
Factual recall
Rationale: This is a terminology question. You need to define all terms to identify the correct answer. There is no such thing as a Hooke's reflex, but there is a Hooke's neurologic law. This misuse of terminology is a common strategy for developing wrong answers.

26. **b**
Application and concept identification
Rationale: The question asks for the physiologic mechanism responsible for the effect of a massage method. You need to define all the terms to identify the correct answer.

27. **d**
Factual recall
Rationale: The question defines crossed extensor reflex.

28. **d**
Application and concept identification
Rationale: Neurologic laws identify consistent patterns of function. Applications of massage need to operate within this structure to have desired outcomes. Read the law carefully, interpret the terminology, and then project application to massage. Answer a is incorrect because massage stimulation can be strong or weak. Technique does not have to be intense to produce a response. Answer c speaks to an entirely different neurologic law.

29. **c**
Application and concept identification
Rationale: Neurologic laws identify consistent patterns of function. Applications of massage need to operate within this structure to have desired outcomes. Read the law carefully, interpret the terminology, and then project application to massage. The law of facilitation speaks to the conservation of energy by repetition of response.

30. **c**
Factual recall
Rationale: Massage applications need to be defined as to effect on the ground substance of connective tissue.

31. **b**
Application and concept identification
Rationale: The question is an example of many different questions that can be written based on application of massage and bodywork methods to affect a body system. The information base in this question includes textbook data about the circulatory system and massage approaches to influence it. Answers a, c, and d are more focused on venous circulation.

32. **d**
Factual recall
Rationale: The correct answer defines gate control.

33. **c**
Factual recall
Rationale: This is an example of the type of question that correlates Eastern and Western theories in bodywork.

34. **a**
Factual recall
Rationale: This is an example of the type of question that correlates Eastern and Western theories in bodywork.

35. **d**
Factual recall
Rationale: This is an example of the type of question that correlates Eastern and Western theories in bodywork.

36. **d**
Factual recall
Rationale: The question is the definition of experiment replication.

37. **b**
Factual recall
Rationale: All research begins with a question to be answered.

38. **a**
Factual recall
Rationale: The discovery phase is when the researcher identifies what exists.

39. **d**
Factual recall
Rationale: Definition of theory.

40. **b**
Factual recall
Rationale: Factors that have an effect on the experiment are called variables.

41. **c**
Factual recall
Rationale: The purpose of an experiment is to test the hypothesis.

42. **c**
Concept identification
Rationale: Choose the variable that is manipulated (i.e., massage is added as the independent variable).

43. **d**
Factual recall
Rationale: The methods section described how the experiment was designed.

44. **b**
Factual recall
Rationale: It is important that a researcher does not influence the research findings but objectively reports on the outcome of the research.

17

Indications and Contraindications for Therapeutic Massage

Review Tips

The indications and contraindications for therapeutic massage are the foundation for safe practice. Massage provides benefits that are justified by research and clinical experience. It is important for massage to benefit clients and not harm them. The major reason for licensing is to protect the public. It would be prudent to test this content extensively on exams. Questions typically are written in all three forms of questions. The best study strategy for factual recall and concept identification questions is memorization of the terminology, using the clinical reasoning process, and identifying wrong answers. Use these questions to help determine whether you have a comprehension of the vocabulary used. Look up any terminology you do not understand.

This content can be tested in the case study type of question assessing for the ability to synthesize the information and use clinical reasoning to identify the best answer based on the facts supplied in the question.

Questions

1. A contraindication means an approach could be harmful. Which of the following is not a type of contraindication?

   a. Support of a treatment modality other than massage

   b. General avoidance of an application: Do not perform any massage techniques (person severely bruised over entire body).

   c. Regional avoidance of an application: Do massage but avoid a particular area (person has broken foot).

   d. Application with caution: Do massage with supervision but carefully select method, duration, and frequency.

2. Which of the following is not a general benefit of massage?

   a. Improvement in circulation

   b. Enhanced elimination

   c. Inhibition of homeostasis

   d. Increased levels of endorphins

3. Massage therapy benefits conditions by encouraging the body through the phases involved in rehabilitation, restoration, and _____ of anatomic and physiologic function.

   a. Secretion

   b. Normalization

   c. Control

   d. Circulation

Correct answers are on pages 173-175.

4. A client is in the exhaustion phase of the general adaptation response. When one is considering a treatment plan for massage, which of the following is not appropriate?

   a. Ability of the client to expend energy for active change
   b. The availability of support and resources during change process
   c. Practitioner must have appropriate knowledge and skills
   d. Completing outcomes in 10 sessions or fewer

5. Condition management involves the use of massage methods to support clients who cannot undergo a therapeutic change but who wish to be as effective as possible within an existing set of circumstances. Which of the following is an example of condition management?

   a. Managing the existing physical compensation patterns
   b. Assisting the client through learning to walk again
   c. Restoring a client's range of motion to preinjury state
   d. Using massage to help a client feel better about self and to change jobs

6. A client enters the massage room complaining of a bad back from working at the computer. There are no stated contraindications. This is a stage 1 dysfunction. The client wants to reverse the condition. Which approach is the best process?

   a. Referral of client to a low-back specialist
   b. Therapeutic change
   c. Condition management
   d. Palliative care

7. Which of the following persons may require only palliative care from a massage therapist?

   a. An athlete with a sprained ankle
   b. A 48-year-old woman with a broken arm
   c. A man with terminal cancer
   d. A pregnant woman in the first trimester

8. The definition of health is _____.

   a. Prepathologic state
   b. Homeostatic and restorative body mechanisms can no longer adapt
   c. Anatomic and physiologic functioning limits
   d. Optimal functioning with freedom from disease or abnormal processes

9. Pathology can be best defined as _____.

   a. The in-between state of not healthy but not sick
   b. Anatomic and physiologic functioning limits
   c. The study of disease
   d. Processes of inflammatory tissue repair

10. Which of the following statements is most correct?

    a. The body has no actual anatomic or physiologic functioning limits.
    b. The body has only anatomic functioning limits.
    c. The body has only physiologic functioning limits.
    d. The body has anatomic and physiologic functioning limits.

11. Disease conditions usually are defined, diagnosed, and identified by signs and symptoms. A sign is _____.

    a. Subjective abnormalities felt only by the patient
    b. Objective abnormalities seen or measured by someone other than the patient
    c. A dysfunctional process noted by the patient
    d. An environmental situation described by the patient

12. Homeostasis can be defined as _____.

    a. The process of counterbalancing a defect in body structure or function
    b. A group of signs and symptoms
    c. The relative constancy of the internal environment of the body
    d. The subjective abnormalities felt by the patient

13. The general adaptation syndrome (the response of the body to stress) _____.

    a. Is always a preexisting condition
    b. Involves three stages: alarm, resistance, and exhaustion
    c. Involves three stages: inflammatory response, swelling, and pain
    d. Is a genetic factor

14. The inflammatory response can occur to any tissue injury. This response has four signs: redness, swelling, pain, and _____.

    a. Stickiness
    b. Liquid
    c. Heat
    d. Mucus

15. What is it called when new cells are similar to those that they replace?

    a. Egestion
    b. Fibrosis
    c. Inflammation
    d. Regeneration

16. Massage has been shown to slow formation of scar tissue and helps keep scar tissue pliable. This assists the healing process by _____.

    a. Blocking the action of antihistamines
    b. Counterbalancing the defect in the body
    c. Promoting regeneration and keeping replacement to a minimum
    d. Keeping the functioning energy reserves in place

17. Therapeutic inflammation can be accomplished most effectively through _____.

    a. Deep frictioning and connective tissue stretching
    b. Gliding
    c. Effleurage
    d. Tapotement and rapid compression

18. Therapeutic inflammation is best used in situations _____.

    a. In which there is a compromised immune function
    b. Resolving a fibrotic connective tissue dysfunction
    c. In which active inflammation is already present
    d. In which a condition such as fibromyalgia exists

19. The generally accepted definition of chronic pain is _____.

    a. A symptom of a disease condition or a temporary aspect of medical treatment
    b. Pain frequently experienced by clients who have had a limb removed
    c. Pain that persists or recurs for indefinite periods, usually longer than 6 months
    d. Pain that often subsides with or without therapy

20. Which of the following is a description of burning pain?

    a. Short-lived but intense and easily localized
    b. Constant but not well localized
    c. Slow to develop, lasts longer, and less accurately localized
    d. Blood supply to the muscle is occluded, and contraction causes pain

21. The origin of pain can be somatic or visceral. Somatic pain is defined as _____.

    a. Pain from only stimulation of receptors in the skin
    b. Pain from only stimulation of receptors in the skeletal muscles, joints, or tendons
    c. Pain resulting from only stimulation of receptors in the internal organs
    d. Pain arising from stimulation of receptors in the skin, skeletal muscles, joints, tendons, and fascia

22. If a client is experiencing pain in a surface area away from the stimulated organ, this is termed _____.

    a. Muscle pain
    b. Referred pain
    c. Deep pain
    d. Acute pain

Correct answers are on pages 173-175.

23. Neck pain on the right side can be indicative of referred pain from what organs?

    a. Appendix and kidney
    b. Colon and bladder
    c. Heart and lungs
    d. Liver and gallbladder

24. Lung and diaphragm pain may be referred to which cutaneous area?

    a. Left side of the neck
    b. Right side of the chest
    c. Right side of the neck
    d. In the hip girdle area

25. Intervention is different for managing acute versus chronic pain. Acute pain is managed _____.

    a. With inhibitory methods
    b. Using aggressive rehabilitation approach
    c. Less invasively and is focused to support the current healing process
    d. By compression on a nerve in a bony structure

26. Nerve impingement syndromes occur primarily in plexus areas. A person experiencing an impingement in the cervical plexus would have _____.

    a. Shoulder pain, chest pain, arm pain, wrist pain, and hand pain
    b. Low back discomfort with a belt distribution of pain, as well as pain in lower abdomen, genitals, and thigh
    c. Gluteal pain, leg pain, genital pain, and foot pain
    d. Headaches, neck pain, and breathing difficulties

27. Sacral plexus nerve impingement is indicated by _____.

    a. Gluteal pain, leg pain, genital pain, and foot pain
    b. Headaches, neck pain, and breathing difficulties
    c. Shoulder pain, chest pain, arm pain, wrist pain, and hand pain
    d. Low back discomfort with a belt distribution of pain and with pain in lower abdomen, genitals, thigh, and medial lower leg

28. The most effective massage methods to work on impingement syndromes are _____.

    a. Tapotement and shaking
    b. Muscle energy and lengthening
    c. Rapid deep compression
    d. Friction

29. Regional contraindications are _____.

    a. Those that require a physician's evaluation to rule out serious underlying conditions before any massage
    b. Present when health is the optimal functioning goal
    c. In effect when a client is in the in-between state of "not healthy" but also "not sick"
    d. Those that relate to a specific area of the body

30. The difference between benign tumors and malignant tumors is _____.

    a. Early detection is easier for benign tumors
    b. Malignant tumors are bigger
    c. Benign tumors remain localized within the tissue from which they arise; malignant tumors tend to spread to other regions of the body
    d. Benign tumors cannot grow rapidly

31. Massage and medication have three general processes in common: they stimulate a body process, they replace a chemical in the body, and _____.

    a. They work on a cure for the problem
    b. They work from a pathologic base
    c. They inhibit a body process
    d. They remove cellular debris

32. What occurs when medication and massage stimulate the same process?

    a. Antagonism
    b. Synergism
    c. Metastasis
    d. Impingement

33. What is the major reason that massage practitioners need to be aware of endangerment sites?

    a. These are soft areas that are unable to tolerate any pressure or movement.
    b. They may be a sign of a life-threatening disorder.
    c. The remaining proximal portions of sensory nerves are exposed here.
    d. These areas are not well protected by muscle or connective tissue, so deep sustained pressure could damage vessels, nerves, or other structures.

34. Intractable pain is _____.

    a. Cutaneous distribution of spinal nerve sensations
    b. A diffuse, localized discomfort that persists for indefinite periods
    c. Chronic pain that persists even when treatment is provided
    d. An abnormality in a body function that threatens well-being

35. Predisposing conditions that may make the development of disease more likely by the client than by another person are called _____.

    a. Metastasis
    b. Pathology
    c. Signs
    d. Risk factors

36. Objective abnormalities that can be seen or measured by someone other than the client are _____.

    a. Stress
    b. State-dependent memory
    c. Signs
    d. Pain

37. The functions of the most abundant tissue of the body include support, structure, space, stabilization, and scar formation. What is this tissue?

    a. Connective tissue
    b. Visceral tissue
    c. Bone marrow
    d. Fibrotic tissue

38. A client is taking an anticoagulant. Which of the following would be contraindicated?

    a. Resting stroke
    b. Friction
    c. Muscle energy
    d. Rocking

39. Which of the following is contraindicated for application of deep sustained compression?

    a. Lymph nodes
    b. Trigger points
    c. Dermatomes
    d. Ground substance

40. A doctor referral is indicated if the _____.

    a. Client has mild edema in the lower legs after a plane flight
    b. Client complains about care at the local outpatient clinic
    c. Client bruises easily
    d. Client is beginning a new medication

Correct answers are on pages 173-175.

Exercise

Using the foregoing questions as examples, now write at least three more questions—one of each type: factual recall and comprehension, application and concept identification, and clinical reasoning and synthesis. Make sure to develop plausible wrong answers, and be sure that the correct answer is clearly correct. Then write a rationale for each question. The more questions you write, the better you will understand the material.

Answers and Discussion

1. **a**
Factual recall
Rationale: The three wrong answers are correct examples of types of contraindications. This question is an example of how the correct answer is wrong information. Read questions written in this form carefully.

2. **c**
Factual recall
Rationale: This question is another example of when the correct answer is wrong information. In this question massage does everything but produce inhibition of homeostasis.

3. **b**
Factual recall
Rationale: This is a terminology question. You need to define all of the terms to answer the question correctly.

4. **d**
Clinical reasoning and synthesis
Rationale: The facts provided in the question indicate that the client has a condition in which the ability to continue to adapt is compromised. A treatment plan needs to be designed to support recovery without placing additional strain on the system. Because this question is asking for which of the possible answers is something that should not be done, attempting to generate outcomes in 10 sessions or fewer would seem to be contrary to the best treatment plan.

5. **a**
Application and concept identification
Rationale: The treatment plan approach of condition management is defined in the question. The correct answer would conform to this definition. Answer a is correct. Answers b and c are therapeutic change, and answer d may be a breach of scope of practice.

6. **b**
Application and concept identification
Rationale: The question presents data, and the answers are asking for a treatment approach in response to the data. Referral in this situation seems overly cautious because there is a reason for the discomfort and it fits the criteria of stage 1, which is easily reversible. Reversible conditions respond to therapeutic change.

7. **c**
Application and concept identification
Rationale: Palliative care reduces suffering and would be most appropriate for the man with terminal cancer. This does not mean that the other three conditions would not respond to palliation, but condition management would be more appropriate.

8. **d**
Factual recall
Rationale: The correct answer defines health. The other three answers indicate that the mechanisms of health are breaking down.

9. **c**
Factual recall
Rationale: The correct answer defines pathology.

10. **d**
Factual recall
Rationale: This question type asks for the identification of terminology used in the correct context.

11. **b**
Factual recall
Rationale: The correct answer defines a sign in relation to the information presented in the question. Signs are objective and observable information. The wrong answers are examples of subjective data.

12. **c**
Factual recall
Rationale: The correct answer is the definition of homeostasis.

13. **b**
Factual recall
Rationale: This is a terminology question. You need to define all the terms to identify the correct answer.

14. **c**
Factual recall
Rationale: This is the type of question in which some of the components are provided in the question and the last component in the sequence needs to be identified.

15. **d**
Factual recall
Rationale: This is a terminology question. You need to define all the terms to identify the correct answer.

16. **c**
Factual recall
Rationale: The question provides information about a benefit of massage in relation to good tissue healing, which involves promoting regulation and keeping replacement minimal.

17. **a**
Factual recall
Rationale: The question provides an outcome for a massage method and then asks for the best approach to achieve this goal.

18. **b**
Application and concept identification
Rationale: The question asks for the situation in which creating therapeutic inflammation would be appropriate. Answers a, c, and d are contraindicated for this approach.

19. **c**
Factual recall
Rationale: The correct answer is the definition of chronic pain.

20. **c**
Factual recall
Rationale: All of the answers describe pain, but it is important to differentiate between types of pain to identify indications and contraindications for massage.

21. **d**
Factual recall
Rationale: The correct answer is the definition of somatic pain. You need to define all the terms. *Soma* means body and is used to describe the soft tissue including skin, muscles, joints, tendons, and fascia.

22. **b**
Factual recall
Rationale: The question presents another pain type—referred pain.

23. **d**
Factual recall
Rationale: You must recognize the viscerally referred pain pattern to identify a need for referral. This question addresses this factual content.

24. **a**
Factual recall
Rationale: You must recognize the viscerally referred pain pattern to identify a need for referral. This question addresses this factual content.

25. **c**
Application and concept identification
Rationale: The question addresses issues pertaining to treatment plans for different types of pain. Chronic and intractable pain are addressed with symptom relief. Chronic pain may be addressed with aggressive methods if the client has adaptive capacity. Answer c is the correct answer for acute pain, and answer d is misuse of terminology.

26. **d**
Factual recall
Rationale: You need to define terms in the question and identify the referred pain patterns of impingement of all the plexuses to identify the correct referred pain pattern, which would be into the head and neck area.

27. **a**
Factual recall
Rationale: You need to define terms in the question and identify the referred pain patterns of impingement of all the plexuses to identify the correct referred pain pattern, which would be into the leg and gluteal area without lumbar pain.

28. **b**
Application and concept identification
Rationale: First, you need to define impingement syndromes. Then you need to choose the proper method to address the condition. Because massage most specifically addresses soft tissue nerve entrapment by increasing the resting length of muscles, answer b is the best method of those listed.

29. **d**
Factual recall
Rationale: The correct answer is the definition of regional contraindication.

30. **c**
Factual recall
Rationale: You need to define *benign* and *malignant* to choose the correct answer.

31. **c**
Factual recall
Rationale: The similarity between medication effect and massage benefit is seen in these three basic interactions: replace, stimulate, and inhibit.

32. **b**
Factual recall
Rationale: You need to define the terms in relation to medication usage. When massage and medication perform a similar function, the relationship is synergistic.

33. **d**
Application and concept identification
Rationale: Various areas on the body are susceptible to pressure damage.

34. **c**
Factual recall
Rationale: The answer provides the definition of intractable pain.

35. **d**
Factual recall
Rationale: The question defines risk factors.

36. **c**
Factual recall
Rationale: The question defines signs.

37. **a**
Factual recall
Rationale: The question defines connective tissue.

38. **b**
Application and concept identification
Rationale: You need to determine the action of the medication to identify which massage application would be detrimental in combination with the medication. This is an example of the many questions that can be written about medication and massage applications for safe practice. An anticoagulant prevents or reduces blood clotting, so friction may cause bruising.

39. **a**
Application and concept identification
Rationale: This question asks about endangerment sites.

40. **c**
Clinical reasoning and synthesis
Rationale: You need to analyze each of the possible answers to determine what would be safe for massage and what needs more expert diagnosis. Answer a provides facts about edema, the severity of the condition, and a logical explanation. No referral would be necessary. Answer b does not represent a condition in relation to massage. Answer c is the correct answer because there is no explanation for the condition and bruising can be a sign of a more serious pathologic condition. Answer d does not represent a contraindication unless there is something contraindicated with the medication.

18
Hygiene, Sanitation, and Safety

Review Tips

Hygiene, sanitation, and safety continues the theme of maintaining a safe massage experience for the client. This content typically is assessed with factual recall questions. Effective study strategy involves review of terminology.

The content covers pathogenic organisms and how to control the spread of these disease-causing agents through hygiene and sanitation. Standard precautions have been developed to maintain a safe environment not only for the client but also for the massage therapist.

Maintaining a safe environment is important as well. Fire safety, environmental safety, and premise safety are main topics.

Questions

1. Pathogenic disease-causing organisms include _____.

   a. Dirt, sweat, and grime
   b. Paint, tar, and dust
   c. Viruses, bacteria, and funguses
   d. Smoking, drinking, and washing

2. A group of simple parasitic organisms that are similar to plants but have no chlorophyll and live on skin or mucous membranes are _____.

   a. Viruses
   b. Funguses
   c. Bacteria
   d. Protozoa

3. Pathogens are spread by three main routes. Which of those below is one of these?

   a. Opportunistic invasion
   b. Clean uniform
   c. Intact skin
   d. Aseptic technique

4. The three primary ways pathogens are spread are person-to-person contact, environmental contact, and _____.

   a. Hand washing
   b. Universal precautions
   c. Shoes
   d. Opportunistic invasion

5. Pressurized steam bath would be an example of what common aseptic technique?

   a. Isolation
   b. Sterilization
   c. Disinfections
   d. Universal precautions

6. The simplest, most effective deterrent to the spread of disease is _____.

   a. Hand washing
   b. Sterilization technique
   c. Using a towel barrier
   d. Keeping shots up-to-date

7. An example of disinfection is _____.

    a. Chemicals such as alcohol or soaps
    b. Extreme temperature
    c. Sanitary disposal of tissues
    d. Pressurized steam bath

8. You are running behind today and your next client has been waiting for 15 minutes. It is most important that you _____.

    a. Maintain your scheduled appointments on time
    b. Have materials and activities available for clients to entertain themselves
    c. Make sure sheets and linens are changed and equipment disinfected between massages
    d. Apologize to the client for being late

9. Acquired immunodeficiency syndrome is _____.

    a. An inflammatory process caused by a virus
    b. Human immunodeficiency virus
    c. A group of clinical symptoms caused by a dysfunction in the immune system
    d. A disease contracted by casual contact such as shaking hands or sharing bathroom facilities

10. Which of the following is not a safe professional practice?

    a. Assisting the elderly on and off the massage table
    b. Burning candles for atmosphere in the massage room
    c. Maintaining good lighting in massage areas
    d. Regularly checking cables of portable massage tables

11. Standard precautions are defined as _____.

    a. Emergency care given to all ill or injured persons before medical help arrives
    b. Procedures developed by the Centers for Disease Control and Prevention to prevent the spread of contagious disease
    c. The process by which all microorganisms are destroyed
    d. The process by which pathogens are destroyed

12. Severe acute respiratory syndrome is _____.

    a. Noncontagious
    b. Spread by person-to-person contact
    c. Not deadly
    d. Controlled with nutrition

Exercise

Using the foregoing questions as examples, now write at least three more questions—one of each type: factual recall and comprehension, application and concept identification, and clinical reasoning and synthesis. Make sure to develop plausible wrong answers, and be sure that the correct answer is clearly correct. Then write a rationale for each question. The more questions you write, the better you will understand the material.

Correct answers are on page 180.

Answers and Discussion

1. **c**
   Factual recall
   Rationale: The correct answer provides examples of pathogenic organisms.

2. **b**
   Factual recall
   Rationale: The question defines funguses.

3. **a**
   Factual recall
   Rationale: This question is an example of how the same information can be tested in an exam question. See question 4. The three wrong answers are methods that prevent the spread of disease.

4. **d**
   Factual recall
   Rationale: This question is an example of how the same information can be tested in an exam question. See question 3. The three wrong answers are methods that prevent the spread of disease.

5. **b**
   Factual recall
   Rationale: The question provides an example of sterilization. You need to define all the terms to identify the correct answer.

6. **a**
   Factual recall
   Rationale: Proper hand washing is essential to sanitary massage therapy practice.

7. **a**
   Factual recall
   Rationale: The correct answer is an example of disinfection.

8. **c**
   Clinical reasoning and synthesis
   Rationale: This type of question asks for a decision. The correct answer is the one that best conforms to standards of sanitary practice. All of the answers are correct, but safety of the client always is a priority.

9. **c**
   Factual recall
   Rationale: The correct answer is the definition of acquired immunodeficiency syndrome.

10. **b**
    Factual recall
    Rationale: The correct answer is the one containing incorrect information. Always read questions written in this style carefully. An open flame is a safety hazard. All safety hazards need to be identified to promote safe professional practice.

11. **b**
    Factual recall
    Rationale: Standard precautions are a specific protocol of sanitary procedures developed by the Centers for Disease Control and Prevention.

12. **b**
    Factual recall
    Rationale: Severe acute respiratory syndrome is a very contagious disease.

19
Body Mechanics

Review Tips

The information on body mechanics varies in different textbooks; therefore writing exam questions on this content is difficult if the exam needs to be legally defensible, such as the National Certification Exam and the National Certification Exam for Therapeutic Massage and Bodywork or licensing exams. The content is important and describes ergonomics.

Because textbooks do not agree, questions are typically general and avoid controversial areas.

One of the best study strategies is to identify why all the wrong answers in the sample question are incorrect. Terminology is not standardized, so studying vocabulary is important but not as effective as in other content areas.

Questions

1. When a practitioner is in a relaxed standing posture supporting the gravitational line with the normal knee-locked position, which muscles are used for balance?

   a. Psoas
   b. Gastrocnemius
   c. Hamstrings
   d. Quadriceps

2. What is the most efficient standing position?

   a. Symmetrical
   b. Wide stance (shoulder length apart)
   c. Asymmetrical
   d. Lead foot with the pressure on it

3. Most massage applications use a force generated _____.

   a. Downward
   b. Forward
   c. Downward and forward
   d. Forward and across

4. When one is applying compressive force down and forward, weight transfer is most efficient when the massage therapist puts weight _____.

   a. On the back leg and foot
   b. On the front leg and knee
   c. On the back foot and toes
   d. On the front foot and toes

5. A massage professional is feeling strain in the shoulders and arms after doing four massage sessions. Which of the following is the most logical reason?

   a. The massage professional is using muscle strength in the arms to exert force.
   b. The massage professional is standing in an asymmetrical stance.
   c. The client is positioned for best mechanical advantage.
   d. The massage professional is effectively leaning at a 45° angle

6. A massage practitioner has been experiencing increasingly severe low back pain. The practice is full time with 20 clients per week. What could the massage practitioner do to reduce back strain?

   a. Bend the knees past 15° of flexion while performing massage.
   b. Raise the table height to prevent torso bending.
   c. Keep the head forward and down to change the center of gravity.
   d. Externally rotate the back foot away from the line of force.

7. A client keeps complaining of discomfort at the end of the massage stroke. What is happening?

   a. The practitioner is pushing with the legs.
   b. The practitioner is off balance and using counterpressure.
   c. The skin is being pulled from lack of lubricant.
   d. The compressive force is distributed over a narrow base at the end of the stroke.

8. A massage professional is complaining of pain in the wrist and near the elbow. Which of the following is an appropriate corrective action?

   a. Maintain the hands in a clenched fist to promote stability.
   b. Increase the movement of the stroke at the shoulder joint.
   c. Relax the hand and fingers during massage.
   d. Shift the compressive force to the fingers and thumb.

9. Observation of a fellow massage practitioner indicates that the shoulder girdle is aligned with the pelvic girdle, the pressure-bearing arm opposite the weight-bearing leg, the fingers relaxed, the head up, the back straight, the elbows bent, and the stance asymmetrical. Which of these areas needs correction?

   a. Elbows
   b. Stance
   c. Back position
   d. Shoulder position

10. A massage professional is feeling strain in the knees. Which of the following is the most logical cause?

    a. Doing massage on hard floors
    b. Working with clients in the side-lying position
    c. Keeping the knees flexed and static
    d. Moving whenever the arm reach is beyond 60 degrees

11. Increasing levels of pressure are achieved by _____.

    a. Moving closer to the massage table
    b. Moving away from the massage table
    c. Standing on the toes
    d. Shifting the weight-bearing foot to the front

12. When stretching the legs of a client by applying a pull against the ankle, the massage practitioner should _____.

    a. Fix the feet and pull with the shoulders
    b. Move to a symmetrical stance and lean back
    c. Maintain asymmetrical stance and lean back, keeping the back straight
    d. Bend the knees and push back

13. The massage therapist needs to have _____ to be effective with body mechanics?

    a. Core stability
    b. Hyperflexibility
    c. Hypoflexibility
    d. Forearm strength

Exercise

Using the foregoing questions as examples, now write at least three more questions—one of each type: factual recall and comprehension, application and concept identification, and clinical reasoning and synthesis. Make sure to develop plausible wrong answers, and be sure that the correct answer is clearly correct. Then write a rationale for each question. The more questions you write, the better you will understand the material.

Correct answers are on page 184.

Answers and Discussion

1. **b**
   Factual recall
   Rationale: The relaxed standing position conserves muscle energy while maintaining balance with the gastrocnemius and soleus muscles.

2. **c**
   Factual recall
   Rationale: The incorrect answers are fatiguing.

3. **c**
   Factual recall
   Rationale: Two directional forces are used with massage: compressive force down with a forward momentum.

4. **a**
   Factual recall
   Rationale: This question is an example of how information presented in the question or the possible answers can relate to other questions in the examination. This question relates to question 3. A person who did not know the answer to question 3 would find it in question 4 by the way it is worded. In this question the correct answer describes proper weight distribution.

5. **a**
   Clinical reasoning and synthesis
   Rationale: Facts in the question suggest that something is incorrect with the delivery of the massage. You need to analyze the answers against the question to make the decision about the cause. The incorrect answers describe appropriate body mechanics, whereas the correct answer is a logical explanation for the strain in the arms and shoulders.

6. **b**
   Clinical reasoning and synthesis
   Rationale: The facts in the question are low back pain that is getting worse and full-time massage practice. You need to analyze the possible answers for the logical reason for this condition and what could be done to correct the problem. Answer a likely would make the condition worse and add knee strain. Answer b is the correct answer. Answers c and d are actions that would increase the strain.

7. **d**
   Application and concept identification
   Rationale: If the massage practitioner shifts the weight to the front foot at the end of the stroke, the focus of the pressure is smaller and would be uncomfortable.

8. **c**
   Clinical reasoning and synthesis
   Rationale: The question indicates that something is wrong with the body mechanics, resulting in pain. All three of the incorrect answers would increase the pain.

9. **a**
   Application and concept identification
   Rationale: The question provides information about correct body mechanics except one area, bent elbows.

10. **c**
    Clinical reasoning and synthesis
    Rationale: The question asks for a decision on the cause of knee pain. After analysis of each answer, the only one that is logical is flexed and static knees.

11. **b**
    Factual recall
    Rationale: The center of gravity changes, resulting in increased pressure if the weight-bearing foot is moved farther away from the table but not to the point that one stands on the toes.

12. **c**
    Application and concept identification
    Rationale: This massage outcome would be accomplished most efficiently by using the method described in the correct answer.

13. **a**
    Concept identification
    Rationale: One of the most important aspects of perpendicularity and weight transfer is core stability.

20
Preparation for Massage

Review Tips

The content for preparation for massage includes massage equipment, draping, sanitation, hygiene, lubricant types, the massage environment—and how to communicate and give and get feedback in the professional setting. The difficulty with this content is that it is more opinion based than fact based, so writing legally defensible questions is difficult. The case study format is common, and the key to finding the correct answer is to eliminate the wrong answers. When reading the content in your textbook, identify those content areas that are not as opinion based. For example, draping of clients and the use of massage lubricant are generally expected. Specifically how the drape is used or how the lubricant is applied is more of an opinion.

As in all the content areas, there is unique terminology to study.

Questions

1. The most important stability feature of a portable massage table is the _____.

   a. Frame
   b. Cable support
   c. Adjustable legs
   d. Center hinge

2. A client is particularly concerned with safety and is afraid of falling. Of the following massage equipment, which would make the client most comfortable?

   a. Mat
   b. Stationary table
   c. Portable table
   d. Chair

3. Regardless of the type of draping material used, which of the following is required?

   a. Disposable
   b. Large
   c. Opaque
   d. Cotton fabric

4. To maintain sanitary practice, draping material must be _____.

   a. Laundered in hot soapy water with a disinfectant such as bleach
   b. Sterilized and heat pressed
   c. Professionally laundered
   d. Warm, large enough to cover the client, and of different colors

5. To prevent allergic reactions, all lubricants should be _____.

   a. Oil based
   b. Water based
   c. Dispensed in sanitary fashion
   d. Scent free

6. The purpose of lubricant is _____.

   a. To moisturize the skin
   b. To reduce drag on the skin
   c. To transport nutrients
   d. Counterirritation

Correct answers are on pages 189-190.

7. A massage professional has just rented office space and fully decorated the area. The massage room has a window and overhead and indirect lighting. The central thermostat is in another area, but the massage room has a fan and an electric heater to adjust temperature. The small waiting area is bright and comfortable, with many sorts of flowering plants. A private restroom is just off the waiting room. The massage room does not have a closet but does have hooks for the clients' clothing. A closed cabinet holds supplies. The business area is small but has a locked file cabinet and small desk.
   What suggestion would you make for improving the massage environment?

   a. Add an aromatherapy atomizer.
   b. Put a lock on the massage room door.
   c. Move the file cabinet into the massage room.
   d. Remove the flowering plants.

8. Which environment is the most difficult for maintaining professional boundaries?

   a. Public events
   b. Private office in a commercial building
   c. On-site at a residence
   d. Home office

9. A massage practitioner has been seeing the same client weekly for 3 months. The client often discusses personal issues with the massage practitioner. Last session the massage professional provided some reading information to help the client and talked with the client about how the practitioner had dealt with a similar issue. The client has canceled the last two appointments. What is the most logical cause?

   a. Feedback about the massage broke down.
   b. Conversation with the client overshadowed the massage session.
   c. Gender issues are influencing the session.
   d. The orientation process needs to be repeated.

10. A massage professional is preparing an orientation process for a new client. The professional has developed the following checklist: Show client massage area, where to change and hang clothes, massage table draping and positioning, how to get on and off the massage table, music choices, and restrooms. Explain charts and equipment, lubricant types, sanitary procedures, and privacy methods. What did the massage professional forget?

    a. To explain the general idea of massage flow
    b. To provide a centering meditation with the client
    c. To provide education on self-help
    d. To introduce the client to products for sale

11. A client complains of a mild general low back pain. Which of the following is appropriate?

    a. Use a side-lying position with knee support.
    b. Work with the client prone, using no support under the ankles.
    c. Work with the client supine, using support only under the neck.
    d. Position the client in a seated position and avoid supports.

12. A client is shy and modest. Which of the following draping methods would be the best choice?

    a. Contoured draping with towels
    b. Partial body towel draping
    c. Full body sheet and towel draping
    d. Sheet draping with no towels

13. In which situation would you stay in the massage room and assist a client on and off the massage table?

    a. A client in the first trimester of pregnancy
    b. A 65-year-old man with diabetes
    c. An elderly woman with high blood pressure
    d. An adolescent with a wrist cast

14. An adolescent athlete is coming for massage with a parent. You have been informed that the client is uncomfortable with disrobing. Which of the following is the most logical alternative?

    a. An educational session
    b. A draping demonstration
    c. Working only with the feet
    d. Having the client wear loose shorts and T-shirt

15. A client regularly lingers after the massage session to talk. The massage professional gets behind schedule because of this. What is the most likely cause of this problem?

    a. Policies regarding leaving promptly after the massage were not addressed and reinforced.
    b. The client requires a longer appointment.
    c. The client needs more frequent appointments.
    d. The massage professional is displaying transference.

Correct answers are on pages 189-190.

Exercise

Using the foregoing questions as examples, now write at least three more questions-one of each type: factual recall and comprehension, application and concept identification, and clinical reasoning and synthesis. Make sure to develop plausible wrong answers, and be sure that the correct answer is clearly correct. Then write a rationale for each question. The more questions you write, the better you will understand the material.

Answers and Discussion

1. **b**
Factual recall
Rationale: The cable support is the structural design component for stability, and the center hinge is the weak point.

2. **a**
Application and concept identification
Rationale: The mat would allow work to be done on the floor, where falling would not be an issue.

3. **c**
Factual recall
Rationale: Draping material provides warmth and modesty, so the material must be opaque.

4. **a**
Factual recall
Rationale: Sanitation is a priority, using disinfection appropriate for linens.

5. **d**
Factual recall
Rationale: The most common reason for allergic reaction to a lubricant is the volatile oils that are used to scent the product.

6. **b**
Factual recall
Rationale: The only reason for lubricant is to reduce skin drag when doing gliding or kneading massage methods. All other reasons, such as medicinal or cosmetic ones, may be a breach in the scope of practice.

7. **d**
Clinical reasoning and synthesis
Rationale: All of the recommendations and cautions for creating a massage environment need to be reviewed to decide what needs to be changed in the massage area described by the question. Answer a is not recommended because scents may cause allergic reactions in sensitive individuals and personal preference varies. A lock on the massage door can be considered entrapment, so it is inappropriate. Because the file cabinet is locked, confidentiality is maintained. It is recommended to remove the plants, again because many persons are allergic to them.

8. **c**
Factual recall
Rationale: Of the four answers provided, going to a client's home presents the most difficult boundary issues.

9. **b**
Clinical reasoning and synthesis
Rationale: A summary of the facts provided in the question indicates that boundary issues have been breached and conversation with the client was inappropriate. To identify the correct answer, one must understand the concepts of feedback, gender issues, and an appropriate orientation process.

10. **a**
Application and concept identification
Rationale: The question reflects a comprehensive, first-client orientation process. Explanation of the massage flow to clients is important so that they are more comfortable with the process. The incorrect answers describe a boundary violation or are not part of the orientation process.

11. **a**
Application and concept identification
Rationale: Prone and supine positioning tend to aggravate low back pain. Even a seated position can be tiring to the low back. Therefore the side-lying position is the best choice.

12. **c**
Clinical reasoning and synthesis
Rationale: The question presents a common massage practice situation. In this situation the wrong answers do not provide enough body coverage to accommodate this client.

13. **c**
Application and concept identification
Rationale: When safety is a concern, the therapist should assist the client on and off the table. When considering the client conditions presented, the elderly woman with blood pressure concerns is correct because she could be dizzy after the massage.

14. **d**
Clinical reasoning and synthesis
Rationale: Massage can be done without the client removing clothing. Methods can be modified to adjust to the situation or the client can wear clothing that is easy to work around. To change the client's beliefs with a demonstration of draping or an educational session is not necessary when having the client wear shorts and loose shirt solves the problem.

15. **a**

Clinical reasoning and synthesis
Rationale: As with all of these types of questions, there is a decision about what to do in a particular situation or what is wrong or right with the situation presented in the question. In this question, a client does not leave after the session, which makes it difficult for the professional to maintain a work schedule. Usually this is because the policies and client rules were not enforced from the beginning, as described in the correct answer. Wrong answers b and c would predispose to future problems, and answer d is an incorrect word usage.

21
Massage Manipulations and Techniques

Review Tips

The chapter on massage manipulations and techniques introduces many new terms to understand. By this time, you should know to look up all terms you do not understand, and you should be able to use the terminology correctly. This content often is found in the factual recall/comprehension question style.

Use of the massage methods in a safe and appropriate way is necessary. This content usually is assessed in the concept identification or the clinical reasoning/synthesis type of questions. Case studies are common.

An effective study strategy is to explain a concept in words different from those in the text or to give an example of what the text is talking about or to develop a metaphor about the content.

Anatomy and physiology terminology is common in these questions. You must be able to interpret the language in the question and possible answers and to use a clinical reasoning process to find the correct answer.

Questions

1. Massage manipulations are _____.

   a. Skillful use of the hands and forearms to affect the soft tissue directly
   b. Skillful use of the hands to affect the joints directly
   c. Application of methods using heat and equipment to affect soft tissue
   d. Application of compressive forces to affect meridians

2. A massage practitioner uses massage manipulations in a brisk and specific way. Which of the following client goals is best served by this approach?

   a. Decreased alertness
   b. Increased parasympathetic response
   c. Decreased sensory awareness
   d. Increased alertness

3. A client has an outcome goal for the massage of increased circulation and range of motion for the knee. Which of the following is the best approach?

   a. Reflexive methods focused on chemical changes
   b. Mechanical methods focused on the area
   c. Mechanical methods to influence neuroactivity reflexively
   d. Reflexive methods to increase compressive force to the viscera

4. A massage client is unhappy with the massage. The main complaint is a feeling of choppiness and lack of continuity. Which of the following qualities of touch is most responsible?

   a. Depth of pressure
   b. Drag
   c. Rhythm
   d. Direction

5. Which of the following methods is most beneficial for abdominal massage to mechanically encourage fecal movement in the large intestine?

   a. Effleurage/gliding
   b. Resting position
   c. Tapotement/percussion
   d. Compression

6. Which of the following methods has as its primary effect a lifting of the tissue away from underlying structures?

   a. Compression
   b. Kneading
   c. Gliding
   d. Vibration

7. A client reports a sensitivity to lubricant during the history and would like a massage in which no lubricant is used. Which method would be inappropriate?

   a. Shaking
   b. Compression
   c. Kneading
   d. Gliding

8. When the outcome for the massage is to produce parasympathetic dominance, which combination of methods would be the best choice?

   a. Gliding, rocking, and passive joint movement
   b. Compression, shaking, and friction
   c. Active joint movement, reciprocal inhibition, and rocking
   d. Tapotement, compression, and vibration

9. A client complains of restricted range of motion in the shoulder. The primary outcome for the massage is to increase shoulder mobility. Which method would be the best choice?

   a. Friction
   b. Muscle energy
   c. Hydrotherapy
   d. Resting stroke

10. A client requests that tapotement be used at the end of the massage to stimulate the nervous system. Which is the best choice for the face?

    a. Hacking
    b. Cupping
    c. Tapping
    d. Slapping

11. Which of the following methods would be best for assessing for the physiologic and pathologic motion barrier?

    a. Passive joint movement
    b. Active resistive movement
    c. Post-isometric relaxation
    d. Concentric isotonic contraction

12. Which of the following is produced voluntarily?

    a. Joint play
    b. Arthrokinematic movement
    c. Osteokinematic movement
    d. Joint end-feel

13. Which component is essential for effective application of joint movement?

    a. Stabilization to isolate the movement to the targeted joint
    b. Tapotement to stimulate the joint kinesthetic receptors
    c. High-velocity manipulative movement
    d. Cross-directional tissue stretching to cause traction on the joint capsule

14. A client's muscles cramp when the massage professional attempts to use post-isometric relaxation to lengthen a shortened group of muscles. Which of the following methods would be a better choice to lengthen the muscle group?

    a. Skin rolling
    b. Active resistive joint movement
    c. Reciprocal inhibition
    d. Stretching

15. A client is feeling fatigued and does not wish to participate during the massage. Instead the client wishes to remain passive and quiet. Which of the following muscle energy methods would be appropriate?

    a. Positional release
    b. Pulsed muscle energy
    c. Integrated approach
    d. Approximation

16. Which method is being described? Isolate the target muscle in passive contraction. Have the client contract the antagonist group. Have the client relax and then lengthen the target muscles.

    a. Post-isometric relaxation
    b. Reciprocal inhibition
    c. Contract-relax antagonist contract
    d. Pulsed muscle energy

17. A client has been receiving massage weekly for 2 months. The main goal for the massage is increased mobility in the lumbar and hip region. The client has experienced stiffness and reduced ability since a fall off a bike 2 years ago. General massage and muscle energy methods with lengthening have produced mild improvement. Which of the following mechanical methods has the potential to increase results?

    a. Lymphatic drainage
    b. Stretching
    c. Contract/relax
    d. Strain-counterstrain

18. A client is ticklish, particularly on the chest. Which method would be the best choice to use in this area?

    a. Compression over the client's own hand
    b. Friction
    c. Gentle gliding
    d. Fingertip compression

19. A client is requesting extensive massage to the neck and upper shoulders. Which is the most efficient client position to massage these areas easily?

    a. Prone
    b. Supine
    c. Seated
    d. Side-lying

20. Which method is beneficial to use on the hands and feet to stimulate lymphatic movement?

    a. Superficial effleurage
    b. Skin rolling
    c. Vibration
    d. Pumping compression

21. A client complains of a stiff and stuck feeling in the lumbar area. Assessment indicates that the fascia in that area is thick and adhered to the underlying tissue. Which method would best restore pliability to this tissue?

    a. Skin rolling
    b. Shaking
    c. Resting position
    d. Vibration

22. A client has a lot of body hair on his back. During the first massage, lubricant was used. At the return visit the client requests that lubricant not be used on his body where there are large amounts of hair. Which method could be used?

    a. Gliding
    b. Kneading
    c. Compression
    d. Petrissage

23. A major contraindication to massage of the legs is _____.

    a. Acne
    b. Brachial nerve compression
    c. Disk compression
    d. Thrombophlebitis

24. A client likes to have the back massaged and asks that most of the massage time be focused on the back. The client continues to complain that the massage is not effective in reducing back pain. What explanation can be given to the client?

    a. The soft tissue of the back often is tight because of extensive pulling and shortening of the tissues in the chest; massage of the chest may help.
    b. Massage to the back limits blood flow, so the soft tissues remain in contracture.
    c. Massage on the extremities would be better to reduce the pain in this area because the mechanical effect is more concentrated.
    d. The connective tissues of the back respond best to reflexive measures, and using a more generalized approach would provide relief.

25. Which of the following methods is best for general broad applications when lubricant is requested?

    a. Petrissage
    b. Compression
    c. Effleurage
    d. Vibration

26. Which of the following is of most concern when massaging the face?

    a. Proximity to mucous membranes and transmission of pathogens
    b. The skin of the face is thin.
    c. Facial muscles are weak.
    d. Compression damages underlying cranial sutures.

27. A client is complaining about pain and stiffness in the neck but is particularly sensitive to pressure used in the neck area, flinching and stiffening in a protective stance whenever the neck is massaged. The current approach is primarily to use kneading with the client in the prone position. What is the best alternative?

    a. Change position to supine and use gliding.
    b. Use side-lying position and broad-based compression.
    c. Combine passive range of motion, muscle energy, and friction with the client seated.
    d. Have the client seated and then use deep kneading.

28. Which of the following body areas requires special attention to draping?

    a. Hand
    b. Leg
    c. Chest
    d. Shoulder

29. Which of the following body areas often is massaged longer than is effective?

    a. Hands
    b. Abdomen
    c. Legs
    d. Back

30. A client arrives late for a massage appointment. The remaining time is 30 minutes. The goal for the session is general relaxation. Which combination is the best choice to achieve desired outcomes in the allotted time?

    a. Back, gluteals, and hips
    b. Face, hands, and feet
    c. Hands, arms, and back
    d. Face, neck, and shoulders

31. The more current term for effleurage is gliding and most effectively applies which mechanical force to the body?

    a. Shear
    b. Tension
    c. Torsion
    d. Resting

32. A massage application that twists tissue creates which of the following?

    a. Bend
    b. Torsion
    c. Gliding
    d. Compression

33. Which of the following creates shear force?

    a. Gliding
    b. Compression
    c. Tapotement
    d. Friction

34. Kneading is effective if creating _____.

   a. Resting stroke

   b. Tapotement

   c. Bend and torsion force

   d. Entrainment

Exercise

Using the foregoing questions as examples, now write at least three more questions—one of each type: factual recall and comprehension, application and concept identification, and clinical reasoning and synthesis. Make sure to develop plausible wrong answers, and be sure that the correct answer is clearly correct. Then write a rationale for each question. The more questions you write, the better you will understand the material.

Answers and Discussion

1. **a**
   Factual recall
   Rationale: The correct answer is the definition of massage manipulations.

2. **d**
   Application and concept identification
   Rationale: This type of massage application would stimulate the body, increasing alertness.

3. **b**
   Clinical reasoning and synthesis
   Rationale: Both goals of circulation enhancement and increased range of motion are achieved though mechanical methods. Analysis of the incorrect answers indicates that the information is flawed or not in context with the question.

4. **c**
   Application and concept identification
   Rationale: To answer the question, you need to define all the terms and then compare terms with the data in the question. The rhythm of the massage was not appropriate to the client's needs.

5. **a**
   Application and concept identification
   Rationale: The question asks for the best methods to achieve an outcome in a specific body area or function. This question is representative of the many types of questions that can be developed around this content. To answer the question, you need to understand the application and physiologic effect of all the massage methods. In this particular question, effleurage/gliding is the best choice.

6. **b**
   Factual recall
   Rationale: The question defines petrissage/kneading. You need to define all the terms to answer the question.

7. **d**
   Factual recall
   Rationale: Only gliding requires the use of lubricant.

8. **a**
   Application and concept identification
   Rationale: To answer this question, you need to define all the terms and determine the physiologic outcome. Only the correct answer lists those methods that do not stimulate a sympathetic response.

9. **b**
   Clinical reasoning and synthesis
   Rationale: You need to evaluate each method for effectiveness in relation to the goal stated in the question. All of the methods listed may provide benefit, but muscle energy methods are used most specifically to increase range of motion by creating a more normal muscle resting length.

10. **c**
    Application and concept identification
    Rationale: You need to define each term and describe its application. Only tapping is appropriate for the face.

11. **a**
    Application and concept identification
    Rationale: You need to define each term and describe its use for assessment. You also need to understand the terms in the question to interpret the question. Passive joint movement is the best choice for assessment of range of motion because all the other methods involve a muscle contraction.

12. **c**
    Factual recall
    Rationale: This information also was covered in the science study, and the overlap of information is apparent. You need to define the terms to identify osteokinematic movement as the correct answer.

13. **a**
    Application and concept identification
    Rationale: Only if proper stabilization is used can joint movement isolate its effects.

14. **c**
    Application and concept identification
    Rationale: You need to define all the terms to understand that post-isometric relaxation methods first have the target muscle contract. In this instance the contraction is causing cramping. Reciprocal inhibition would make use of the antagonist contracting, bypassing the tendency to cramp.

15. **d**
    Factual recall
    Rationale: After you define the terminology and application of the methods, you realize that only approximation uses direct application by the massage professional to affect the receptors and does not require that the client actively contract muscle groups.

16. **b**
Factual recall
Rationale: The question describes reciprocal inhibition. To answer the question, you must understand how to apply the other muscle energy methods listed.

17. **b**
Clinical reasoning and synthesis
Rationale: First, you need to analyze the question to identify the reasons for the client's symptoms. The question describes reflexive methods and indicates that there has been a small improvement. The question asks for the mechanical application that would improve results based on the goal. Lymphatic drainage is not focused on the goal. Answer b is correct because stretching mechanically affects the connective tissue. Answers c and d are other types of muscle energy methods. This question is an example of the hundreds of questions that can be written to test this type of content.

18. **a**
Factual recall
Rationale: The incorrect answers may increase the tickle sensation.

19. **d**
Application and concept identification
Rationale: Any of the possible answers would allow the neck to be massaged, but the side-lying position provides the best mechanical advantage for the massage therapist to use body mechanics.

20. **d**
Application and concept identification
Rationale: Compression on the lymphatic plexuses located in the hands and feet would provide the best outcome of the methods listed as possible answers.

21. **a**
Application and concept identification
Rationale: Skin rolling is the best method of those listed to affect the connective tissue.

22. **c**
Application and concept identification
Rationale: Compression does not require lubricant.

23. **d**
Factual recall
Rationale: The veins in the legs are more susceptible to blood clot development.

24. **a**
Clinical reasoning and synthesis
Rationale: You need to answer each of the possible answers to understand them in relation to the question posed. The wrong answers in this question present misinformation. Requesting massage focused on the back is a common occurrence in massage. Usually back tension is caused by shortening of the soft tissue structures of the chest.

25. **c**
Factual recall
Rationale: The question describes a common application of effleurage/gliding.

26. **a**
Factual recall
Rationale: Pathogen transmission through the mucous membranes in the face is a concern. The delicate nature of the facial structures is less of a concern.

27. **b**
Clinical reasoning and synthesis
Rationale: The key to the correct answer is sensitivity to pressure. Only the correct answer provides a method that can be applied lightly, although the side-lying position allows the client to see more of what is happening, making the client more comfortable.

28. **c**
Factual recall
Rationale: The chest area should be draped carefully because of breast tissue.

29. **d**
Factual recall
Rationale: This content was addressed in a previous question and is an example of how content often appears in different forms in an examination. This can be helpful because the different wording may trigger the correct answer in a question that posed difficulties in some other area of the exam.

30. **b**
Clinical reasoning and synthesis
Rationale: The problem presented by the question is which body areas to massage in a limited time to achieve the strongest relaxation effect. You need to review each combination to assess for physiologic effects when applying massage. Face, hands, and feet have the largest nervous system distribution.

31. **b**
Factual recall
Rationale: Gliding effectively creates tension force.

32. **b**
Factual recall
Rationale: Twisting creates torsion force.

33. **d**
Factual recall
Rationale: Definition of friction.

34. **c**
Factual recall
Rationale: Kneading/petrissage results in bending and torsion forces.

22
Assessment Procedures for Developing a Care Plan

Review Tips

The content for assessment procedures for developing a care plan has new terms, but it is more concerned with integration of all the previous textbook content into the actual application of massage. The clinical reasoning and synthesis case study question is the most effective way to assess proficiency in the knowledge.

The best study strategy for factual recall and concept identification questions is memorization of the terminology, use of the clinical reasoning process, and identification of wrong answers. Use the sample questions to help you determine whether you comprehend the vocabulary. Look up any terminology you do not understand.

This content can be tested in the case study type of question assessing for the ability to synthesize the information and use clinical reasoning to identify the best answer based on the facts supplied in the question.

Questions

1. A massage practitioner identifies an area of restricted tissue and immediately uses skin rolling to increase connective tissue pliability. How did this interfere with assessment processes?

   a. The localized treatment did not prove effective.
   b. The pattern was changed before it was understood.
   c. The therapist did not chart the area before the massage.
   d. The method was not appropriate to the condition.

2. A client seems nervous and unwilling to provide information during the history-taking process. The massage therapist is becoming impatient. What is lacking?

   a. Rapport between client and practitioner
   b. Prior information from the physician
   c. State-dependent memory status
   d. Proper clinical reasoning skills

3. When are data collected during the assessment process interpreted as to patterns of dysfunction and methods of massage application?

   a. As the history taking progresses
   b. During the physical assessment
   c. As the information is charted in the subjective section
   d. After the data have been collected and analyzed

4. During the initial greeting, a client seems generally healthy and in good spirits; however, when the client is speaking, the breathing pattern seems strained. What assessment process is being used?

   a. Palpation
   b. Physical assessment
   c. Interviewing
   d. Observation

5. A massage practitioner asks a client the following question, "Please explain to me how you would like to feel after the massage." What is correct about this communication?

   a. The massage practitioner used an open-ended question.
   b. The massage practitioner directed the response to reduce rapport.
   c. The practitioner was formulating a response during listening to the answer.
   d. A closed-ended interview was used to use time effectively.

6. A massage practitioner carefully listens to a client during the interview portion of the assessment process and then proceeds to the physical assessment. What communication step was forgotten?

   a. Open-ended questions and analysis
   b. Charting and treatment plan development
   c. Summarizing and restating information
   d. Using understandable language

7. A vacationing client will have only one massage from the massage practitioner. Which is the appropriate assessment process?

   a. Subjective history taking for possible referral combined with a physical assessment for symmetry and gait assessment for optimal movement patterns
   b. Palpation assessment of soft tissues to identify treatment areas
   c. Subjective and objective assessment for contraindications
   d. Interviewing for client's quantitative goals

8. During postural assessment, the massage professional observes that the client's shoulder girdle is rotated to the left. Which of the following histories is most likely to be the cause?

   a. The client regularly reaches to the left when answering the phone.
   b. The client often wears boots when riding horses.
   c. The client does weight-bearing exercise with machines 3 times a week.
   d. The client wears tight clothing.

9. A regular client has a grade 2 left ankle sprain and is using a crutch to maintain balance when walking. During assessment of posture, the massage therapist notices an elevated right shoulder. What is happening to cause this?

   a. The client is closing an open kinetic chain pattern.
   b. The muscles of the right lower leg are inhibited.
   c. The symmetrical stance is enhanced.
   d. The body is displaying compensation patterns.

10. When one is observing for symmetry, which of the following is correct?

    a. The shoulders should roll forward evenly, leveling the clavicles.
    b. The circumference of the muscle mass in the legs should be similar.
    c. The ribs should be fixed more on the left and springy on the right.
    d. The patella should be pointed more medially.

11. Which of the following is part of a normal gait pattern?

    a. The arms swing freely opposite the leg swing.
    b. The knee is maintained in the "screw-home" mechanism.
    c. The toes contact the floor first and then roll to the heel.
    d. During push-off, the foot is dorsiflexed.

12. While observing a client walk, the massage professional notices that the pelvis does not move evenly. The client complains of focused pain in the right sacral area. Which of the following is most correct?

    a. Create a massage treatment plan describing specific treatment for sacroiliac dysfunction.
    b. This information combined with other data may indicate the need for referral, with current massage focused on general nonspecific approaches.
    c. Design a massage to lengthen the left leg to balance the pelvic rotation.
    d. Immediately refer the client to a chiropractor for sacroiliac dysfunction.

13. During the massage, the massage professional notices a temperature difference in the tissue of the lumbar area. One area the size of a quarter is warmer than the surrounding area. Which type of assessment is being used?

    a. Postural assessment
    b. Gait assessment
    c. Palpation
    d. Muscle testing

14. Which of the following is the most effective way to assess for potential areas of muscle hyperactivity when the focus of the palpation is on the surface of the skin?

    a. Compressing until the striations of the underlying muscles are felt
    b. Light fingertip stroking to assess for areas of dampness or drag
    c. Skin rolling to assess for any adherence of superficial fascia to the skin
    d. Moving the skin on top of the superficial fascia to locate areas of bind

15. When one is using passive joint movement as an assessment method, which of the following is being identified?

    a. End-feel
    b. Viscosity
    c. Vessels
    d. Pilomotor reflex

16. Bilateral assessment of the dorsalis pedis pulse would provide information about _____.

    a. Respiration
    b. Abdominal viscera
    c. Lymph nodes
    d. Arterial circulation

17. During palpation assessment, the massage practitioner wishes to assess for the status of the acupuncture meridians. Where would the practitioner focus the assessment?

    a. Tendons at the proximal attachment
    b. Ligament of synovial joints
    c. Grooves in fascial sheaths
    d. Myotomes

18. Which of the following is incorrect when using muscle strength testing?

    a. Isolate muscles and position attachments as close together as is comfortable.
    b. Use a force sufficient to recruit a full response of the tested muscles and the surrounding muscles.
    c. Use a slow and even counterpressure to pull or push the muscle out of the isolated position.
    d. Compare muscle tests bilaterally for symmetry.

19. A client is complaining of weakness and heaviness in the muscles that flex the left thigh. During muscle testing, the muscle group is found to be inhibited. Based on gait patterns, which of the following muscle groups also should be inhibited?

    a. Right arm flexors
    b. Left arm flexors
    c. Right thigh flexors
    d. Left thigh extensors

20. During muscle strength testing, the flexors and the extensors of the elbow seem equally strong. Why is this a dysfunctional pattern?

    a. Gait patterns should inhibit the flexors.
    b. Flexors should be about 25% stronger than extensors.
    c. Extensors should be 30% stronger than adductors.
    d. Postural muscles are inhibited by gait reflexes.

21. A client is experiencing spasms in the left thigh flexor muscles. An attempt to muscle test the area could result in a cramp. The massage professional remembers that activation of the gait reflexes can facilitate or inhibit muscle contraction. Which group of muscles would the massage professional have the client contract to inhibit the left thigh flexors?

    a. Left arm flexors
    b. Right arm flexors
    c. Left arm extensors
    d. Right thigh extensors

Correct answers are on pages 207-209.

22. If the area between C7 and T12 is pulled forward, making the chest concave, with a right rotation pattern making the right shoulder more forward than the left, where are the shortened soft tissues?

    a. Anterior thorax on the right
    b. Right lumbar posterior
    c. Left thorax posterior
    d. Lower abdominal on the right

23. During the interview process, a client continues to grab the tissue at the back of the neck and pull it. What is the most logical explanation for this gesture?

    a. Nerve entrapment
    b. Joint compression
    c. Trigger point
    d. Connective tissue shortening

24. A client has increased internal rotation of the right shoulder. Which of the following is the best massage approach to reverse the condition?

    a. Frictioning and traction to the external rotators
    b. Muscle energy with lengthening and then stretching of the internal rotators
    c. Compression and tapotement to the internal rotators
    d. Stretching of the flexors and extensors with lengthening to the external rotators

25. A physician refers a client for massage for circulation enhancement to the limbs. The client complains of cold hands and feet. Assessment indicates decreased pliability of the tissues around the elbows and knees. Work-related activities require repetitive movement in these areas. The massage professional presents three main approaches for the physician to consider:

    1. General massage and rest
    2. General massage with connective tissue stretching in the restricted areas
    3. Compression focused specifically to the arteries to encourage circulation

After considering all three options, the physician eliminates option 1 as too time consuming. Option 2 seems viable, but the client does not respond well to methods that may be painful. Option 3 seems too limited an approach to the massage professional. The decision is to begin with option 3 and expand to connective tissue methods when the client is able to tolerate them. Which part of this process best reflects brainstorming possibilities?

    a. Data collection
    b. Analysis of outcomes based on pros and cons
    c. Generating the options
    d. Assessment for more facts

26. A client experienced an episode of severe low back pain 3 years ago. The diagnosis was a compressed disk at L4. The condition has stabilized and pain is experienced only occasionally. Assessment indicates shortened lumbar fascia, increased lateral flexion to the right, and a high shoulder on the right. The massage professional specifically addressed these areas and noted improvement following the massage. The next day the client called complaining that the low back was in spasm. What is the most logical reason for what happened?

    a. The phasic muscles were too weak to maintain posture.
    b. The gait shifted so that there was a more normal heel strike.
    c. Facilitated segments in the skeletal muscles went into spasm.
    d. Resourceful compensation patterns were disturbed.

27. An objective measurement of connective tissue shortening in the lumbar area would be _____.

    a. Measuring a skinfold by lifting the tissue
    b. Placing the client in the prone position and having her lift her chest off the table into extension
    c. Measurements of hot and cold skin temperature
    d. Palpation of adjacent pulse points for evenness

28. When one is evaluating a treatment plan for successful client compliance, which of the following would provide the best information?

    a. Any referral information from the health care provider
    b. Completing a comprehensive physical assessment
    c. Generating multiple treatment options
    d. Indications of enthusiasm for the plan by the client and any support system

29. During range of motion assessment, if full extension of the shoulder has a hard end-feel, what would be a logical conclusion?

    a. The shoulder assesses as normal.
    b. The shoulder has a firing pattern dysfunction.
    c. The anatomic range of movement is dysfunctional.
    d. The shoulder has joint dysfunction.

30. During walking and running, the upper and lower limbs function contralaterally for counterbalance. This being the case, if the shoulder flexion on the right is activated and the hip flexors on the left are assessed, what would be the most logical result?

    a. The muscles should be inhibited.
    b. The muscles should be facilitated.
    c. The muscles should be functioning eccentrically.
    d. The muscles should be fibrotic.

31. A client has recurring hamstring strain and currently is experiencing low back pain. Which of the following is the most logical cause?

    a. Hip extension firing pattern dysfunction
    b. Soft end-feel of the hip joint
    c. Scapular fixation with external rotation
    d. Overpressure of the symphysis pubis

32. During assessment, the massage therapist identifies that the rectus abdominis is firing first during trunk flexion. What does this mean?

    a. This is a normal firing pattern for hip abduction.
    b. Trunk flexion firing pattern is normal.
    c. Trunk flexion firing pattern is synergistic dominant.
    d. The psoas is normal and hip extension is abnormal.

Correct answers are on pages 207-209.

Exercise

Using the foregoing questions as examples, now write at least three more questions—one of each type: factual recall and comprehension, application and concept identification, and clinical reasoning and synthesis. Make sure to develop plausible wrong answers, and be sure that the correct answer is clearly correct. Then write a rationale for each question. The more questions you write, the better you will understand the material.

Answers and Discussion

1. **b**
   Application and concept identification
   Rationale: Assessment seeks to understand the reason for how the body is responding. The immediate application of an intervention method changed the condition before there was a chance to gather more information to understand the rest of the pattern.

2. **a**
   Factual recall
   Rationale: The question is providing an example of a breakdown in rapport.

3. **d**
   Factual recall
   Rationale: The sequence of assessment places interpretation of the data after data collection.

4. **d**
   Factual recall
   Rationale: The question provides an example of assessment by observation.

5. **a**
   Factual recall
   Rationale: The question provides an example of an open-ended question.

6. **c**
   Factual recall
   Rationale: The therapist needs to confirm the information received during the subjective assessment with the client to make sure the therapist understands it.

7. **c**
   Factual recall
   Rationale: Single-session massage applications do not require an extensive assessment process but do need to identify possible contraindications.

8. **a**
   Clinical reasoning and synthesis
   Rationale: This is an example of a question that is asking for cause and effect. The effect is presented in the question, and the correct answer would present a logical explanation for the condition. The correct answer describes a repetitive movement pattern that, over time, could affect shoulder girdle position.

9. **d**
   Clinical reasoning and synthesis
   Rationale: This is an example of a question that is asking for cause and effect. The effect is presented in the question, and the correct answer would present a logical explanation for the condition. The correct answer describes a common compensation pattern.

10. **b**
    Factual recall
    Rationale: Symmetry means the same on both sides, as reflected in the correct answer.

11. **a**
    Factual recall
    Rationale: Knowledge about a normal gait pattern is necessary to answer this question.

12. **b**
    Clinical reasoning and synthesis
    Rationale: The question provides symptoms that need to be correlated with the data in the correct answer. Answers a and d diagnose instead of assess the problem, which is outside the scope of practice for massage. There is no indication of leg imbalance. Through this elimination process, answer b emerges as the correct answer.

13. **c**
    Factual recall
    Rationale: The question gives an example of palpation.

14. **b**
    Factual recall
    Rationale: The only answer that focuses the palpation to the skin surface as explained in the question is answer b.

15. **a**
    Factual recall
    Rationale: End-feel of joints would be the only logical answer.

16. **d**
    Factual recall
    Rationale: You need to define the terms to correlate the data from the question with the correct answer. Pulses assess arterial circulation.

17. **c**
    Factual recall
    Rationale: This question addresses assessment and traditional Chinese medicine theory.

18. **b**

Application and concept identification
Rationale: The question asks for the wrong information, so three of the answers are accurate information. Do not let this be confusing. You must understand muscle testing procedures to answer the question. Synergistic or fixator muscles should not be recruited. If this happens, the pressure is excessive.

19. **a**

Clinical reasoning and synthesis
Rationale: Normal gait pattern would determine a counterbalancing effect of the opposite arm and leg. If one group is inhibited, it is likely that the paired group also is inhibited.

20. **b**

Factual recall
Rationale: Flexors are typically stronger than extensors.

21. **a**

Clinical reasoning and synthesis
Rationale: The question is asking for a decision based on reflex patterns. The information about interactions of muscle groups during walking is necessary to answer the question.
The counterbalancing arm swing during gait facilitates left arm and right leg muscles and right arm and left leg muscles whether the action is flexion or extension. If the leg is flexed, then the opposite-arm flexors also are activated. If the leg is extended, then the extensors of the paired arm also are activated. Based on these interactions and on reciprocal inhibition of the antagonist group, the activated agonist is inhibited. To inhibit the left thigh flexor muscle groups, the client should contract the same-side left arm flexors. Many questions can be written using this basic information about muscle group interactions.

22. **a**

Clinical reasoning and synthesis
Rationale: The question asks for the causal factor when symptoms are present. Also necessary for these types of questions is a strong anatomy and physiology base. The area described is the thorax. The facts of the question report the dysfunction as a pulling, which typically is contracted muscles or shortened connective tissue and often both. The shortened tissues described in the wrong answers would not result in the postural change.

23. **d**

Application and concept identification
Rationale: The client is gesturing. Pulling on tissue usually indicates connective tissue shortening.

24. **b**

Clinical reasoning and synthesis
Rationale: The facts state that assessment has identified an internal rotation of the right shoulder. To answer the question, you must know information about muscle and joint function and the physiologic effect of various massage methods. If internal rotation is increased, the muscles that produce this movement are overly tense with inhibited external rotators or the connective tissue of the area is shortened, pulling the shoulder into internal rotation. If the condition is recent, it is probably neuromuscular; if it is chronic, there likely will be a myofascial shortening aspect to the dysfunction. Local intervention to the area is best achieved by combining muscle-energy methods to restore a normal resting length and stretching to increase pliability of the connective tissue in the area. Answers a and d would increase the weakness of the external rotators. Answer c would increase the contraction of the internal rotator.

25. **c**

Application and concept identification
Rationale: The question presents an example of a clinical reasoning process. Knowledge of the four-step process is necessary to answer the question. Brainstorming generates options.

26. **d**

Application and concept identification
Rationale: The question asks for intelligent application of methods with respect for the existing compensation pattern. The client has resourceful compensation that was disturbed by the massage intervention.

27. **a**

Factual recall
Rationale: You need to define the terms, and quantify assessment as much as possible.
All of the possible answers would result in a measurement, but only answer a would identify connective tissue shortening.

28. **d**
    Application and concept identification
    Rationale: Evaluating a treatment plan is an analytic process that involves the use of the clinical reasoning model. One area that is considered is the feelings of the persons involved, and this is the area being targeted by the question. Answers a and b are fact gathering, and answer c is brainstorming. Only answer d indicates the feelings of the persons involved because compliance is all about feelings.

29. **d**
    Clinical reasoning synthesis
    Rationale: The shoulder should not have a hard end-feel. Typically a hard end-feel indicates joint dysfunction.

30. **b**
    Concept identification
    Rationale: This is an example of the gait aspect of kinetic chain reflex interactions.

31. **a**
    Clinical reasoning synthesis
    Rationale: The question describes a firing pattern problem. Soft end-feel of the hip would be normal. The scapula is the wrong location, and the symphysis pubis is not a synovial joint, so applying overpressure would be illogical.

32. **c**
    Concept identification
    Rationale: The rectus abdominis should not fire first because it is a synergist.

23
Complementary Bodywork Systems

Review Tips

This information surveys bodywork systems generally not considered therapeutic massage but often included as part of the massage. This distinction is becoming less apparent as massage methods targeting fluids, connective tissue, and trigger points commonly are included in the general type of massage.

Again there is new terminology to understand, and so the factual recall and comprehension question is common. Questions often cover safe and appropriate inclusion of the methods into the general massage application.

You must understand the pertinent anatomy and physiology involved with these methods. You also may need to review science content that is relevant.

Asian bodywork methods are controversial content on therapeutic massage exams. The conflict involves presenting this vast and unique knowledge as a part of massage when many consider it a sepa-rate and unique system that should be tested separately. It is prudent to investigate just how much of this content is covered on the exams you will take. The study aids located in Section V and the companion textbooks (*Mosby's Fundamentals of Therapeutic Massage* and *Mosby's Essential Sciences for Therapeutic Massage*) cover this content in sufficient depth to prepare you for typical questions.

Questions

1. Bodywork methods that focus on meridians and points fall into which category?

   a. Eastern and Asian
   b. Reflex
   c. Energetic
   d. Structural

2. A client has been receiving massage for a mild peripheral arterial circulation problem. Which of the following would be an appropriate self-help method to teach the client?

   a. Lymphatic drainage
   b. Skin rolling
   c. Alternating applications of hot and cold
   d. Frictioning

3. Cold applications of hydrotherapy to reduce swelling are called _____.

   a. Analgesic
   b. Antipyretic
   c. Antispasmodic
   d. Antiedemic

4. The secondary effect of a local cold application is _____.

   a. Sedative
   b. Increased localized circulation
   c. Diaphoretic
   d. Decreased systemic circulation

5. What is the water temperature for a neutral bath?

   a. 65° to 92° F

   b. 98° to 104° F

   c. 92° to 98° F

   d. 56° to 65° F

6. A folded towel soaked in water of the desired temperature and placed on a large area of skin is called a _____.

   a. Tonic friction

   b. Vaporizer

   c. Sponge

   d. Pack

7. PRICE applications for first aid are appropriate for _____.

   a. Primary care of abrasion

   b. Grade 2 and 3 sprains and strains

   c. Neural injury

   d. Shock

8. A client has mild edema in her lower legs from a long plane fight the previous day. Which of the following is an appropriate treatment plan?

   a. Short, light gliding strokes focused on the legs. Compression to the soles of the feet. Active and passive joint movement for the ankle, knee, and hip. Placing the legs above the heart.

   b. Compression to the legs focused on the medial side from proximal to distal. Muscle energy and lengthening combined with stretching in the area of the most accumulation of fluid.

   c. Deep gliding strokes from proximal to distal on the legs. Placing the legs above the heart. Limiting movement to encourage drainage.

   d. Superficial and deep compression along the vessels in the lateral leg. Active resistive joint movement combined with shaking.

9. A client is getting ready to play a tournament tennis game in 60 minutes. She wants to increase circulation and prepare her muscles for the game. Which of the following treatment plans is the best option?

   a. Long gliding strokes from distal to proximal focused toward the heart combined with rocking. Duration of the massage: 45 minutes.

   b. Broad-based compression to the soft tissue of the limbs generally focused from proximal to distal combined with shaking and tapotement. Duration of the massage: 20 minutes.

   c. Full-body massage with muscle energy methods and lengthening. Duration of the massage: 45 minutes.

   d. Compression, superficial myofascial release, and trigger point work focused on the limbs combined with passive joint movement and shaking. Duration of the massage: 15 minutes.

10. Because of a skin condition, general massage is contraindicated for a client, but he is allowed to have his feet and hands worked on. He complains of neck stiffness. If using foot reflexology theory, where would the massage practitioner focus massage on the foot to affect the neck?

    a. Heel

    b. Tips of the toes

    c. Base of the large toe

    d. Sole of the foot

11. Reflexology can be beneficial because _____.

    a. The complex structure of the foot is highly innervated and sensitive to changes in pressure and position, making it highly responsive to massage manipulation

    b. The flexor withdrawal mechanism of the foot is inhibited with pressure to the foot, and this inhibits neural activity in the dorsal horn of the spinal cord

    c. The specific mapped areas of reflex activity in the foot to organs have a direct relationship to visceral/cutaneous responses

    d. Stimulation of the zone therapy points on the bottom of the foot activates meridian energy movement in the chakra system

12. A client injured his right shoulder 3 years ago. Assessment indicates decreased mobility of the skin surrounding the shoulder coupled with a painful but normal range of motion. Which is the best treatment option for this client?

    a. Deep transverse friction
    b. Superficial myofascial release
    c. Compression
    d. Lymphatic drainage

13. Myofascial methods are focused most specifically on change in the _____.

    a. Motor point
    b. Lymph nodes
    c. Gait control mechanism
    d. Ground substance

14. Deep transverse friction applied correctly will ____.

    a. Inhibit circulation
    b. Create controlled inflammation
    c. Provide broad-based application
    d. Replace broadening contractions

15. Which of the following is correct in application of trigger point therapy?

    a. 15-minute application in combination with lengthening and stretching
    b. 45-minute application with hydrotherapy cold applications
    c. Limiting application to latent trigger points only
    d. Using pressure methods first and limiting lengthening

16. An active trigger point that is left untreated for 6 months often will _____.

    a. Become an ashi point
    b. Become hot to the touch
    c. Have fibrotic changes
    d. Only elicit referred pain

17. Trigger points commonly are located in _____.

    a. Ligaments
    b. Tendons
    c. The joint capsule
    d. Muscles

18. When treating trigger points, _____.

    a. Direct pressure methods and squeeze methods should be used first
    b. Positional release with lengthening is the first application method
    c. Connective tissue stretching needs to accompany muscle energy application
    d. Lengthening of the tissue housing the trigger point is only effective with a local tissue stretch

19. In shiatsu the points are called _____.

    a. Hara
    b. Meridians
    c. Jitsu
    d. Tsubo

20. In shiatsu, a qi energy flow that is under energy is called _____.

    a. Tao
    b. Kyo
    c. Jitsu
    d. AhShi

21. In yin/yang theory, if yang is over energy, which is correct?

    a. Meridians are in balance.
    b. Stimulate yin and sedate yang.
    c. Sedate yin and stimulate yang.
    d. Apply acupressure to jitsu points.

22. Which of the following meridians is yin?

    a. Gallbladder
    b. Stomach
    c. Lung
    d. Large intestine

23. Which of the following meridians is located on the lateral side of the body beginning at the ear and ending at the toes?

    a. Pericardium
    b. Bladder
    c. Liver
    d. Gallbladder

Correct answers are on pages 219-222.

24. Which of the following meridians is most medial?

    a. Central
    b. Spleen
    c. Liver
    d. Large intestine

25. A client is experiencing pain on palpation of many points along the kidney meridian. Which element of the five elements contains the kidney meridian?

    a. Fire
    b. Water
    c. Wood
    d. Earth

26. Which is a correct way to sedate a hyperactive acupuncture point?

    a. Tap the point.
    b. Vibrate the point.
    c. Place sustained pressure on the point.
    d. Stimulate the meridian containing the point.

27. In the earth element, if the stomach is yang, then what is yin?

    a. Spleen
    b. Bladder
    c. Liver
    d. Triple heater

28. Going clockwise on the five-element wheel, which element is adjacent to the fire element?

    a. Earth
    b. Metal
    c. Water
    d. Wood

29. In the five-element theory, what is the relationship of water to fire?

    a. Yin
    b. Yang
    c. Inhibiting
    d. Facilitating

30. A client has a cough and nasal mucus, diarrhea, and intestinal cramping. The large intestine meridian is tender to the touch. Which other meridian that is part of the metal element is involved directly?

    a. Pericardium
    b. Lung
    c. Bladder
    d. Heart

31. A system of health and medicine developed in India is called _____.

    a. Prana
    b. Elements
    c. Polarity
    d. Ayurveda

32. Which of the following is considered an Ayurvedic dosha?

    a. Pitta
    b. Marma
    c. Governing
    d. Ch'i

33. In Ayurvedic theory, bones, flesh, skin, and nerves belong to which element?

    a. Ether
    b. Air
    c. Earth
    d. Water

34. A dosha is physiologically a(n) _____.

    a. Nerve pathway
    b. Chemical pattern
    c. Electrical pattern
    d. Dietary pattern

35. A client complains of increased hunger and thirst, feels hot, and has been in a bad temper lately. Which of the Ayurvedic elements is out of balance?

    a. Earth
    b. Fire
    c. Water
    d. Ether

36. In Ayurveda, the chakras are considered _____.

    a. Seven centers of prana located in the aura
    b. Seven centers of qi located on the central meridian
    c. Seven centers of prana located along the spinal column
    d. Six locations of kyo corresponding to centers of consciousness

37. Massage in Ayurvedic theory concentrates on _____.

    a. Manipulation of the doshas
    b. Tapping, rubbing, and squeezing points called kappa
    c. Movement of fluid along the Vata centers
    d. Tapping, rubbing, and squeezing points on the body called marmas

38. A system that combines the theory of Asian medicine and Ayurveda is _____.

    a. Polarity
    b. Rolfing
    c. Shiatsu
    d. Reflexology

39. The main therapeutic focus of polarity therapy is to _____.

    a. Balance the tridosha system
    b. Restore balance in the yin/yang system
    c. Remove structural imbalance
    d. Locate blocked energy and release it

40. In polarity theory the left side of the body is considered _____.

    a. Ether
    b. Negative
    c. Neutral
    d. Positive

41. In polarity theory, how many major body currents exist?

    a. Two
    b. Three
    c. Five
    d. Seven

42. In polarity theory, the color green is associated with which body current?

    a. Ether
    b. Air
    c. Fire
    d. Water

43. If an area of blocked energy is located, a simple polarity method is to _____.

    a. Place the left hand on the painful area and the right hand opposite the painful area
    b. Rub the area with specialized oil preparations
    c. Press into the area with the fire finger and hold
    d. Stimulate the corresponding marma

44. In polarity therapy, the joints are considered _____.

    a. Chakra areas
    b. Serpentine brain wave currents
    c. Neutral
    d. Negative

45. In polarity therapy, the heel of the foot is in a reflex relationship with the _____.

    a. Shoulders and chest
    b. Pelvis
    c. Head and brain
    d. Abdomen

46. Which of the following would be an indication for using lymphatic drainage during the massage?

    a. A client has edema in the lower extremities but no logical reason for the fluid retention.
    b. A client has premenstrual bloat and edema.
    c. A client has kidney disease although the client does not need dialysis.
    d. A client has a fever and is generally lethargic and achy.

Correct answers are on pages 219-222.

47. Which is the most correct about the application of lymphatic drainage methods?

    a. The pressure levels are only sufficient to drag the skin.
    b. The direction is toward the heart.
    c. The rhythm is variable and moderate to fast.
    d. Pressure is variable toward slow and rhythmic drain patterns.

48. How does the tensegritic form involve the application of connective tissue methods during massage application?

    a. A tensegrity model of the body combines the tension of the soft tissue and the compression of the bones to create an interconnected resilient structure that responds to the mechanical forces of massage.
    b. The body is separated into independent functional units. The tensegritic form compartmentalizes the body so massage can isolate application.
    c. The compression elements (bones) are manipulated at the joints with direct methods to normalize the tension elements of the soft tissue.
    d. Fluid movement follows channels created by the tensegritic line of the fascial form, and the lines of force introduced by massage are cross-directional to pump the fluid.

49. Which of the following are all yin meridians?

    a. Bladder, kidney, liver
    b. Heart, spleen, kidney
    c. Wood, earth, metal
    d. Stomach, gallbladder, large intestine

50. Which of the following meridians can be accessed when massaging the arms?

    a. Liver
    b. Kidney
    c. Large intestine
    d. Stomach

51. Which of the following meridians has beginning points on the fingers?

    a. Heart
    b. Triple heater
    c. Governing
    d. Spleen

52. Which of the following meridians has the most acupuncture points?

    a. Lung
    b. Liver
    c. Gallbladder
    d. Bladder

53. A client has been diagnosed with imbalance in the water element. The bladder is over energy and the kidney is under energy. Which cluster of symptoms is most correct?

    a. Dry throat and pain in the arm
    b. Headache and edema
    c. Low back pain and bloat
    d. Neck and shoulder aching

54. The term used to describe assessment is _____.

    a. lui qi
    b. Si Zhen
    c. Wu wei
    d. Doa Yin

55. Which of the following is an essential element of the spa environment?

    a. Medical assessment
    b. Acupuncture
    c. Pampering
    d. Mat massage

56. Which of the following is likely to involve medical intervention?

    a. Luxury spa
    b. Resort spa
    c. Day spa
    d. Weight loss spa

57. Which of the following typically is found in some from in the spa environment?

    a. Shiatsu
    b. Stone ritual
    c. Hydrotherapy
    d. Color therapy

58. Aromatherapy often is used during massage or hydrotherapy treatments in the spa environment. Which of the following essential oils would be used often in the spa environment?

    a. Clove
    b. Lavender
    c. Spirulina
    d. Paraffin

59. A spa treatment that is said to stimulate circulation is _____.

    a. Body polish
    b. Dry brush
    c. Mud mask
    d. Mylar wrap

Correct answers are on pages 219-222.

Exercise

Using the foregoing questions as examples, now write at least three more questions—one of each type: factual recall and comprehension, application and concept identification, and clinical reasoning and synthesis.

Make sure to develop plausible wrong answers, and be sure that the correct answer is clearly correct. Then write a rationale for each question. The more questions you write, the better you will understand the material.

Answers and Discussion

1. **a**
   Factual recall
   Rationale: You need to define the terms to identify the correct answer.

2. **c**
   Application and concept identification
   Rationale: The key to this question is self-help. The one approach that most lends itself to this is hydrotherapy.

3. **d**
   Factual recall
   Rationale: You need to define the terms to identify the correct answer.

4. **b**
   Factual recall
   Rationale: The question describes an effect of cold after the primary effect.

5. **c**
   Factual recall
   Rationale: You need to define the terms to identify the correct answer.

6. **d**
   Factual recall
   Rationale: You need to define the terms to identify the correct answer.

7. **b**
   Application and concept identification
   Rationale: The question asks first for a definition of PRICE to be able to identify when it is most appropriate. Then you need to define the possible answers to correlate the best answer with the recommended application of protection, rest, ice, compression, and elevation.

8. **a**
   Clinical reasoning and synthesis
   Rationale: The facts presented in the question present a logical explanation for mild edema. The question asks for safe and beneficial treatment application. Knowledge about anatomy, physiology, and physiologic effect of massage methods is necessary to choose the correct answer. The correct answer describes the recommended combination of methods to support normal lymphatic function. The incorrect answers present misinformation or less effective application of methods.

9. **b**
   Clinical reasoning and synthesis
   Rationale: Accumulated knowledge is necessary to answer the question. The main focus is increasing arterial blood flow without interfering with performance. Any massage over 30 minutes would be fatiguing, which eliminates answers a and c. Any work that would substantially change muscle tone or create pain is contraindicated before athletic performance, so the only logical answer is answer b.

10. **c**
    Factual recall
    Rationale: The question asks for the area on the foot that would affect the condition based on reflexology theory.

11. **a**
    Factual recall
    Rationale: The correct answer provides a scientific explanation for the benefits of foot massage.

12. **b**
    Application and concept identification
    Rationale: You need to define all of the methods presented as possible answers and then analyze for best application based on the information in the question. Deep transverse friction is too aggressive. Compression and lymphatic drain are likely to be less effective than the correct answer, which is superficial myofascial release.

13. **d**
    Factual recall
    Rationale: You need to define all the terms to identify ground substance as the correct answer.

14. **b**
    Factual recall
    Rationale: The correct answer describes the physiologic effect of deep transverse friction-controlled inflammation.

15. **a**
    Factual recall
    Rationale: Muscles containing trigger points need to be lengthened to restore normal resting length. No more than 15 minutes of this type of intervention is recommended.

16. **c**
    Application and concept identification
    Rationale: The changes that occur when a condition such as trigger points becomes chronic instead of acute involve fibrotic changes.

17. **d**
    Factual recall
    Rationale: Trigger points are found in muscles.

18. **b**
    Application and concept identification
    Rationale: Recommendation of treatment of
    trigger points is to use least invasive measures
    first. The wrong answers are too aggressive
    (answers a and c) or misinformation (answer d).

19. **d**
    Factual recall
    Rationale: This question is an example of how
    terminology describing Eastern and Asian
    methods can be presented in text questions.
    You need to define all the terms.

20. **b**
    Factual recall
    Rationale: This question is an example of how
    terminology describing Eastern and Asian
    methods can be presented in text questions.
    You need to define all the terms.

21. **b**
    Application and concept identification
    Rationale: You need to understand the
    relationship of yin to yang along with all the
    terminology to identify the correct answer.
    In yin/yang theory, over energy is sedated
    and under energy is stimulated.

22. **c**
    Factual recall
    Rationale: You need to define all terms and
    categorize the meridians as yin or yang to
    answer the question.

23. **d**
    Factual recall
    Rationale: You need to identify the location of all
    the meridians to answer the question.

24. **a**
    Factual recall
    Rationale: You need to identify the location of all
    the meridians to answer the question.

25. **b**
    Factual recall
    Rationale: The relationship of the meridians to
    the five elements is necessary to answer the
    question.

26. **c**
    Application and concept identification
    Rationale: The question is asking for the
    application that would calm down an
    acupuncture point. The three wrong answers
    would result in increased energy in the point.

27. **a**
    Factual recall
    Rationale: The relationships of the meridians to
    the five elements are necessary to answer the
    question.

28. **a**
    Factual recall
    Rationale: The relationships of the five elements
    to each other are necessary to answer the
    question.

29. **c**
    Application and concept identification
    Rationale: The metaphor of the five elements for
    the qualities represented by fire and water would
    indicate that water inhibits fire.

30. **b**
    Factual recall
    Rationale: Lung and large intestine make up the
    metal element.

31. **d**
    Factual recall
    Rationale: Define the terms to identify the
    correct answer.

32. **a**
    Factual recall
    Rationale: Define the terms to identify the
    correct answer.

33. **c**
    Factual recall
    Rationale: You need to define the physiology
    represented by the Ayurvedic elements to
    answer the question.

34. **b**
    Factual recall
    Rationale: You need to define the relationships
    of the dosha to physiology to answer the question.

35. **b**
    Application and concept identification
    Rationale: The question is representative of how
    many questions can be developed to test
    knowledge about complementary bodywork.
    You need to define each of the Ayurvedic
    elements to identify the symptoms that would
    indicate dysfunction.

36. **c**
    Factual recall
    Rationale: The question is testing terminology.
    The incorrect answers are not part of the
    language used in Ayurveda or present incorrect
    information.

37. **d**
    Factual recall
    Rationale: You need to define all the terminology to identify the answer that makes sense. A dosha is a chemical pattern, not a physical part of the body to be massaged. The marmas are points on the body.

38. **a**
    Factual recall
    Rationale: This is a definition question.

39. **d**
    Factual recall
    Rationale: The wrong answers describe modalities other than polarity.

40. **b**
    Factual recall
    Rationale: The right side is positive energy flow, and the left side is negative energy flow.

41. **c**
    Factual recall
    Rationale: Five currents exist: ether, air, fire, water, earth.

42. **b**
    Factual recall
    Rationale: Each body current has a color sense, food, and other qualities. You need to understand these to answer the question.

43. **a**
    Application and concept identification
    Rationale: Polarity theory indicates that placing a negative energy flow over the pain and a positive energy flow opposite the pain will move and balance the energy.

44. **c**
    Factual recall
    Rationale: The flexibility of the joints indicates that they are neutral.

45. **b**
    Factual recall
    Rationale: Study a diagram to identify foot reflexes in the polarity system.

46. **b**
    Clinical reasoning and synthesis
    Rationale: The only clear indication for lymphatic drain is the client described in the correct answer. The other scenarios are risky unless there is physician support.

47. **d**
    Concept identification
    Rationale: Various levels of pressure are used, and direction can vary as well. Fluid movement in the lymphatic system is slow, and the massage mimics a pump.

48. **a**
    Clinical reasoning and synthesis
    Rationale: The wrong answers are flawed in different ways. Answer b is the opposite of the interconnected network of the body design. Answer c is accurate but not within the scope of practice for massage, and d is a nonsense answer.

49. **b**
    Factual recall
    Rationale: Bladder, stomach, gallbladder, and large intestine are yang. Answer c lists aspects of the five elements.

50. **c**
    Factual recall
    Rationale: The wrong answers list meridians that begin and end on the torso and legs.

51. **b**
    Factual recall
    Rationale: Location of meridians. Yang meridians begin distal and flow proximal; yin meridians begin proximal and flow distal.

52. **d**
    Factual recall
    Rationale: When you begin to study meridians, concentrate on location: yin or yang and location of points.

53. **b**
    Concept identification
    Rationale: Each meridian and the yin and yang pair represented in the five elements have symptoms relating to function. Headache and edema are consistent with common symptoms of water element imbalance.

54. **b**
    Factual recall
    Rationale: This is a terminology question. It is respectful to use the correct language when discussing various concepts. Asian methods are no different. The textbooks and study helps in this text provide language that interfaces with massage. Flash cards are a good study strategy.

55. **c**
    Factual recall
    Rationale: A standard component of the spa environment is pampering.

56. **d**
    Concept identification
    Rationale: Weight loss is a health care intervention that commonly involves medical expertise.

57. **c**

Concept identification

Rationale: Although spas are innovative and creative, a common theme is various applications of hydrotherapy.

58. **b**

Factual recall

Rationale: Lavender is a safe and commonly used essential oil. Clove is not. Spirulina is a sea weed used in thalassotherapy baths, and paraffin is a heat application.

59. **b**

Factual recall

Rationale: Dry brush is specific for circulation. Answers a and c are more for exfoliation, and Mylar is a material used for wraps.

CHAPTER

24
Serving Special Populations

Review Tips

The content on serving special populations is more about unique circumstances involving individuals. The relevance is how the massage therapist needs to adapt to the specific needs of individuals that have unique challenges.

Again there is terminology to study, but by this time you should know the various study strategies to learn vocabulary.

This content usually is assessed by the case study type of question to identify whether the massage practitioner knows how to make the appropriate accommodations in the environment and alterations in massage delivery to benefit and not harm the client.

Questions

1. In which area would additional study be required when working with any population with special needs?

   a. Massage methods
   b. Special situations
   c. Psychology
   d. Relaxation methods

2. An adult male client has many surgical scars on his chest and abdomen. History indicates that the client had surgical intervention as a child to repair congenital malformations. The client enjoys massage on the limbs and back in the prone position but appears distant and unsettled when turned to the supine position. What is the most logical explanation for this response?

   a. An abusive family history
   b. Reenactment
   c. Dissociation
   d. Integration

3. A college football player is seeking massage as part of a healing program for an injured knee that required surgical intervention. The athletic trainer is supervising the massage. The massage consists of general full-body massage that addresses any developing compensation caused by the gait change while the knee is healing. Specific applications of kneading and myofascial release are being used to maintain pliability in the soft tissue of the upper and lower leg. What type of massage is being performed?

   a. Postevent massage
   b. Recovery massage
   c. Remedial massage
   d. Rehabilitation massage

4. In which of the following circumstances would breast massage be most appropriate?

   a. General massage
   b. Adjunct to breast cancer treatment
   c. Scar tissue management
   d. Examination for lumps

5. In which of the following circumstances would massage without supervision by a health care professional best benefit children?

 a. Growing pains
 b. Anxiety disorder
 c. Touch sensitivity
 d. Attention deficit disorder

6. A massage professional has been working with a client who has chronic pain syndrome. The massage helps when combined with physical therapy, judicious use of pain medications, and support group attendance. Improvement in the condition began after 6 or 7 massage sessions. After 10 to 12 sessions the client missed 3 or 4 sessions and then returned for massage and indicates that she is right back where she started. She states that she does not feel like the situation will ever improve. What is the most logical explanation for this behavior?

 a. State-dependent memory
 b. Increase in hardiness
 c. Secondary gain
 d. Acute pain

7. What would be the most challenging counter-transference situation a massage professional faces when working with clients with chronic illness?

 a. Understanding combined effects of massage and medications
 b. Managing frustration with a client whose condition does not improve
 c. Maintaining boundaries with a client who sees massage as the answer to all physical problems
 d. Managing acute episodes of chronic illness

8. A massage professional has been working with an 86-year-old female client. The client still lives independently with some outside support. Family lives in a nearby state. The client is unable to drive. In which way does this client most likely benefit from a weekly massage?

 a. Physical and emotional stimulation
 b. Increased circulation
 c. Friendship
 d. Spiritual support

9. A parent massaging an infant encourages _____.

 a. Hardiness
 b. Dissociation
 c. Developmental disabilities
 d. Bonding

10. A massage therapist has just started a job at a family practice medical center. The center deals with many clients who exhibit stress-related symptoms. Which of the following professional skills will the massage therapist need to perfect?

 a. Muscle energy methods
 b. Restorative massage
 c. Charting and record keeping
 d. Lymphatic drainage

11. A client just began working with a massage professional who specializes in massage for those with physical disability. Which of the following would be a likely accommodation the client would notice?

 a. The building is barrier free.
 b. Special massage methods are used.
 c. All clients have guardians.
 d. All clients set quantifiable and qualifiable goals.

12. A massage practitioner has been asked by a group of mental health professionals to begin working at a residential facility. She would need to be most concerned over which of the following?

 a. Types of mental health issues
 b. Obtaining informed consent
 c. Learning specific massage protocols for each condition
 d. Frequency and duration of the massage

13. A massage therapist has developed a referral network with a group of physicians and physiologists dealing with anxiety and panic disorders. Which of the following will he need to be effective in managing with massage?

 a. Exercise protocols
 b. Nutrition
 c. Support group interactions
 d. Breathing pattern dysfunction

14. A massage client is in the first trimester of her third pregnancy. Which of the following is contraindicated?

   a. Prone position
   b. Massage of the feet
   c. Deep abdominal massage
   d. Lymphatic drainage

15. A long-term client has just notified you that he has a terminal illness. Which of the following can massage best offer?

   a. Therapeutic change
   b. Palliative care
   c. Remedial massage
   d. Rehabilitation massage

16. Which of the following complaints by athletes can be addressed with lymphatic drainage?

   a. Muscle guarding
   b. Laceration
   c. Delayed-onset muscle soreness
   d. Cramp

17. Which of the following athletic injuries is addressed most effectively with massage?

   a. Grade 3 acute strain
   b. Dislocation
   c. Stress fracture
   d. Chronic tendinitis

18. Which of the following is a medical emergency?

   a. Heat rash
   b. Heat stroke
   c. Capsulitis
   d. Heat cramp

19. A massage therapist specializes in prenatal massage. Which of the following would she need to be aware of in the second trimester?

   a. Breast changes
   b. Constipation
   c. Preeclampsia
   d. Positioning

Exercise

Using the foregoing questions as examples, now write at least three more questions—one of each type: factual recall and comprehension, application and concept identification, and clinical reasoning and synthesis. Make sure to develop plausible wrong answers, and be sure that the correct answer is clearly correct. Then write a rationale for each question. The more questions you write, the better you will understand the material.

Answers and Discussion

1. **b**
   Factual recall
   Rationale: Massage methods do not change, but the persons being served do.

2. **c**
   Application and concept identification
   Rationale: The question describes dissociation and provides a logical explanation for why the client might respond in such a way.

3. **d**
   Application and concept identification
   Rationale: The client is an athlete, so the approach is sports massage. Sports massage has categories of treatment you need to define to answer the question.

4. **c**
   Application and concept identification
   Rationale: Ethical concerns exist for breast massage for the female client. Scar tissue massage is the most relevant form of massage to the breast area.

5. **a**
   Clinical reasoning and synthesis
   Rationale: You need to define each of the conditions listed and then analyze them in relationship to massage for children without the supervision of a medical professional. Answers b, c, and d are more complex conditions than growing pains.

6. **c**
   Clinical reasoning and synthesis
   Rationale: The question describes a pattern often seen in those with chronic pain. As soon as improvement is seen, clients seem to sabotage themselves. In such a situation, secondary gain may be present.

7. **b**
   Application and concept identification
   Rationale: You need to define the terms. Dealing with those with chronic pain can cause frustration for the massage professional.

8. **a**
   Factual recall
   Rationale: For many, massage is the professional structure for human contact.

9. **d**
   Factual recall
   Rationale: Pleasurable and secure touch supports bonding.

10. **c**
    Factual recall
    Rationale: Working with special populations in a health care setting requires special attention to record keeping.

11. **a**
    Factual recall
    Rationale: The most common accommodation for those with physical disability is barrier-free access to the facility.

12. **b**
    Application and concept identification
    Rationale: With mental health issues, the ability of the client to make an informed decision is a priority.

13. **d**
    Factual recall
    Rationale: A common factor that can be managed with massage in this population is breathing in excess of demand, which triggers a sympathetic nervous system dominance pattern contributing to the anxiety symptoms.

14. **c**
    Factual recall
    Rationale: You need to define the three trimesters of pregnancy to identify the correct answer in relation to massage application.

15. **b**
    Factual recall
    Rationale: You need to define the terms in the question and possible answers to identify the correct answer.

16. **c**
    Concept identification
    Rationale: Laceration is a wound type. Muscle guarding and cramp is a neurologic issue, but delayed-onset muscle soreness is a fluid and inflammation issue.

17. **d**
    Clinical reasoning and synthesis
    Rationale: Grade 3 strain is a regional contraindication in the acute phase. Answers b and c do not respond to massage as a primary treatment, but the tight and rubbing structures involved in tendinitis can be addressed by massage.

18. **b**
    Factual recall
    Rationale: Capsulitis is not a heat injury, and rash and cramp are not medical emergencies, but heat stroke is life threatening.

19. **c**
    Concept identification
    Rationale: Breast changes and constipation are common in the first trimester. Positioning is for comfort, but preeclamspia is a medical emergency.

25
Wellness Education

Review Tips

The content concerning wellness education is important in ensuring that the massage professional has a broad base of understanding of the different factors that support wellness and health. Massage is an important part of health maintenance, illness and injury prevention, and well-being. This content is interesting, but exams typically contain only a few questions involving this information and how massage is a part of the health practice. Therefore, do not overemphasize this content.

All three question types are used to assess this content. Study all the terminology. Develop examples and metaphors, and explain the content in words different from those used in your textbooks.

Questions

1. During the massage, a client often speaks of problems with his children respecting house rules. This is a _____.

   a. Body issue
   b. Mind issue
   c. Spiritual issue
   d. Core issue

2. A massage practitioner notices that he becomes a bit aloof if he gets behind and is late for scheduled massage sessions. This is a(n) _____.

   a. Denial measure
   b. Defensive measure
   c. Exhaustion phase response
   d. Lack of purpose

3. Wellness programs usually include methods to improve communication. Which of the following best explains why communication is more difficult to improve than diet?

   a. Diet and nutrition are more concrete and objective than subjective communication.
   b. Diet is much more dependent on others, whereas communication is independent of others.
   c. Stress focuses change toward healthful food choices.
   d. Communication skills are highly genetically influenced, but diet is not.

4. Wellness usually involves simplification of lifestyle to reduce demands. A stressful outcome of this process is often _____.

   a. Hyperventilation syndrome
   b. Financial stability
   c. Dealing with loss and letting go
   d. Increased social support

5. When breathing in the normal relaxed pattern, _____.

    a. The inhale is longer than the exhale
    b. Deep inspiration is accentuated
    c. Accessory muscles only work on exhalation
    d. The exhale is longer than the inhale

6. When one is considering the wellness components of balanced body, mind, and spirit, in which of the following intervention areas is massage most effective?

    a. Promoting exercise
    b. Restoration of an appropriate eating and sleep cycle
    c. Normalization of breathing mechanisms
    d. Promoting belief system changes

7. A client feels fatigued all the time. She explains that she does not seem to sleep all night. Which of the following may improve her situation?

    a. An afternoon cup of coffee
    b. Taking a long nap in the afternoon
    c. Going to bed and watching television
    d. Spending at least 30 minutes outdoors

8. When one feels confident with commitment, control, and challenge in life, one is _____.

    a. Coping well
    b. Using behavior modification
    c. Functioning from an external locus of control
    d. Reliant on defense mechanisms

9. A client has been relatively inactive. Recently, the client had been diagnosed with diabetes and needed to begin an exercise program. Which of the following best describes the client's level of fitness?

    a. Deconditioned
    b. Endurance
    c. Flexibility
    d. Aerobic

10. A client has begun a walking exercise program. She is walking an hour per day. Which of the following best describes her program?

    a. Stretching and flexibility
    b. Aerobic continuous training
    c. Circuit-interval training
    d. Metabolic anaerobic

Exercise

Using the foregoing questions as examples, now write at least three more questions—one of each type: factual recall and comprehension, application and concept identification, and clinical reasoning and synthesis.

Make sure to develop plausible wrong answers, and be sure that the correct answer is clearly correct. Then write a rationale for each question. The more questions you write, the better you will understand the material.

Answers and Discussion

1. **b**
   Factual recall
   Rationale: The question provides an example of mind issues.

2. **b**
   Factual recall
   Rationale: The question provides an example of defensive measures.

3. **a**
   Application and concept identification
   Rationale: All three of the wrong answers present incorrect information. The strategy in developing the incorrect answers is to pair conflicting statements together. The correct answer states a logical connection.

4. **c**
   Factual recall
   Rationale: The reduction of demand means letting go of something to lighten the stress load.

5. **d**
   Factual recall
   Rationale: You need to understand the entire breathing cycle to answer the question. Only the correct answer presents correct breathing when relaxed.

6. **c**
   Application and concept identification
   Rationale: Massage cannot do everything. Wellness is multidimensional. Although massage can support various lifestyle changes, it can influence breathing function directly.

7. **d**
   Factual recall
   Rationale: Various activities can support or interfere with sleep patterns. The three wrong answers can interfere with sleep.

8. **a**
   Factual recall
   Rationale: The question defines effective coping.

9. **a**
   Concept identification
   Rationale: The client has not exercised extensively and is likely deconditioned.

10. **b**
    Concept identification
    Rationale: A walking program would stimulate aerobic function and is continuous.

26
Business Considerations for a Career in Therapeutic Massage

Review Tips

The content on standard business practices is what most commonly appears on exams. Legally defensible exams cannot present questions based on opinion. Therefore questions typically take the factual recall and comprehension format presented in the case study style.

There is business terminology to learn to be able to decipher the meaning of the question and possible answers. Make sure that you know why the wrong answers are incorrect.

Questions

1. A massage professional is considering a position at a local day spa. The owner of the business offered an employee position at a salary or a subcontractor position based on commission. Which would be an advantage of the employee position?

   a. Variable income
   b. Stable income
   c. Subject to employer's regulations
   d. Independent ability to set work hours

2. A massage professional has been working 12-hour days, 6 days a week, for 2 years. She is seeing 40 clients per week. Lately, she finds herself tired and out of sorts. She does not attempt to rebook clients who cancel. What is the most logical explanation for her behavior?

   a. Motivation
   b. Coping mechanisms
   c. Burnout
   d. Infection

3. Expenses used to begin new business operations are called _____.

   a. Business plan
   b. Reimbursement
   c. Investments
   d. Start-up costs

4. A massage therapist is involved with developing a promotional campaign to increase his massage business since taking on a part-time massage employee. What is this called?

   a. Marketing
   b. Business plan
   c. Resume
   d. Management

Correct answers are on page 236.   **233**

5. A massage practitioner has just redesigned his brochure and has included the types of massage provided, what the massage is like, information about the practitioner's qualifications, and client responsibilities. What did he forget?

   a. Tax structures
   b. Type of premise liability insurance
   c. Fees
   d. Client-practitioner agreement

6. A client notices that the massage office is clean, neat, and efficient and that licenses and certifications are posted on the wall. The client is impressed with the massage practitioner's abilities in _____.

   a. Applications of massage
   b. Communication skills
   c. Marketing
   d. Management

7. A massage professional wants to check to see whether the location for an office being considered for rental is in an appropriate business distinct. Where does one find this information?

   a. Local zoning office
   b. Facility rental agreement
   c. State licensing bureau
   d. County clerk's office

8. Gross income minus expenses equals _____.

   a. Deductions
   b. Deposits
   c. Net income
   d. A draw

9. The type of insurance needed to protect in case a client falls while in the business location is _____.

   a. Malpractice
   b. Premise liability
   c. Independent contractor liability
   d. Disability

10. A massage practitioner has obtained required licenses and permits for her business location. The type of business set up was a sole proprietorship with a DBA. She has her business checking account and tax plan developed with an attorney. She also contacted a local insurance agent for appropriate insurance. She is a member of a professional organization that supplies professional liability insurance. She has a marketing plan and client practitioner agreements. What did she forget?

    a. Retirement investment plan
    b. Zoning approval
    c. Salary structure
    d. Business plan

Exercise

Using the foregoing questions as examples, now write at least three more questions—one of each type: factual recall and comprehension, application and concept identification, and clinical reasoning and synthesis. Make sure to develop plausible wrong answers, and be sure that the correct answer is clearly correct. Then write a rationale for each question. The more questions you write, the better you will understand the material.

Answers and Discussion

1. **b**
   Factual recall
   Rationale: Standard comparison of the two types of positions indicates that stable income is considered an advantage.

2. **c**
   Application and concept identification
   Rationale: When considering all the information provided in the question against the implications of the possible answer, burnout seems the most likely situation.

3. **d**
   Factual recall
   Rationale: As with all questions of this type, you need to define the terminology to answer the question. The question is the definition of start-up costs.

4. **a**
   Factual recall
   Rationale: The question provides an example of marketing.

5. **c**
   Factual recall
   Rationale: You need to compare the common elements included in a brochure with the list provided in the question to identify the missing element.

6. **d**
   Factual recall
   Rationale: The question provides an example of management.

7. **a**
   Factual recall
   Rationale: The government department that deals with zoning would determine whether the business was in the proper district.

8. **c**
   Factual recall
   Rationale: The question is the definition of net income.

9. **b**
   Factual recall
   Rationale: The question defines premise liability insurance.

10. **a**
    Factual recall
    Rationale: All the components of a business plan have been identified in the question except for a retirement plan.

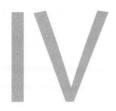

27

Integration Questions Covering Multiple Content

Review Tips

The following questions are very complex—some are quite long and involved. These types of questions are not usually found on exams. However, they are excellent resources for challenging your problem-solving skills. It is prudent to spend sufficient time to dissect the question and each possible answer. This exercise will tone your test-taking skills and boost your confidence.

Questions

1. A massage professional is relocating the massage practice from a city to a rural area. The population is primarily farm workers and factory workers who commute to a nearby city. After interviewing some of the residents from the town, the massage professional discovers that low back pain and fatigue are chief complaints and that the average income is $35,000 per year. Which combination of methods and marketing would be the best to build the new business quickly?

   a. General massage with energetic specialization provided in the client's home at a cost of $75 per session. Newspaper advertising used.

   b. General massage with myofascial and trigger point specialization in a one-person office. Massage rate set at $40 for a 1-hour massage, with an introductory offer of a free 30-minute massage when a package deal of five massage sessions is purchased for $150.

   c. A multiperson office providing space for three full-time massage practitioners and two part-time practitioners, with each practitioner having a particular specialty. Massage fees set at $55 per session. A radio campaign with $5 coupon offered.

   d. Subleasing a room in the local cosmetology business and providing general massage for relaxation. Fees set at $45 per session. Advertising done by word of mouth and free 15-minute chair massages on Saturdays.

2. A client had a severe viral infection 4 years ago and continues to have episodes of relapse. She just recently has been diagnosed with fibromyalgia. During assessment, the massage professional notices that the client inhales longer than she exhales and that most of the movement during breathing happens in the upper chest. Her physician has suggested massage as part of a total management program but is asking for a treatment plan. Which of the following is the most reasonable expectation in terms of benefit, cost, and compliance?

   a. Weekly massage for 3 months
   b. Monthly massage for 12 months
   c. Weekly massage indefinitely
   d. Massage 3 times a week for 6 months

3. A massage professional has experienced a substantial increase in client base in the last 3 months because of skills in soft tissue mobilization with massage. He books 25 clients per week and has a waiting list of 15 clients wishing to get appointments. He has attempted to squeeze in an additional four or five clients by extending evening appointments. He charges $40 for a 1-hour massage. He nets $600 per week and would like to increase his income by $100 per week. During the last month, he has been experiencing fatigue and mild shoulder pain, which disturbs him. One of the reasons he became a massage professional was to be able to work independently without personnel problems. Which of the following would be the best suggestion from a mentor?

   a. Raise prices by $5 per session and review application of body mechanics.
   b. Increase client load by three clients and switch from general massage to energetic methods.
   c. Raise prices by $10 and reduce client load to 20 clients.
   d. Hire a massage practitioner and increase client load in the business by 15 clients.

4. A client seeks massage to support parasympathetic dominance and reduce a tendency toward high blood pressure. The client responds best to applications of broad-based heavy compression or deep gliding strokes. Skin mobility and flexibility are good, as is range of motion. The client prefers to be nonparticipative during the massage. The client prefers weekly appointments in the evening. The massage professional has been working with this client for 3 months, and while the client is pleased with the work, the massage professional is exhausted after the session. What is the most likely cause?

   a. The client is emotionally draining, and the therapist has issues with countertransference.
   b. The massage professional finds the sessions complex and interactive, and the constant challenge is fatiguing.
   c. The nonparticipation by the client is unrealistic in terms of client goals, requiring the massage professional to work too hard.
   d. The client's needs are basic and nonchallenging, and the therapist is using poor body mechanics to maintain the pressure and repetitive nature of the massage.

5. A client is seeking reimbursement for massage fees from his insurance company. He was injured in a car accident, and the massage is primarily palliative. He has requested a summary report from the massage therapist describing the massage care received over the past 6 months. Where will the massage professional obtain the data to write this report?

   a. Treatment plan
   b. Client history
   c. Informed consent
   d. SOAP charts

6. A client requested a relaxation massage. The client then complained that the massage felt uncomfortable and that the skin on her back was warm and itching. Post-procedure assessment indicated a histamine response midthorax in the area between T6 and T12. Which of the following components of massage was incorrect in relation to the client's goals?

   a. Direction
   b. Drag
   c. Duration
   d. Rhythm

7. A massage professional is experiencing shoulder pain and has the sensation of tingling and numbness in the arms. The massage professional can identify various trigger points in the trapezius and scalenes when palpating the area. The massage practice has doubled from 10 clients per week to 20 clients per week, and although the massage therapist enjoys the increased income and is pleased now to have a full-time practice, she feels pressured to perform. Instead of relaxing at the end of the day, she feels anxious, restless, and fatigued. She also recognizes that she is breathing more shallowly and yawns often. Which of the following would be the best intervention?

   a. Reduce the number of massage clients to 10 sessions per week, and take a month sabbatical.
   b. Reduce the number of massage clients to 15 sessions per week, and see her physician for antianxiety medication.
   c. Have a peer check body mechanics to look for overuse of shoulder muscles, and speak to her mentor about managing business pressures.
   d. Raise rates so that 10 clients provide the same income as 20 clients.

8. A massage professional recently relocated the business to work in partnership with a mental health professional who refers patients for stress management. The massage practitioner is now required to write monthly reports on client progress and meet with the psychologist. The clients are progressing, and the massage professional and the psychologist can observe the changes, but the reports provided are vague and confusing to the psychologist. Which of the following is the most likely cause?

   a. Use of too many abbreviations in the narrative report
   b. Lack of preassessment and post-assessment in relation to quantitative and qualitative goals
   c. Ineffective informed consent procedures
   d. Subtle physiologic changes that cannot be measured

9. A massage professional has been working with a college football player to increase endurance and reduce tendency toward muscle strains. The massage professional uses a combination of methods to influence both motor and muscle tone, connective tissue pliability, and fluid dynamics, particularly blood exchange in the capillary beds on the lower legs. The massage professional recently has taken a class on muscle energy methods and has been using them to lengthen the muscles of the athlete's legs. The athlete feels looser, but his performance has decreased, and the coach and athletic trainer are not pleased. They feel that something with the massage may be the cause. Which of the following would support the coach and athletic trainer's position?

   a. The training effect on the leg muscles has been disrupted by the introduction of the muscle energy methods.
   b. The massage has caused increased inflammation in the tissues.
   c. The client is fatigued after participating in the muscle energy methods.
   d. The massage professional has not performed the methods correctly.

10. A student of massage is preparing to take final examinations. She has been informed that the exam is comprehensive, timed, and multiple choice. She has been diligent in her studies and practicum and feels confident to begin working on clients once she graduates. She feels nervous about remembering all of the details she has studied, especially scientific terminology and clinical reasoning methods. She wants to be alert while taking the examination but not anxious. Which of the following would be good advice for this student?

    a. Cram study just before the exam to make sure of all the terminology.
    b. Drink coffee while studying to keep awake, but not before the exam.
    c. Breathe deeply with long inhale and short exhale patterns to decrease anxiety.
    d. Get a massage the day before the exam, sleep well, and remember to exhale slowly while taking the exam.

11. A massage practitioner is preparing to work with a client who has been referred by a peer who is moving to another state. The client is a 54-year-old woman who has had successful treatment for breast cancer. The massage practitioner is concerned about meeting the expectations of the client because she was with the referring practitioner for many years. Which of the following areas of professional practice are the most important considerations for the massage practitioner for working with this new client?

    a. Caution for age and hormone dysfunction, professional boundaries, and treatment plan development
    b. Rapport, comprehensive assessment, and alteration of massage application for possible areas of fragile bone structure
    c. Contraindications for cancer treatment, gender concerns, and ongoing mentor-driven rapport issues
    d. Charting, physician referral, deep tissue massage over scar tissue in cancer treatment area.

Correct answers are on pages 249-253.

12. A massage therapist has just completed a needs assessment for a client who is 37 years old, who is pregnant with her first child, and who has diabetes. This is a complex case because of the pregnancy at a relatively advanced age for first pregnancy and the complications that diabetes can present. The client is in her first trimester. She has had some nausea and increased fatigue. At this point the pregnancy is progressing normally, and the diabetes is controlled with diet, exercise, and medication. She has had massage in the past and wants to resume receiving massage during the pregnancy to manage stress and promote sleep. She disclosed during the history that she is anxious about the potential complications of her pregnancy and wants to do whatever is possible to have a normal delivery and healthy baby. Which of the following treatment plans is most appropriate based on this information?

a. The massage should be short and should be done frequently. The pressure would vary depending on the body area being addressed. Fluid movement methods should be avoided.

b. The massage application specifically should target lymphatic drainage. Deep pressure should be avoided. The massage would occur weekly.

c. The massage focus should target parasympathetic dominance and local muscle aching as it presents. Aggressive stretching should be avoided. Fluid movement methods would be used as needed.

d. The massage application should be scheduled as needed and typically in the evening. The massage should be general and avoid any use of trigger point application or acupressure to avoid the potential for miscarriage.

13. A 27-year-old male client is embarking on a weight management program. The program includes a balanced diet with portion control, appropriate use of nutritional supplements, a well-designed exercise program that combines aerobic and weight-bearing activity, and a support group system for emotional support. He wonders what massage may have to offer during this major lifestyle change. Which of the following would be the best and most accurate response to his inquiry?

a. Massage can stimulate similar pleasure and satisfaction centers in the brain as food does and can help with the craving that may occur. Massage also can support the exercise program by managing any exercise-related soreness that might occur.

b. Massage can restructure the fascial tensegrity network and support the release of accumulated fat from the tissues. Massage can alter the metabolism and support exercise.

c. Massage is relaxing and can be used as a reward for progress. It also influences metabolic rate and aerobic capacity, supporting heart health.

d. Massage can be used to stimulate appetite suppression by increasing dopamine and adrenocorticotropic hormone. Massage also influences the thyroid in such a way as to decrease the fat-storing tendency.

14. A massage professional is struggling with balancing a successful massage career with personal responsibilities. One client in particular is demanding. The client is a local television anchor, and the schedule is somewhat erratic. She feels that she cannot maintain a confirmed appointment schedule and needs to be able to call at the last minute for massage. She has combination tension, sinus, and vascular headaches and irritable bowel syndrome. Both of these conditions are aggravated by stress. She notices significant relief after a massage. The massage practitioner has tried to refer her, but she has been unhappy with the massage results. Although the client is demanding, she is also generous and will increase the gratuity substantially when she feels she has received special treatment by the massage therapist. Which of the following best describes the complex nature of this relationship?

    a. The massage therapist does not wish to create conflict and is avoiding confronting the client about the client's demanding behavior.

    b. The client is displaying transference to the point that the professional relationship is compromised, and the massage professional does not know how to reestablish boundaries.

    c. The severity of the client's condition makes it difficult for the massage therapist to refer, and the randomness of the illness makes regular scheduling impossible.

    d. The massage therapist finds the irregular appointment schedule disrupting to her personal life and has attempted alternative action, and the client has not been satisfied.

15. A client often travels for business. The client travels with carry-on baggage that consists of one carry-on piece of luggage and one computer briefcase. Both are packed tight and are heavy. The computer case fits on top of the luggage, and the client pulls them around the airport. The client has a slight short-term memory problem and becomes a bit anxious when checking in and going through security. The client becomes somewhat confused during this process and is afraid of misplacing an item such as the boarding pass or photo identification. This client often receives massage while traveling. Which of the following would be the most logical outcome goals requested by this client, and what treatment plan would best achieve these goals?

    a. Stress management and relief from fatigue. Massage would be targeted to generate sympathetic dominance and sleep enhancement.

    b. Stress management and muscle aching in arm and shoulders. Massage would be targeted to generate parasympathetic dominance and decrease muscle tension in the shoulder girdle muscles.

    c. Breathing restrictions and low back pain. Massage would be targeted to reverse breathing pattern disorder and related sleep disturbances.

    d. Headache and relaxation. Massage would be targeted to shift vascular circulation and increase parasympathetic dominance.

Correct answers are on pages 249-253.

16. A young father is taking an active role in carrying for his infant daughter. The baby is occasionally fussy, and the dad would like to increase his skills in soothing his baby. He occasionally gets a massage to manage tension headache. While receiving a massage, the father asks the massage practitioner if there is anything that massage can do to calm the baby. Which of the following responses is most appropriate for this inquiry?

   a. The massage practitioner suggests that the father bring the baby in for a few sessions and that she will teach him how to calm the baby with massage methods of compression and range of motion.

   b. The massage practitioner suggests that the baby receive massage when the baby is fussy and that she will be able to use energy-based modalities and entrainment applications to calm the baby.

   c. The massage practitioner indicates that she can teach the father a rhythmic breathing technique, and once he perfects the method, if he does it while holding the baby, the baby will relax.

   d. The massage practitioner suggests that the father take a class in infant massage or that she would be willing to give him a few lessons with the baby. Rhythmic massage using a moderate and pain-free depth of pressure has been shown to be calming for infants.

17. A recreational softball player has begun to receive massage for management of fluid retention because of hormone fluctuations. She has responded well to general lymphatic drainage methods and part of the full-body massage application. She reports that her performance while playing ball has improved and that the improvement coincides with the time frame when she started to get regular massage. She asks the massage therapist for an explanation as to why massage targeted to reducing generalized edema has resulted in improved athletic performance. Which of the following is the most logical response?

   a. General massage nonspecifically addresses various aspects of tissue pliability, muscle length-tension relationships and range of motion. The lymphatic drainage application within a general massage supports the restorative mechanism supporting recovery time.

   b. The correlation is likely a coincidence and not directly related. Only specific sports massage should increase athletic performance, and the massage practitioner is not trained in sports massage.

   c. The relationship of the massage application to increase in athletic performance specifically involves increased arterial circulation following the lymphatic drainage method. Increase in circulation supports muscle strength but not recovery after exercise.

   d. The client is sleeping longer and therefore is less fatigued. Being more energetic tends to support the movement strategies required to play ball. Lymphatic drainage also has a secondary effect of restoring gait reflexes and normalizing firing patterns involved in muscle activation sequences.

18. A massage practitioner is finding it increasingly difficult to work with another massage practitioner who shares the massage area. The co-worker does not maintain the environment in a safe and sanitary way in the opinion of the massage practitioner; however, the supervisor does not think that the concerns are serious and will not intervene in the conflict. In addition, scheduling conflicts are increasing because both want to work more hours and the client base is available to support an expanded appointment schedule. The conflict is escalating, and either something has to be done about the problem or the massage therapist will leave the job. The supervisor does not want this to happen. The owner of the business likes the work of both massage therapists and has tasked the supervisor to solve the problem and will support the solution so long as it can be justified. Which of the following has the most likely potential to solve the problem?

    a. The two massage professionals should be brought together for a problem-solving session using collaboration and should come to agreement about the care of the shared environment and scheduling. A checklist would be developed, and each worker would have to complete the tasks on the checklist at the end of each work period.

    b. Each massage practitioner should be provided individual space to maintain as they see fit so long as the safety and sanitation requirements of management are met. Space is available in the facility that can be remodeled at a reasonable cost as long as it also can continue to provide long-term storage of supplies.

    c. A cleaning service can be employed to maintain the environment, and the two therapists can continue to share space. The therapist with the most clients will be allowed first scheduling options but must have the schedule approved each week.

    d. The conflict between the two professionals has escalated to the point that they will not be able to work together regardless of the solution offered. A decision will have to be made by the owner about which massage professional to ask to leave.

19. A day spa owner is looking to increase business and intends to expand the massage offerings. The business recently has added stone massage and is looking to add more modalities. A massage professional suggests that they combine stone massage with aromatherapy and sound vibration to cause a harmonic resonance effect during the session. The policy of the owner is only to offer services that can be justified. Can the massage application suggested be reasonably justified, and what would be the most accurate explanation?

    a. No, this combination of methods would not be synergistic and actually would negate the effects of modalities being combined.

    b. Yes, this combination of methods has research to validate that the methods enhance each other and support entrainment.

    c. Yes. Each method had a logical mechanism of benefit, and these physiologic mechanisms appear to be synergistic if not actually validated by research.

    d. No. There is no such thing as harmonic resonance, and sound is not caused by vibration, so the explanation is not valid.

Correct answers are on pages 249-253.

20. A massage therapist is looking at various career options. The therapist has completed an entry-level educational program and has passed the licensing exam for therapeutic massage. Now the therapist wants to continue his education with advanced training. The therapist enjoys science studies and problem solving. The therapist likes to work independently but appreciates the expertise of other professionals for peer support and mentoring. The therapist is 32 years old and has a 10-year-old child and reliable child care except for weekends. The therapist has a grandparent in long-term care and feels a strong connection with the elderly. Which of the following career tracks would best support the needs of this person and why?

    a. Massage in the medical environment, primarily hospice, because the therapist can determine the hours and work independently yet still be around other professionals. The terminally ill population would satisfy the client's need for connection with the elderly.

    b. Fitness massage targeted to cardiac rehabilitation in a fitness center that works cooperatively with a medical center and a senior citizen assisted-living complex. The flexibility of the environment allows for scheduling, professional interaction, and work with the senior population.

    c. Work in a spa setting in a vacation area that serves the retired population. The clients would be elderly, and the flexibility of the spa environment allows for independent practice and interaction with other professionals.

    d. Independent practice in a private office with a varied population but offering senior discounts. This environment offers the most scheduling flexibility. The business location is within walking distance of a long-term care facility and would allow residents to walk to the office for massage appointments.

21. A client is being treated for a chronic low back condition related to soft tissue dysfunction. The client also has diabetes and generalized anxiety. The client believes that massage will help, and during the interview with the massage therapist, the client has difficulty identifying outcome goals for the massage. The client asks the massage therapist for assistance and wants the therapist to explain what the massage would entail for each of the major conditions and what the therapist thinks would be a reasonable set of goals and why. Which of the following is most accurate for responding to this client?

    a. Massage can provide symptom relief and management of symptoms of low back pain of soft tissue origin. Many of the same methods used for low back treatment also are used to normalize breathing. Normal breathing function may help ease the anxiety. The suggested treatment plan is massage to address soft tissue dysfunction in the thorax as it relates to low back pain and observe for changes in breathing function.

    b. Massage for stress management especially increasing sympathetic dominance has been shown to be helpful in a diabetic treatment process. The same massage application would reduce anxiety but would not treat the low back dysfunction effectively, although generalized pain management would be possible. The suggested treatment plan is to address the diabetic condition with components of pain management.

    c. The low back pain can be addressed mechanically with soft tissue methods, but no other outcomes are reasonable. In addition, the diabetes presents contraindications that would limit the ability of the massage therapist to use some of the most effective massage applications for the low back condition. Taking this into consideration, the massage therapist only feels comfortable recommending a general massage application targeted at pain management.

    d. The anxiety disorder is likely the underlying cause of the low back condition, and the increased production of serotonin by the adrenal glands is contributing to the diabetes. Massage potentially could reverse both anxiety and low back disorder and substantially improve the diabetic condition. The massage treatment plan would involve breathing retraining, myofascial release, and acupressure to rebalance the energy mechanism in the body, thus improving homeostasis.

22. A client is in generally good health and enjoys massage. The client is extremely value conscious and asks the massage professional to explain the benefits of regular massage for a healthy individual so as to determine the cost versus benefit of regular massage treatment. The client also is seeking to determine optimal frequency of massage. The client also wonders about various durations of massage application and wonders what are the benefits of 30-, 60-, or 90-minute sessions. Which of the following would be most accurate in response to the client's inquiry?

    a. Massage is best used weekly for 90 minutes. The approach would be therapeutic change with aspects of palliative care to address the client's desire for a pleasant experience. The outcome of the regular massage application would be to treat identified conditions as they occur. The benefit is to prevent disease from becoming worse and requiring medical intervention.

    b. Massage can be used periodically, changing frequency and duration as needed to address specific concerns. The massage would be targeted to condition management with specific applications that reverse existing health conditions. The benefit would be to meet relaxation and restorative needs.

    c. Massage is best used regularly as a restorative and maintenance system. Frequency of once a week is ideal for these outcomes. Sessions every 2 weeks are adequate. Duration of 60 minutes is typically sufficient to achieve these benefits. The outcome should be prevention of stress-related symptoms and treatment of mild muscular skeletal conditions as they occur.

    d. Massage benefits are increased with frequency of use. The 30-minute massage 3 times per week is ideal with occasional 60-minute massage sessions once per week if time does not permit scheduling of the more frequent application. Benefits are stress management and immune system support. Frequent application for shorter duration allows for a slow and relaxing full-body approach to encourage parasympathetic dominance.

23. A massage practitioner is changing from a sport and fitness career track for massage to a spa environment massage career. The therapist has a solid fundamental educational background in the sciences and theory and practice of therapeutic massage and the science studies that support that practice. Much of the therapist's anatomy studies involved kinesiology and biomechanics with an emphasis in movement. In previous education the therapist had begun an exercise science program and completed most of the science studies and so is naturally strong in that area. As the exercise science education progressed, the therapist realized a desire for a more eclectic career and felt massage could provide more options. The spa at which the therapist will be working targets skin care, pampering, and various combinations of massage and hydrotherapy. Which of the following would best describe what additional science and methods studies the massage therapist would need to increase the therapist's skill for this career change?

    a. It would be helpful to increase science study of the integument and the effects of skin care products. The physiologic effects and application of hydrotherapy also would be beneficial. The study of essential oils also is indicated. Further study of the effects of environment design and client care in a service industry would support career development.

    b. It would be important to study Asian massage methods and thermotherapy and to become a cosmetologist to be cross-trained in skin care. Communication skills necessary for human services and negotiation and mediation are also important. Increased science study on mental health benefits would be beneficial.

    c. Additional science studies on the effects on aging and nutrition would be helpful. Esoteric study involving energy-based modalities also is necessary, especially in the area of meditation and mindfulness. Continuing education classes should target connective tissue methods and shiatsu. Business management and human resources studies would enhance marketing skills.

    d. A comprehensive study of the circulatory system prepared for using lymphatic drainage to treat various skin conditions and pathologic conditions. The methods studies include various ancillary methods such as paraffin treatment, waxing, and débridement. Hot stone massage proficiency is necessary as well. Communication skills for sales would be beneficial.

Correct answers are on pages 249-253.

24. Assessment indicates that a client has muscle imbalances consistent with lower crossed syndrome. What would be the client's main symptoms? Which firing pattern (muscle activation sequence) most likely is involved, and what is the most logical treatment for the condition?

    a. Leg pain with heaviness, shoulder abduction main firing pattern. Treatment includes connective tissue stretching and facilitation of the upper trapezius.

    b. Low back pain and headache of the vascular type. Firing pattern imbalance is trunk flexion, and treatment involves lymphatic drainage and meridian massage.

    c. Kyphosis and flattened lower back with deep abdominal aching. Firing pattern dysfunction includes kinetic chain limb counterbalancing, and treatment involves muscle energy methods and lengthening.

    d. Low back pain and leg heaviness. Main firing patterns involve trunk flexion and hip extension. Main treatment is inhibition of rectus abdominis and hamstring and core training.

25. A student is preparing to take final exams to graduate from massage training and then take the state licensing exam and national certification exam. The student is overwhelmed with what to memorize, what to analyze, and in general how to study. Which of the following is the best recommendation for success in passing the various exams?

    a. Purchase various study guides and make sure to know the answers to the questions in the study guides. Memorize all the attachments of all the muscles, but it is less important to know the functions.

    b. Concentrate on theory and practice content and spend a lot less time on the science studies. Use flash cards for clinical reasoning activities.

    c. Read the various textbooks used to develop the exams, and then memorize all the terminology. Once this is done, use checklists to eliminate the irrelevant information and concentrate on definitions and factual recall.

    d. Reread the textbooks and concentrate on understanding the content. Study the glossaries to perfect language skills. Write test questions, developing plausible wrong answers and right answers.

Answers and Discussion

1. **b**
   Clinical reasoning and synthesis
   Rationale: The question covers special populations issues, specific massage outcomes, methods of massage, complementary bodywork, and marketing. All the pieces have to come together to create a successful practice. The population is blue collar and would have to justify the cost versus benefit, especially because the average income is less than $40,000 per year. The potential clients have typical low back pain and fatigue, which respond well to general massage and the more mechanical methods of myofascial and trigger point applications. The correct answer addresses these issues, whereas the business plans offered in the wrong answers would better serve a different population and target market.

2. **c**
   Clinical reasoning and synthesis
   Rationale: The question combines information about pathology, contagious diseases, assessment, breathing patterns, treatment plan development, and clinical reasoning skills. Each of the possible answers addresses frequency and duration of the massage, and the best choice for the condition listed is condition management, which would be based on weekly sessions indefinitely.

3. **a**
   Clinical reasoning and synthesis
   Rationale: Content covered includes business practices, motivation, massage skills and application, body mechanics, ethics and professional skills, and support by a mentor. You need to evaluate all of the possible answers against the information presented in the question. Answer a is the correct answer. Answer b is incorrect because it shifts methods from what is working to a form unfamiliar to the client base. Answer c is incorrect because the practitioner did not experience problems until he began to increase his workload, indicating that 25 appointments per week is manageable and a $10 raise actually may decrease clients. Answer d is incorrect because the massage professional states he does not want to work with anyone.

4. **d**
   Clinical reasoning and synthesis
   Rationale: Content covers anatomy and physiology, application and physiologic outcome of massage methods, assessment application and interpretation, business structure, body mechanics, professional dynamics and ethics, and burnout. The question asks about the condition of the massage professional in relationship to this client. Answer a is incorrect because the client is not emotionally draining. Answer b is incorrect because the session is based on repetitive application of basic skills. Answer c is incorrect because the goals are realistic. Answer d is correct because the massage professional is likely to be bored with the client and to be using poor body mechanics.

5. **d**
   Application and concept identification
   Rationale: Content covered is charting, insurance reimbursement, type of care, and content of a narrative summary. The SOAP notes best describe the ongoing care information necessary to write the narrative.

6. **b**
   Clinical reasoning and synthesis
   Rationale: Content covered is physiology of relaxation and methods used to achieve this outcome, histamine response symptoms and what would cause them, assessment, and analysis of effectiveness of methods used. The four answers present the qualities of massage. Because the client did not request connective tissue work, the drag was too intense for the outcome.

7. **c**
   Clinical reasoning and synthesis
   Rationale: Content covered is assessment, trigger points, muscle anatomy and physiology, business practices, body mechanics, and symptoms of hyperventilation. Self-care and a change in business structure are provided in the correct answer. The incorrect answers do not address the fact that the client likes what is being done. Only answer c provides information that pertains to the question.

8. **b**

   Clinical reasoning and synthesis
   Rationale: Content covered includes business environment, mental heath affiliation requirements, referral, stress response, record keeping, communication skills, justification process skills, development of quantitative and qualitative goals, and outcome measurement. The correct answer identifies the confusion related to unclear outcomes for the massage sessions.

9. **a**

   Clinical reasoning and synthesis
   Rationale: Content covered includes athletic population and massage approaches, outcomes, massage methods, physiologic effects, resourceful compensation patterns, and professional dynamics with supervising professionals. This question points out complex situations and the bigger picture in terms of massage application as presented in the correct answer.

10. **d**

    Clinical reasoning and synthesis
    Rationale: This question may be describing you. If you have been a committed student, used the textbooks as suggested, reviewed with this study guide, and have a heart's desire to do massage, it will all work out. There is no way you will remember everything. The goal is not to be perfect. The goal is to be a compassionate and skilled massage professional who continues to learn for a lifetime. Remember to take care of yourself, get a massage, breathe from your diaphragm instead of your chest, sleep, eat and relax before the exam, and put the whole process in perspective.

11. **b**

    Clinical reasoning and synthesis
    Rationale: The main concerns between this client and massage practitioner are establishing a professional relationship and developing rapport. The client had been through a difficult time with the breast cancer treatment while seeing the previous massage therapist, possibly leading to an increased dependency and potential boundary concerns. Typically it is difficult for the client when the massage practitioner leaves. In addition, because of the cancer history, a comprehensive assessment and understanding of the types of treatment she had received are necessary. If radiation was one of the treatments, then the bones in the chest may be fragile. The wrong answers target areas that may be of concern but are not clustered together to target the main areas or present irrelevant information or suggest contraindicated treatment.

12. **c**

    Clinical reasoning and synthesis
    Rationale: Although the client's condition is complex, at this point she is experiencing a normal pregnancy and the massage would be applied for a normal pregnancy. Her goals are stress management and sleep, and the massage described in the correct answer supports these outcome goals. The wrong answers do not target the client's goals. Answer a would not promote relaxation and sleep. Answer b is too concentrated on fluid movement when the facts in the question do not indicate that this is a concern at this point. Answer d is too conservative because during the pregnancy, postural shifts may result in some localized trigger point activity that can be addressed safely.

13. **a**

    Clinical reasoning and synthesis
    Rationale: Only answer a presents research-validated outcomes for massage related to weight management. The wrong answers are based on speculation and nonjustifiable massage benefits. Elements of the wrong answers are applicable, but in combination with the inaccurate information the total statement is incorrect. Specifically in answer b, massage can support an exercise program but does not affect fat cells. Answer c is flawed because massage does not influence aerobic heart capacity directly, and answer d is flawed because the thyroid is not stimulated to decrease fat storage.

14. **d**

Clinical reasoning and synthesis
Rationale: This is an ethical dilemma question that has no easy solution. The question does not ask for an answer to the problem, but an analysis of the problem. This is an aspect of the clinical reasoning process: facts, possibilities, analysis, plan. The facts of the question indicate that there are reasonable explanations for the dilemma. This makes decision making more difficult. The client is demanding but her professional schedule would make this reasonable. She does have health concerns that are stress related and would be helped by regular massage to manage stress and appointments as needed when symptoms increase. The massage professional is skilled in the massage application that helps this client and has attempted referral, but the client has not had good outcomes. The client did go to the other massage practitioners when referred, so she was willing to be cooperative. She also responds to the extra efforts of the massage therapist by increasing the gratuity, so there is a financial issue as well. The wrong answers do not effectively analyze the problem posed by the question. This is not a conflict issue or a severe boundary issue because the reasons for the problems are reasonable. The health concerns mentioned do respond to regular massage, so answer d is flawed.

15. **b**

Clinical reasoning and synthesis
Rationale: This question involves the clinical reasoning process and asks for logical outcomes matched with appropriate treatment plan. The question describes symptoms of situational anxiety likely caused by increase in sympathetic dominance and muscle aching from managing heavy luggage. Fatigue and headache are not mentioned; therefore, eliminate answers a and d. Answer b or c is possible, and a decision would need to be made between the two as to which one best meets the facts presented in the question. Although breathing disruption is often a factor in anxiety, it is not always a concern. The client history did not mention breathing symptoms, so a more general approach to stress management is more appropriate. In addition, the lifting and pushing of the heavy luggage is more apt to strain the arms and shoulders than the low back, although low back aching is also possible, but the question asks for the most logical response. Clinical reasoning would indicate that answer b is the best response.

16. **d**

Clinical reasoning and synthesis
Rationale: This question is more complex that it may seem. Ethical concerns and massage application concerns factor into the appropriate decision about the correct answer. The father asks for information about how massage might help him calm the baby. The response that the massage practitioner actually does the massage does not address the intent of the question; therefore answer b is incorrect and may indicate a boundary concern. Teaching the client a breathing method does not respond to the question, which is about massage. This also could be a scope of practice issue because breathing training may not be an aspect of massage practice in certain jurisdictions; therefore this would not be the best answer even though the approach suggested may be affected. Answer a is correct in suggesting that the massage therapist teach the father massage application, but the approach to the massage may not be calming because the research indicates that the rhythmic application of gliding with a comfortable depth of pressure is what produces the calming affect on infants. Answer d suggests that the father learn infant massage techniques and suggests more validated methods.

17. **a**

Clinical reasoning and synthesis
Rationale: Answer a is the only answer that presents logical and reasonable explanations for the increase in performance. General massage can support more optimal movement and promote recovery. Training specifically in sports massage is not necessary. Answer c is flawed because normalization of circulation does support recovery after exercise, and answer d is flawed because lymphatic drainage does not affect gait reflexes and firing patterns sufficiently to make this claim.

18. **b**

Clinical reasoning and synthesis

Rationale: The problems posed by the question involve two areas: actual use of the room for massage, which is a logistical issue, and values about what is clean and safe. The complaining massage practitioner has higher standards than the management and wants to impose those standards on others. Collaboration or cleaning by a third party is unlikely to work, and even if it does, both professionals are experiencing an increase in clients and want more time in the area. Because space is available and remodeling costs are reasonable and the owner has indicated that support is available, this would appear to be the best way to manage the situation. Although some personality conflict may linger between the two professionals, the interaction between the two would be substantially limited, and the cause of the conflict would be eliminated.

19. **c**

Clinical reasoning and synthesis

Rationale: Each method can be explained in a reasonable way but not necessarily validated by research. Essential oils used in aromatherapy appear to be able to enter the bloodstream by coming in contact with the mucous membranes during inhalation of the vapors and by coming in contact with the capillaries in the skin. Sound is a vibration, and harmonics are entrained vibrations. Again the research is scant, but the explanations are reasonable.

20. **b**

Clinical reasoning and synthesis

Rationale: The medical environment and the spa environment typically do not offer scheduling flexibility or extensive independent practice. These are team environments with structured scheduling. The facts in the question did not indicate that the massage therapist wanted to work with the terminally ill population. It did indicate that the massage therapist enjoyed working with the elderly. Those in long-term care usually are not able to travel independently, so the reasoning for locating a massage office where this population could walk to appointments is flawed. Also independent practice is often isolated and does not easily offer interaction with other professionals. The fitness environment best seems to meet all the client's criteria.

21. **a**

Clinical reasoning and synthesis

Rationale: The other answers are flawed. Refer back to the section that describes how wrong answers are developed. In answer b, stress management typically involves parasympathetic dominance—not sympathetic—and massage can be helpful in the multidisciplinary treatment of low back pain. In answer c, massage reasonably can address some of the breathing dysfunction involved with anxiety, and reducing stress can be part of managing diabetes. In answer d the hormones related to glandular function are wrong: serotonin is not produced by the adrenal glands. Also the claims made are unlikely in terms of condition reversal.

22. **c**

Clinical reasoning and synthesis

Rationale: This is a complex question requiring that each possible answer be accurate in the information content and relevant to the client's inquiry. The wrong answers are flawed in either or both of these areas. Answer a indicates a duration of 90 minutes and a therapeutic change process for existing conditions. Massage is usually 60 minutes with 90 minutes used in unusual circumstances such as a large client or if multiple goals exist and the client is healthy in general; otherwise, the adaptive demand is too extensive. Also the client is healthy and does not have existing conditions to treat. Answer b is flawed because massage as a maintenance system is best used regularly much like body housekeeping: keep the body healthy as opposed to cleaning up big messes. Also the answer then goes on to say that condition management is targeted, and this outcome is not addressed effectively with random appointments. Pleasure needs and simple relaxation goals are better achieved with random massage. Answer d is flawed because slow full-body massage is not reasonable in 30 minutes. Sixty minutes is the more typical time for relaxation or restorative massage. The 30-minute session 3 times a week may be applicable for a fragile client with pain or similar issues, but this is not the condition of this client.

23. **a**
    Clinical reasoning and synthesis
    Rationale: The wrong answers are flawed as follows:
    b. Becoming a cosmetologist is somewhat extensive for retraining, but the real flaw is in scope of practice: for example, negotiation and mental health.
    c. Again, scope of practice issues flaw the answer, particularly nutrition and potential mental health areas. Connective tissue methods also are more involved in therapeutic change application as opposed to the spa environment.
    d. Lymphatic drainage as presented is more of a medical application requiring health care supervision. Débridement is the removing of damaged skin such as when burns are being treated.

24. **d**
    Clinical reasoning and synthesis
    Rationale: This question requires the student to understand symptom identification, assessment, and treatment application. Answer a is flawed because firing pattern does not relate to lower crossed syndrome, and even if firing pattern is involved, the treatment is incorrect. The upper trapezius would be inhibited. Answer b is flawed because vascular headache has different causal patterns than those related to serial muscle distortion pattern. Answer c is flawed because gait assessment is described when addressing the segment on firing pattern. A lower crossed syndrome pattern also would result in an increased lordosis.

25. **d**
    Clinical reasoning and synthesis
    Rationale: When studying, seek to understand, and then use thinking and problem-solving skills to solve the puzzle of each question. You must know the language of the topic, or you cannot analyze the question. Writing good questions that are more complex than the factual recall questions is effective for study.

SECTION

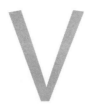

V

28
Labeling Exercises

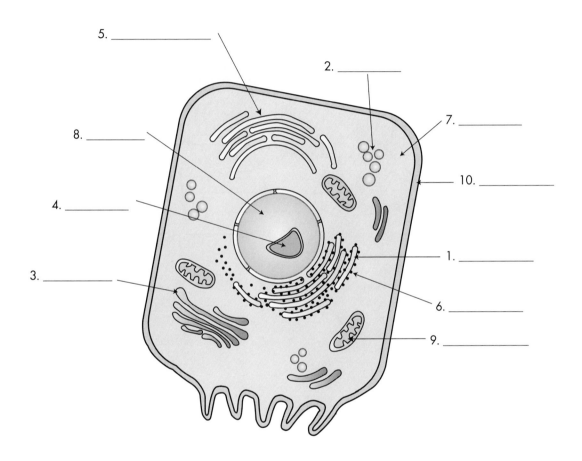

5. _____

2. _____

7. _____

8. _____

10. _____

4. _____

3. _____

1. _____

6. _____

9. _____

Labeling Exercise 1
Generalized Cell

Choices

Cell (plasma) membrane	Mitochondrion	Rough endoplasmic reticulum
Cytoplasm	Nucleolus	Smooth endoplasmic reticulum
Golgi apparatus	Nucleus	
Lysosome	Ribosomes	

Modified from Fritz S: *Mosby's essential sciences for therapeutic massage*, ed. 2, St. Louis, 2004, Mosby.

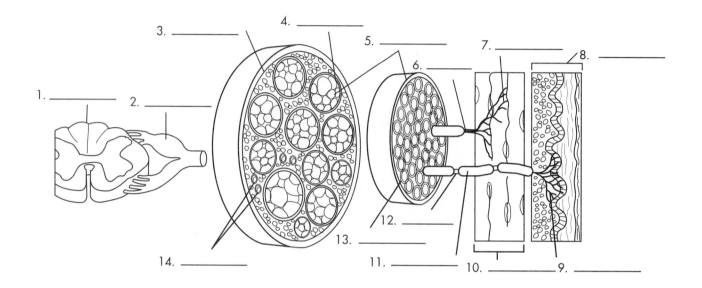

Labeling Exercise 2
Peripheral Nerve Trunk and Coverings

Choices

Axon	Muscle	Perineurium
Blood vessels	Myelin sheath	Skin
Endoneurium	Nerve bundle (fasciculus)	Spinal cord
Epineurium	Node of Ranvier	Spinal ganglion
Motor end plate	Pain receptors	

Answers are on pages 297-306.

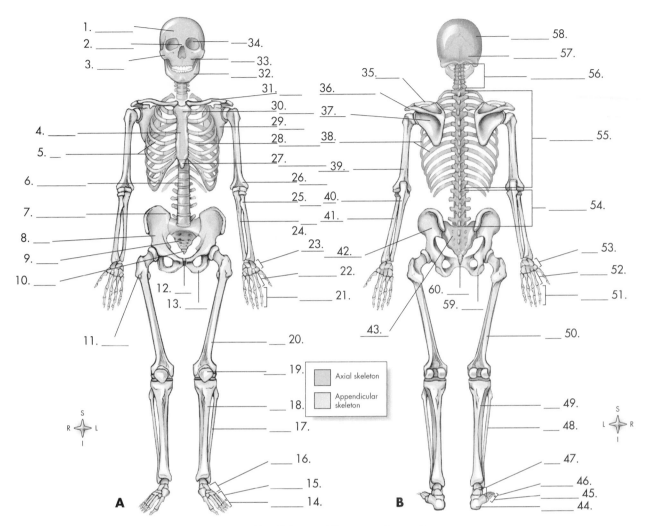

Labeling Exercise 3
Skeleton. A, Anterior View. B, Posterior View.

Choices

Acromion process
Calcaneus
Carpals (2 times)
Cervical vertebrae (7)
Clavicle (2 times)
Coccyx (2 times)
Costal cartilage
Coxal (hip) bone (2 times)
Femur (2 times)
Fibula (2 times)
Frontal bone
Greater trochanter
Humerus (2 times)
Ilium

Ischium (2 times)
Lumbar vertebrae (5)
Mandible
Manubrium
Maxilla
Metacarpals (2 times)
Metatarsals (2 times)
Nasal bone
Occipital bone
Orbit
Parietal bone
Patella
Phalanges (4 times)

Pubis
Radius (2 times)
Ribs (2 times)
Sacrum (2 times)
Scapula (2 times)
Sternum
Tarsals (2 times)
Thoracic vertebrae (12)
Tibia (2 times)
Ulna (2 times)
Vertebral column
Xiphoid process
Zygomatic bone

Answers are on pages 297-306.

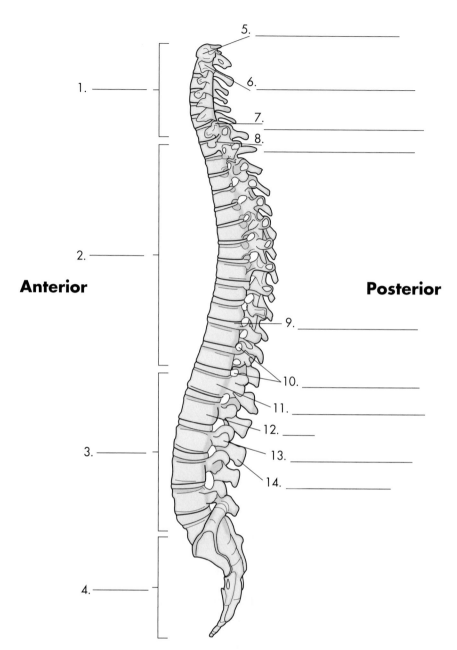

Labeling Exercise 4
Vertebral Column

Choices

Body	Intervertebral disk	Seventh cervical vertebra
Cervical curve	Intervertebral foramina	Spinous process
First cervical vertebra (atlas)	Lumbar curve	Thoracic curve
First lumbar vertebra	Sacral curve	Transverse process
First thoracic vertebra	Second cervical vertebra (axis)	

Answers are on pages 297-306.

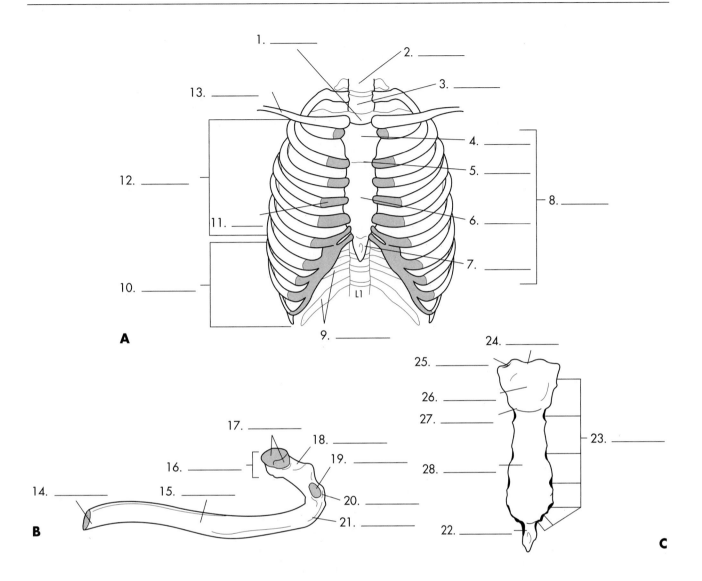

Labeling Exercise 5
A, Ribcage. B, Typical Rib. C, Sternum.

Choices

Angle
Articular facets for body of
    vertebrae
Articular facet for transverse
    process of vertebrae
Body (3 times)
Clavicle
Clavicular notch
Costal cartilage

Facets for attachment of costal
    cartilages 1 to 7
False ribs
First thoracic vertebra
Floating ribs
Head
Jugular notch (2 times)
Manubrium (2 times)
Neck

Seventh cervical vertebra
Sternal angle (2 times)
Sternal end
Sternum
True ribs
Tubercle
Xiphoid process (2 times)

Modified from Fritz S: *Mosby's essential sciences for therapeutic massage*, ed. 2, St. Louis, 2004, Mosby.

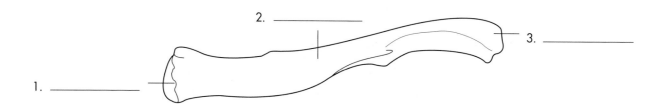

2. ⎯⎯⎯⎯⎯⎯⎯⎯⎯

3. ⎯⎯⎯⎯⎯⎯⎯⎯⎯

1. ⎯⎯⎯⎯⎯⎯⎯⎯⎯

Labeling Exercise 6
Clavicle

Choices

Acromial end
Body
Sternal end

Modified from Fritz S: *Mosby's essential sciences for therapeutic massage*, ed. 2, St. Louis, 2004, Mosby.

Answers are on pages 297-306.

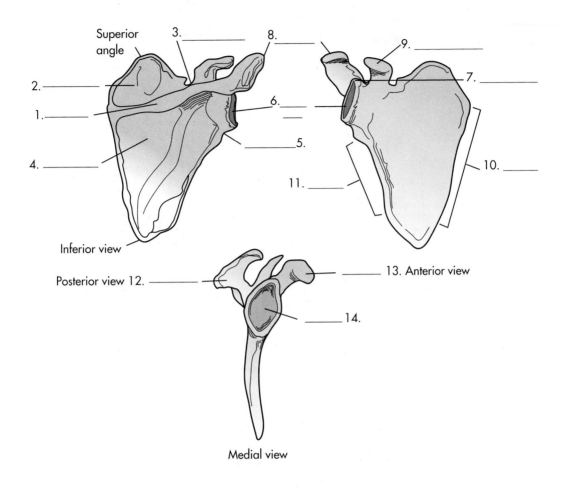

Superior angle

3.

8.

9.

2.

1.

4.

6.

5.

7.

10.

11.

Inferior view

Posterior view 12.

13. Anterior view

14.

Medial view

Labeling Exercise 7
Scapula: Three Views

Choices

Acromion	Infraglenoid tubercle	Supraglenoid tubercle
Coracoid fossa	Infraspinous fossa	Suprascapular notch
Coracoid process	Lateral border	Supraspinous fossa
Glenoid fossa (2 times)	Scapular spine (2 times)	Vertebral border

Answers are on pages 297-306.

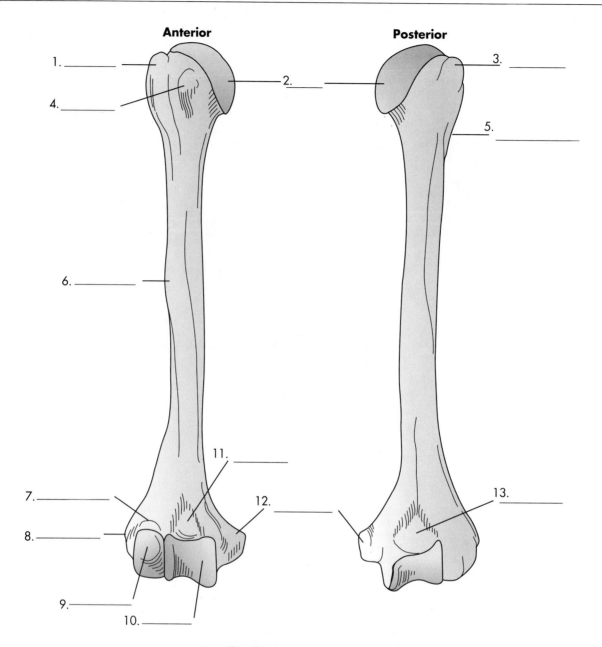

Anterior

Posterior

1. _____

2. _____

3. _____

4. _____

5. _____

6. _____

11. _____

7. _____

12. _____

13. _____

8. _____

9. _____

10. _____

Labeling Exercise 8
Humerus: Anterior and Posterior Views

Choices

Capitulum	Lateral epicondyle	Surgical neck
Coronoid fossa	Lesser tubercle	Trochlea
Deltoid tuberosity	Medial epicondyle	
Greater tubercle (2 times)	Olecranon fossa	
Head	Radial fossa	

Modified from Fritz S: *Mosby's essential sciences for therapeutic massage*, ed. 2, St. Louis, 2004, Mosby.

Answers are on pages 297-306.

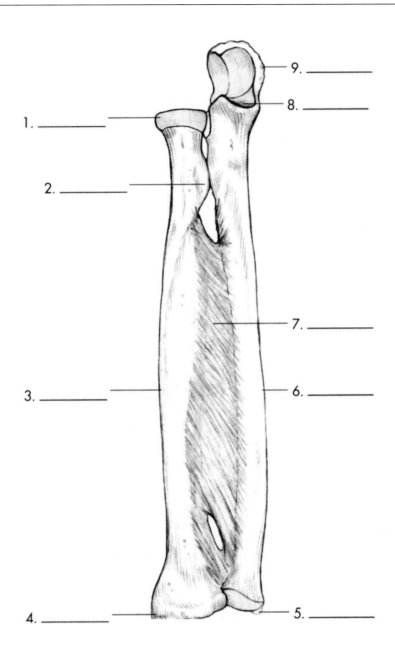

Labeling Exercise 9
Forearm Bones

Choices

Interosseous membrane	Radial styloid	Trochlear notch
Olecranon process of ulna	Radial tuberosity	Ulna
Radial head	Radius	Ulnar styloid

Answers are on pages 297-306.

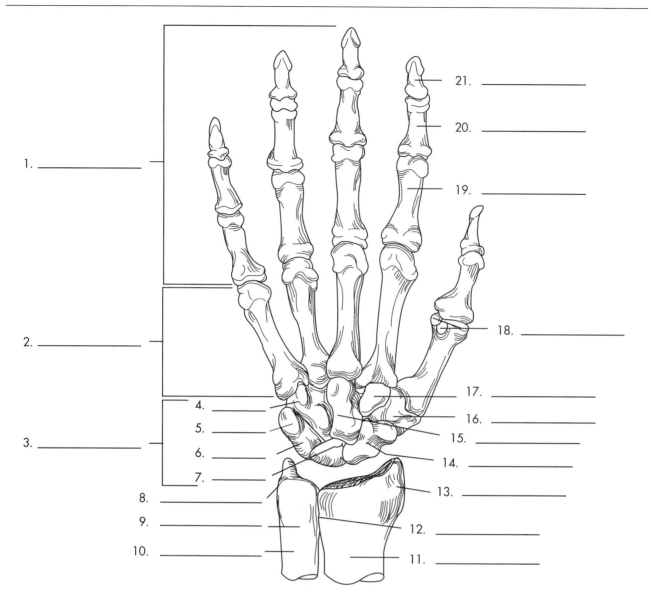

1. _____
2. _____
3. _____
4. _____
5. _____
6. _____
7. _____
8. _____
9. _____
10. _____
11. _____
12. _____
13. _____
14. _____
15. _____
16. _____
17. _____
18. _____
19. _____
20. _____
21. _____

Labeling Exercise 10
Hand Skeleton: Volar View

Choices

Capitate	Phalanges	Trapezium
Carpus	Pisiform	Trapezoid
Distal	Proximal	Triquetrum
Hamate	Radius	Ulna
Lunate	Scaphoid	Ulnar head
Metacarpus	Sesamoids	Ulnar notch of radius
Middle	Styloid process (2 times)	

Modified from Fritz S: *Mosby's essential sciences for therapeutic massage*, ed. 2, St. Louis, 2004, Mosby.

Answers are on pages 297-306.

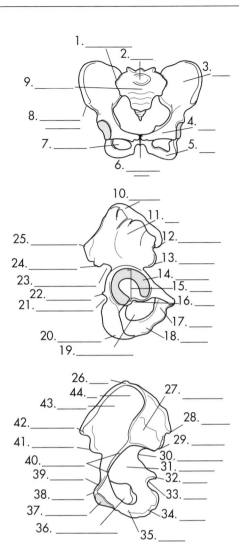

Labeling Exercise 11
Pelvis

Choices

Acetabular notch
Acetabulum
Anterior inferior iliac spine
  (2 times)
Anterior superior iliac spine
  (3 times)
Auricular surface
Body of ischium
Greater sciatic notch (2 times)
Iliac crest (2 times)
Iliac fossa
Iliopectineal line

Ilium (3 times)
Inferior pubic ramus
  (2 times)
Ischial ramus (2 times)
Ischial spine (2 times)
Ischial tuberosity
Ischium
Lesser sciatic notch (2 times)
Lunate surface
Obturator foramen (3 times)
Posterior inferior iliac spine
  (2 times)

Posterior superior iliac spine
  (2 times)
Pubic crest
Pubis
Sacral promontory
Sacroiliac joint
Sacrum
Superior pubic ramus
Symphysis pubis (2 times)

Modified from Fritz S: *Mosby's essential sciences for therapeutic massage*, ed. 2, St. Louis, 2004, Mosby.
Copyright © 2006, 2002 by Mosby, Inc., an affiliate of Elsevier, Inc. All rights reserved.

Answers are on pages 297-306.

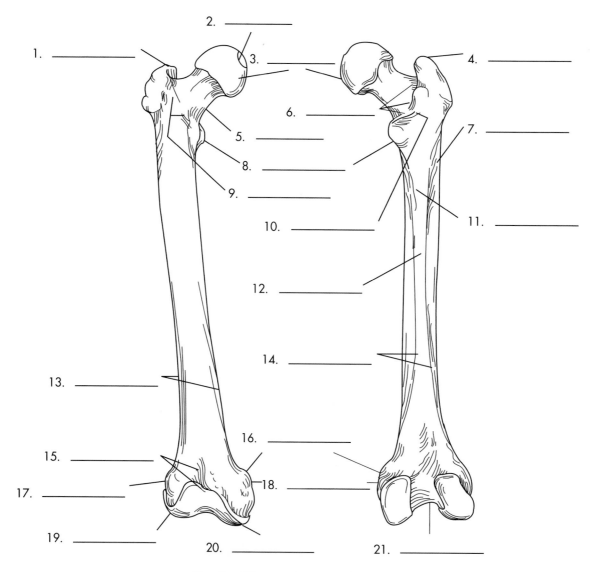

Labeling Exercise 12
Right Femur: Anterior and Posterior Views

Choices

Adductor tubercle	Intertrochanteric line	Medial and lateral supracondylar
Fovea capitis	Lateral and medial supracondylar	lines
Gluteal tuberosity	ridges	Medial condyle
Greater trochanter (2 times)	Lateral condyle	Medial epicondyle
Head of femur	Lateral epicondyle	Neck
Intercondylar fossa	Lesser trochanter	Patellar groove
Intertrochanteric crest	Linea aspera	Pectineal line
Intertrochanteric fossa		

Modified from Fritz S: *Mosby's essential sciences for therapeutic massage*, ed. 2, St. Louis, 2004, Mosby.

Answers are on pages 297-306.

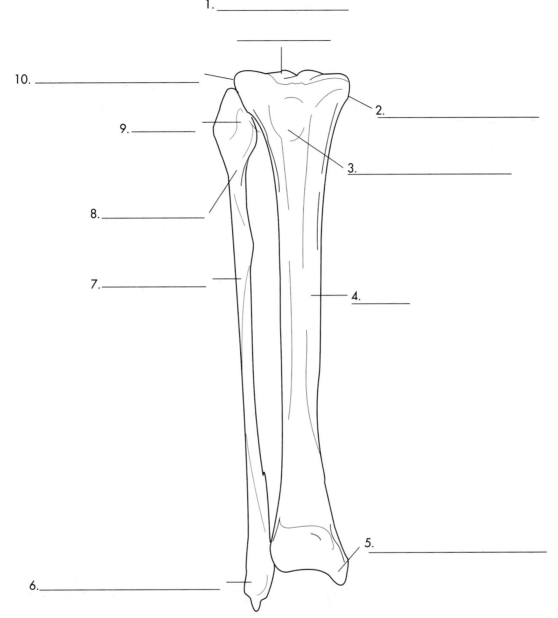

1. _____

10. _____

9. _____

8. _____

7. _____

6. _____

2. _____

3. _____

4. _____

5. _____

Labeling Exercise 13
Tibia and Fibula

Choices

Fibula	Lateral malleolus	Tibia
Head	Medial condyle	Tibial tuberosity
Intercondylar eminence	Medial malleolus	
Lateral condyle	Neck of fibula	

Modified from Fritz S: *Mosby's essential sciences for therapeutic massage,* ed. 2, St. Louis, 2004, Mosby.
Copyright © 2006, 2002 by Mosby, Inc., an affiliate of Elsevier, Inc. All rights reserved.

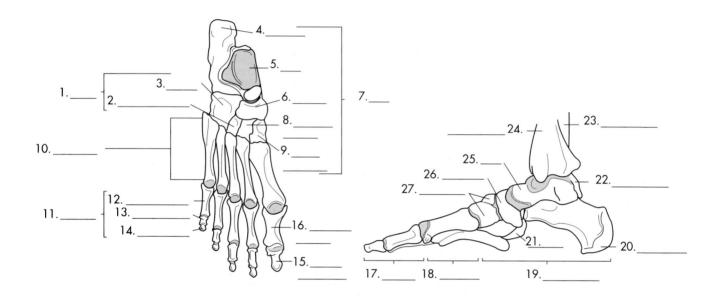

Labeling Exercise 14
Bones of Foot and Ankle

Choices

Calcaneus (2 times)
Cuboid (2 times)
Cuneiforms
Distal phalanx
Distal phalanx of great toe
Fibula

Intermediate cuneiform
Lateral cuneiform
Medial cuneiform
Metatarsals (2 times)
Middle phalanx
Navicular (2 times)

Phalanges (2 times)
Proximal phalanx
Proximal phalanx of great toe
Talus (3 times)
Tarsals (3 times)
Tibia

Modified from Fritz S: *Mosby's essential sciences for therapeutic massage*, ed. 2, St. Louis, 2004, Mosby.

Answers are on pages 297-306.

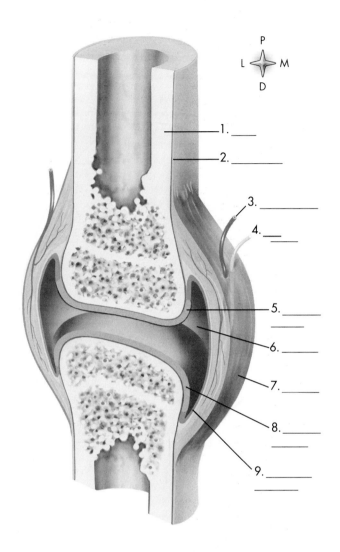

1. ____
2. _____
3. _____
4. ____
5. ____
6. _____
7. ____
8. ____
   ____
9. ____
   _____

Labeling Exercise 15
Structures of a Synovial Joint (Knee)

Choices

Articular cartilage (2 times)	Joint capsule	Periosteum
Blood vessel	Joint cavity	Synovial membrane
Bone	Nerve	

Modified from Vidic B, Suarez FR: *Photograhic atlas of the human body,* St. Louis, 1984, Mosby.

Answers are on pages 297-306.

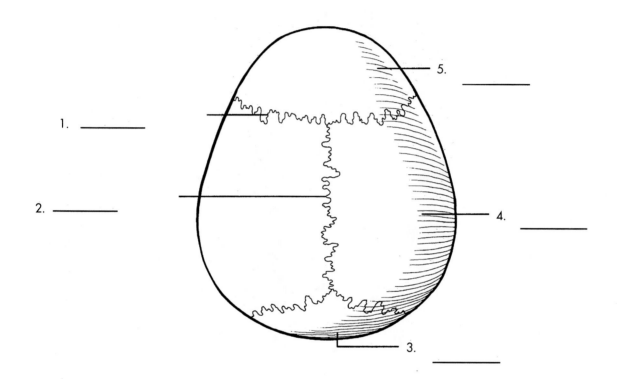

1. _____

2. _____

3. _____

4. _____

5. _____

Labeling Exercise 16
Skull: Top View

Choices

Coronal suture   Parietal bone
Frontal bone   Sagittal suture
Occipital bone

Answers are on pages 297-306.

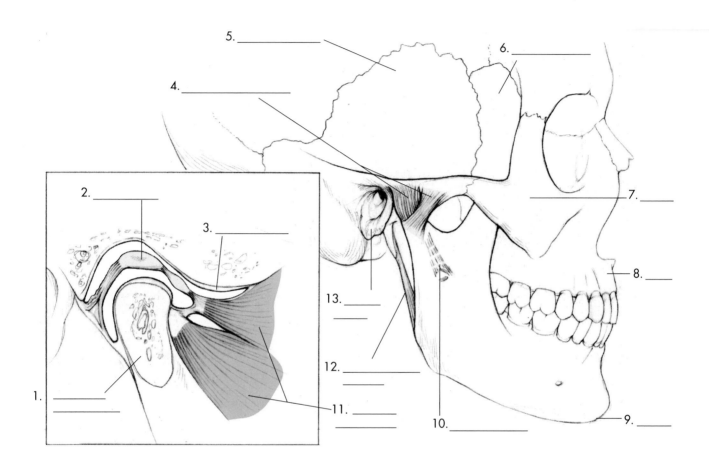

Labeling Exercise 17
Temporomandibular Joint and Inset of Articular Disk

Choices

Anterior tubercle, zygoma
Articular disk
Condylar process of mandible
External auditory meatus
Lateral temporomandibular
    ligament

Mandible
Maxilla
Pterygomandibular septa
Sphenoid, greater wing
Stylomandibular ligament
Temporal bone, squamous part

Two heads of lateral pterygoid
    muscle
Zygoma

Answers are on pages 297-306.

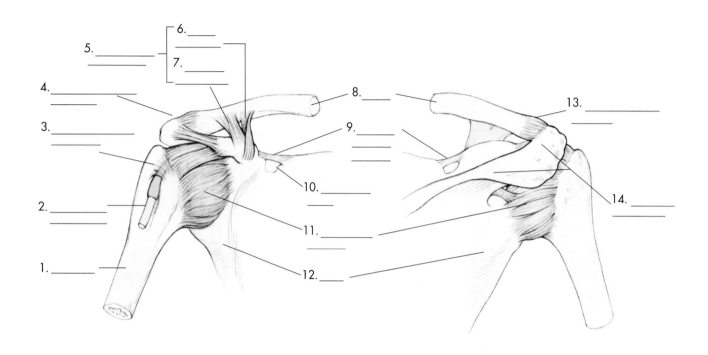

5.____

6.____

7.____

4.____

3.____

2.____

1.____

8.____

9.____

10.____

11.____

12.____

13.____

14.____

Labeling Exercise 18
Ligaments of Shoulder: Anterior and Posterior Views

Choices

Acromioclavicular ligament
  (2 times)
Clavicle
Conoid ligament
Coracoclavicular ligament

Glenohumeral ligament
Humerus
Long head of biceps muscle
Scapula
Scapular spine and acromion

Suprascapular notch
Transverse humeral ligament
Transverse scapular ligament
Trapezoid ligament

Answers are on pages 297-306.

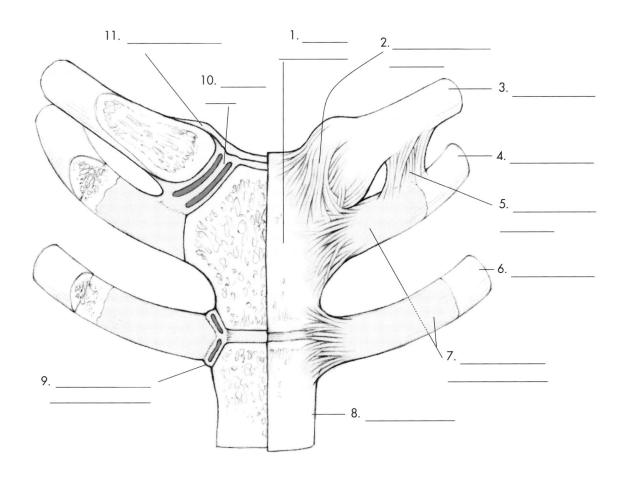

11. _____

1. _____

2. _____
   _____

10. _____

3. _____

4. _____

5. _____
   _____

6. _____

7. _____
   _____

9. _____
   _____

8. _____

Labeling Exercise 19
Joints of Sternum

Choices

Articular disk
Body of sternum
Clavicle
Costal cartilages

Costoclavicular ligament
First rib
Manubrium of sternum
Second rib

Sternoclavicular joint
Sternoclavicular ligament
Synovial chondrosternal joint

Answers are on pages 297-306.

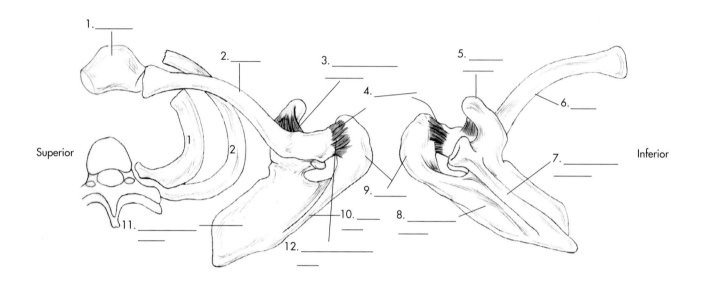

Labeling Exercise 20
Acromioclavicular Joint of Shoulder Girdle.
A, Superior View. B, Inferior View.

Choices

Acromioclavicular joint	Coracoclavicular ligament	Scapular spine
Acromioclavicular ligament	Coracoid process	Sternum
Acromion	Inferior border of scapula	Subscapular fossa
Clavicle (2 times)	Infraspinous fossa	

Modified from Mathers LH et al: *Clinical anatomy principles,* St. Louis, 1996, Mosby.

Answers are on pages 297-306.

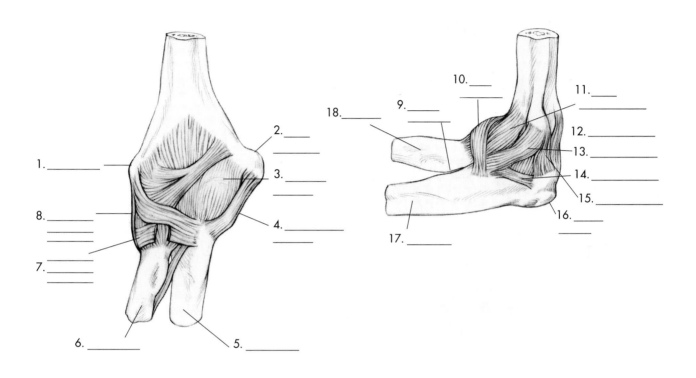

Labeling Exercise 21
Ligaments of Elbow Joint: Anterior and Lateral Views

Choices

Annular ligament
Annular ligament of radius
Anterior band
Anterior elbow capsule
Elbow joint capsule
Lateral epicondyle

Medial epicondyle
Medial (ulnar) collateral ligament
Oblique band
Olecranon of ulna
Posterior band
Radial collateral ligament

Radial tuberosity
Radius (2 times)
Ulna (2 times)
Ulnar collateral ligament

Answers are on pages 297-306.

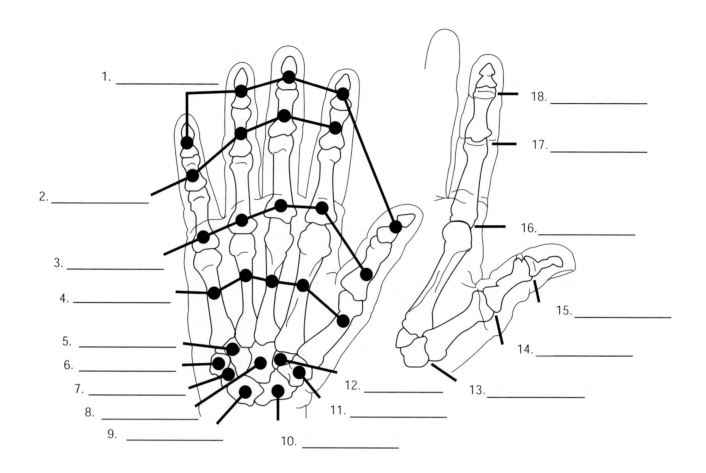

1. _____

2. _____

3. _____

4. _____

5. _____

6. _____

7. _____

8. _____

9. _____

10. _____

11. _____

12. _____

13. _____

14. _____

15. _____

16. _____

17. _____

18. _____

Labeling Exercise 22
Joints of Hand and Wrist

Choices

Capitate	Lunate	Proximal interphalangeal (PIP)
Carpometacarpal	Metacarpals	Proximal phalanges
Distal interphalangeal (DIP)	Metacarpophalangeal	Scaphoid
Distal phalanges	Metacarpophalangeal (MCP)	Trapezoid
Hamate	Middle phalanges	Trapezium
Interphalangeal	Pisiform	Triquetrum

Answers are on pages 297-306.

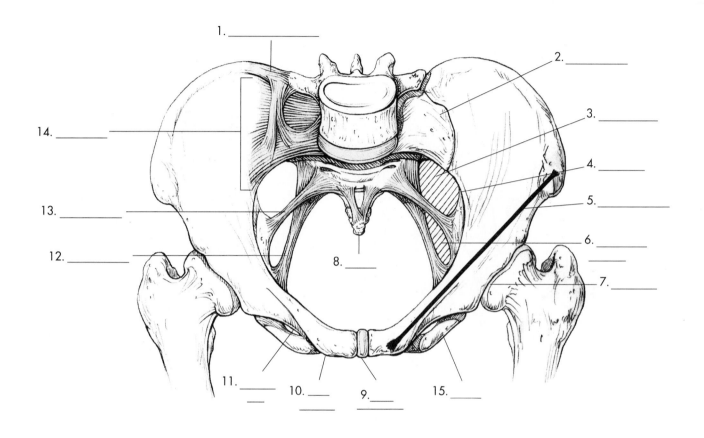

Labeling Exercise 23
Pelvic Ligaments: Superoanterior View

Choices

Acetabulum	Inguinal ligament	Pubic tubercle
Arcuate line	Ischium	Sacroiliac joint
Coccyx	Lesser sciatic foramen	Sacroiliac ligament
Greater sciatic foramen	Pectineal line	Sacrospinous ligament
Iliolumbar ligament	Pubic symphysis	Sacrotuberous ligament

Answers are on pages 297-306.

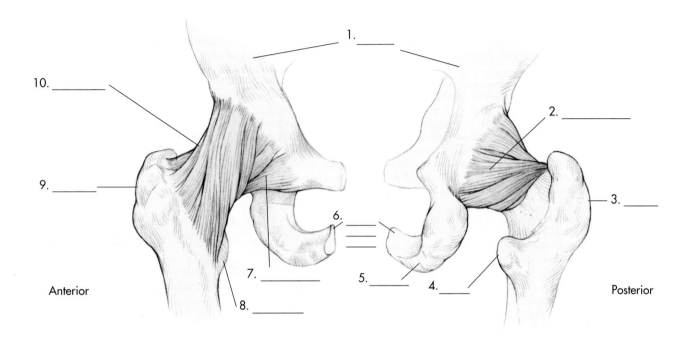

Anterior

Posterior

Labeling Exercise 24
Ligaments of Hip Joint

Choices

Greater trochanter (2 times)   Ischial tuberosity
Iliofemoral ligament   Ischiofemoral ligament
Ilium   Lesser trochanter (2 times)
Inferior pubic ramus   Pubofemoral ligament

Answers are on pages 297-306.

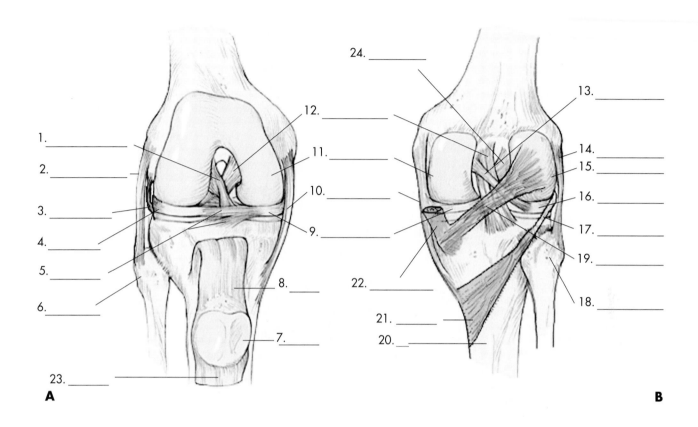

Labeling Exercise 25
Knee Joint Opened. A, Anterior View. B, Posterior View.

Choices

Anterior cruciate ligament (2 times)
Fibular collateral ligament
Fibular head (2 times)
Fibular (lateral) collateral
    ligament
Lateral condyle
Lateral meniscus (2 times)
Medial condyle

Medial meniscus
Oblique popliteal ligament
Patella
Patellar ligament
Patallar tendon
Popliteus muscle
Popliteus tendon
Posterior cruciate ligament

Posterior meniscus femoral
    ligament
Semimembranous tendon
Tendon of popliteus muscle
Tibia
Tibial (medial) collateral ligament
Transverse ligament

Answers are on pages 297-306.

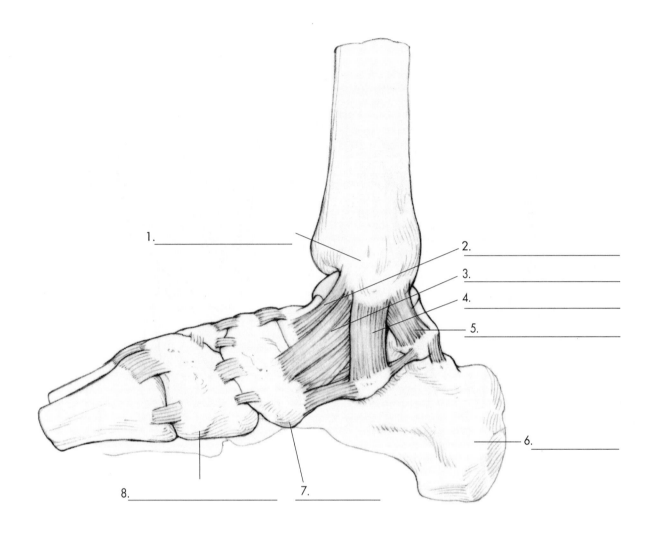

1._____

2._____

3._____

4._____

5._____

6._____

7._____

8._____

Labeling Exercise 26
Deltoid Ligament

Choices

Anterior tibiotalar   Posterior tibiotalar
Calcaneus   Tibiocalcaneal
Medial cuneiform   Tibionavicular
Medial malleolus
Navicular

Answers are on pages 297-306.

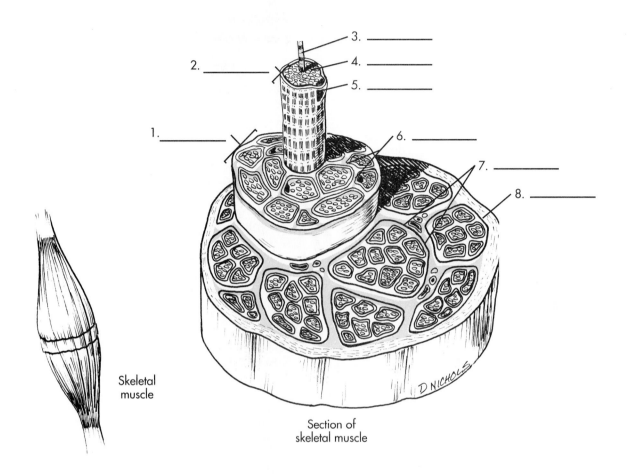

1. _____
2. _____
3. _____
4. _____
5. _____
6. _____
7. _____
8. _____

Skeletal
muscle

Section of
skeletal muscle

D. NICHOLS

Labeling Exercise 27
Section of Skeletal Muscle with Contractile and Noncontractile Connective Tissue

Choices

Endomysium	Myofibril
Epimysium	Nucleus
Fascicle	Perimysium
Muscle fiber	Sarcolemma

Answers are on pages 297-306.

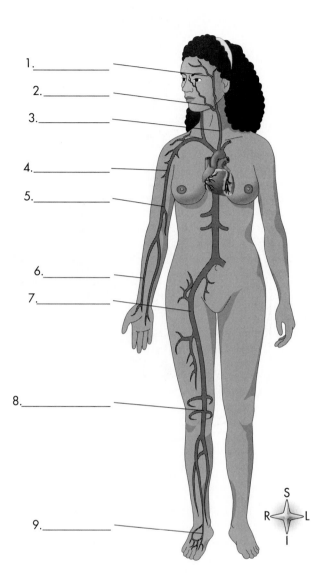

1._____

2._____

3._____

4._____

5._____

6._____

7._____

8._____

9._____

S
R—L
I

Labeling Exercise 28
Pulse Points

Choices

Axillary artery	Dorsalis pedis	Popliteal (posterior to patella)
Brachial artery	Facial artery	Radial artery
Carotid artery	Femoral artery	Superficial temporal artery

Answers are on pages 297-306.

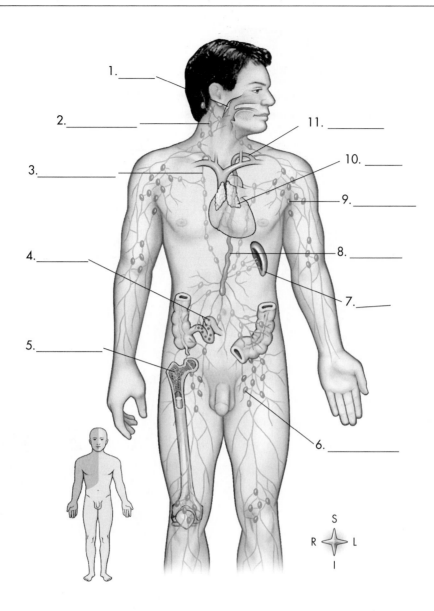

1. _____
2. _____
3. _____
4. _____
5. _____
6. _____
7. _____
8. _____
9. _____
10. _____
11. _____

S
R ✛ L
I

Labeling Exercise 29
Major Organs and Vessels of Lymphatic System

Choices

Axillary lymph node	Inguinal lymph node	Spleen
Cervical lymph node	Peyer's patches in intestinal wall	Tonsils
Entrance of thoracic duct into subclavian vein	Red bone marrow	

Answers are on pages 297-306.

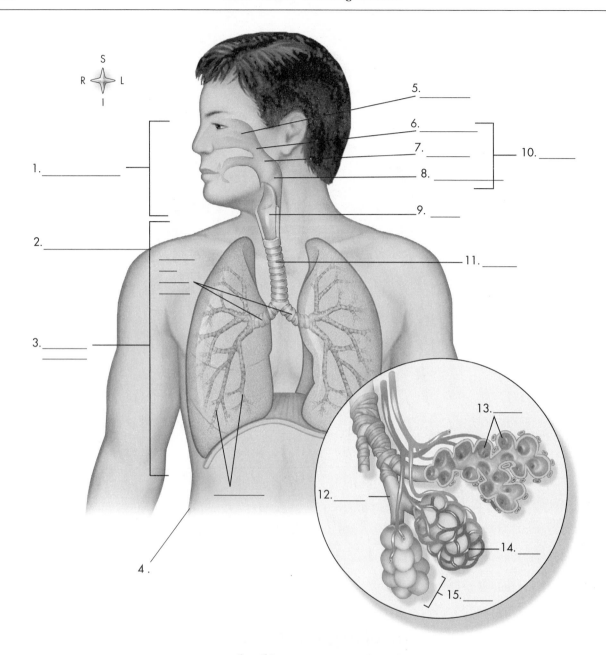

Labeling Exercise 30
Pharynx, Trachea, and Lungs, with Alveolar Sacs in Inset

Choices

Alveolar duct	Larynx	Oropharynx
Alveolar sac	Left and right primary bronchi	Pharynx
Alveoli	Lower respiratory tract	Right main bronchus
Bronchioles	Nasal cavity	Trachea
Laryngopharynx	Nasopharynx	Upper respiratory tract

Answers are on pages 297-306.

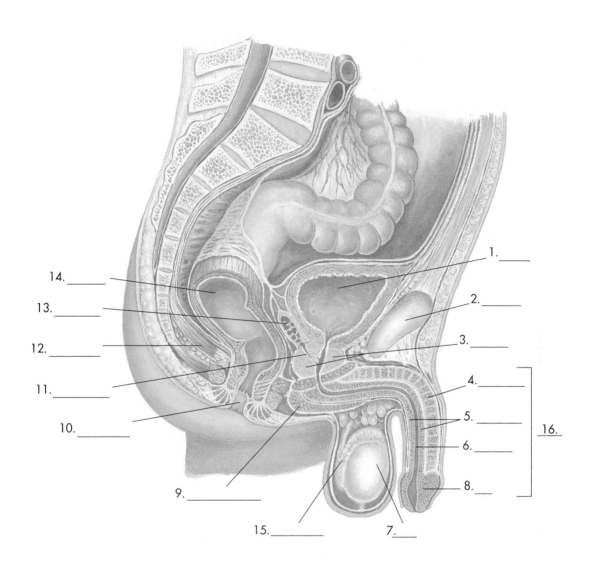

Labeling Exercise 31
Male Pelvic Organs

Choices

Anus	Glans	Symphysis pubis
Bulbocavernosus muscle	Levator ani muscle	Testis
Corpus cavernosum	Penis	Urethra
Corpus spongiosum	Prostate gland	Urinary bladder
Ejaculatory duct	Rectum	
Epididymis	Seminal vesicle	

Answers are on pages 297-306.

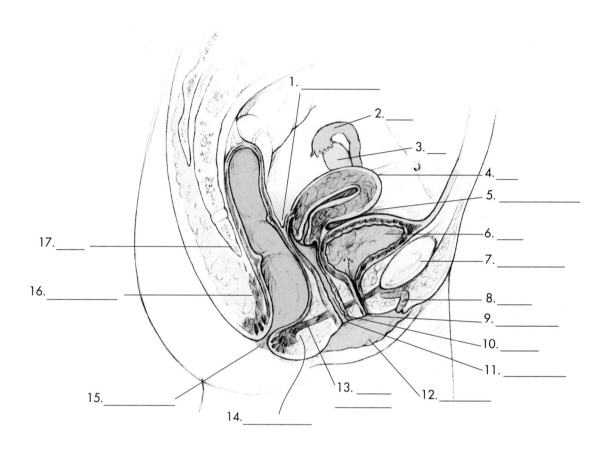

Labeling Exercise 32
Female Pelvic Floor: Midsagittal View

Choices

Anal orifice	Ovary	Urogenital diaphragm
Anococcygeal raphe	Oviduct	Uterus
Bladder	Perineal body	Vagina
Clitoris	Pubic symphysis	Vaginal introitus
Coccyx	Rectouterine fossa	Vesicouterine fossa
Labium minus	Urethral orifice	

Answers are on pages 297-306.

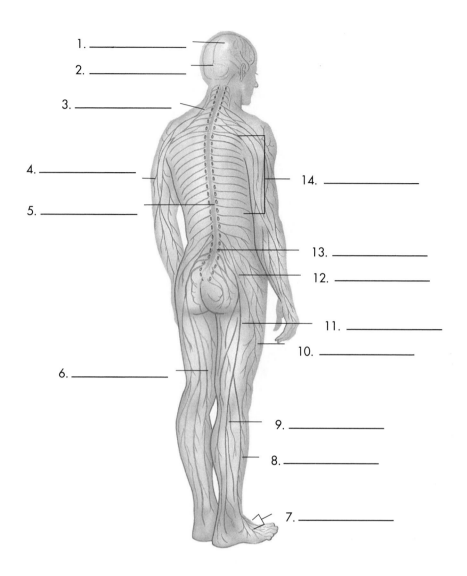

1. _____
2. _____
3. _____
4. _____
5. _____
6. _____
7. _____
8. _____
9. _____
10. _____
11. _____
12. _____
13. _____
14. _____

Labeling Exercise 33
Nervous System: Simplified View

Choices

Brachial plexus
Cauda equina
Cerebellum
Cerebrum
Digital nerves

Femoral cutaneous nerve
Femoral nerve
Intercostal nerves
Ischial nerve
Musculocutaneous nerve

Perineal nerve
Saphenous nerve
Spinal cord
Tibial nerve

Answers are on pages 297-306.

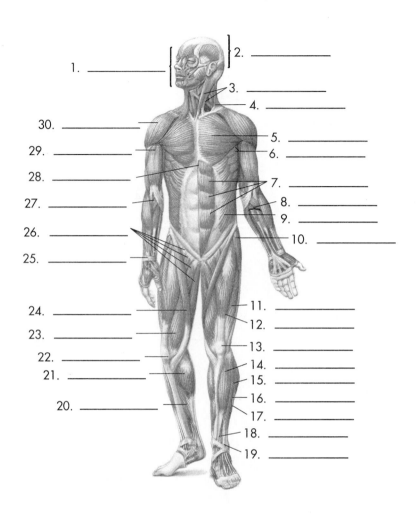

1. _____
2. _____
3. _____
4. _____
5. _____
6. _____
7. _____
8. _____
9. _____
10. _____
11. _____
12. _____
13. _____
14. _____
15. _____
16. _____
17. _____
18. _____
19. _____
20. _____
21. _____
22. _____
23. _____
24. _____
25. _____
26. _____
27. _____
28. _____
29. _____
30. _____

Labeling Exercise 34
Muscular System: Anterior View

Choices

Adductors of thigh	Gastrocnemius	Sartorius
Biceps brachii	Linea alba	Serratus anterior
Cranial muscles	Obliquus externus	Soleus
Deltoideus	Patella	Sternocleidomastoideus
Extensor digitorum longus	Patellar tendon	Superior extensor retinaculum
Extensor hallucis longus tendon	Pectoralis major	Tensor fasciae latae
Extensors of wrist and fingers	Peroneus brevis	Tibialis anterior
Facial muscles	Peroneus longus	Trapezius
Flexor retinaculum	Rectus abdominis	Vastus lateralis
Flexors of wrist and fingers	Rectus femoris	Vastus medialis

Modified from LaFleur-Brooks M: *Exploring medical language: a student-directed approach*, ed. 4, St. Louis, 1998, Mosby.

Answers are on pages 297-306.

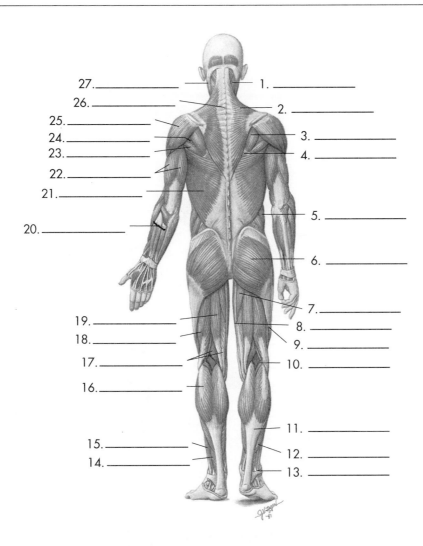

Labeling Exercise 35
Muscular System: Posterior View

Choices

Adductor magnus	Infraspinatus	Soleus
Biceps femoris	Latissimus dorsi	Splenius capitis
Deltoideus	Obliquus externus	Sternocleidomastoideus
Extensors of the wrist and fingers	Peroneus brevis	Superior peroneal retinaculum
Gastrocnemius	Peroneus longus	Teres major
Gastrocnemius tendon (Achilles	Plantaris	Teres minor
tendon)	Portion of rhomboideus	Trapezius
Gluteus maximus	Semimembranosus	Triceps
Gracilis	Semitendinosus	
Iliotibial tract	Seventh cervical vertebra	

Answers are on pages 297-306.

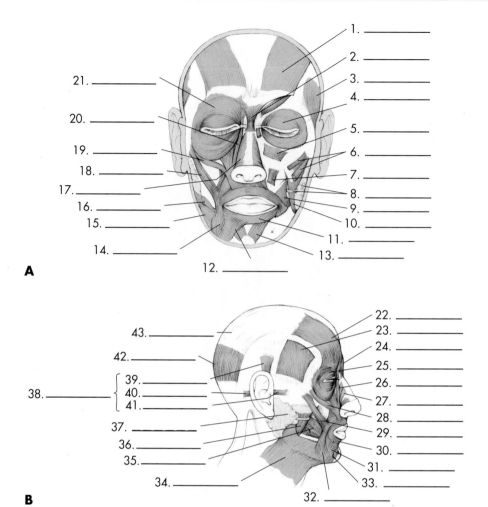

21. _____
20. _____
19. _____
18. _____
17. _____
16. _____
15. _____
14. _____

A

1. _____
2. _____
3. _____
4. _____
5. _____
6. _____
7. _____
8. _____
9. _____
10. _____
11. _____
13. _____
12. _____

43. _____
42. _____
38. _____ { 39. _____
40. _____
41. _____
37. _____
36. _____
35. _____
34. _____

B

22. _____
23. _____
24. _____
25. _____
26. _____
27. _____
28. _____
29. _____
30. _____
31. _____
33. _____
32. _____

Labeling Exercise 36
Facial Muscles. A, Anterior View. B, Lateral View.

Choices

Anterior	Masseter muscle (2 times)	Platysma
Auricular muscles	Mentalis	Platysma muscle
Buccinator muscle (2 times)	Mentalis muscle	Posterior
Depressor anguli oris	Nasalis	Procerus muscle (2 times)
Depressor anguli oris muscle	Nasalis muscle	Risorius
Depressor labii inferioris (2 times)	Occipitalis muscle	Superior
Frontalis muscle (2 times)	Orbicularis oculi muscle	Temporalis muscle (2 times)
Galea aponeurotica	Orbicularis oculi muscle	Zygomaticus major muscle (2 times)
Levator anguli oris	(palpebral part)	Zygomaticus minor muscle
Levator labii superioris	Orbicularis oculi (orbital part)	(2 times)
Levator labii superioris alaeque	Orbicularis oris muscle (2 times)	Zygomaticus major and minor
nasi muscle (2 times)	Parotid gland and duct (2 times)	muscles

Answers are on pages 297-306.

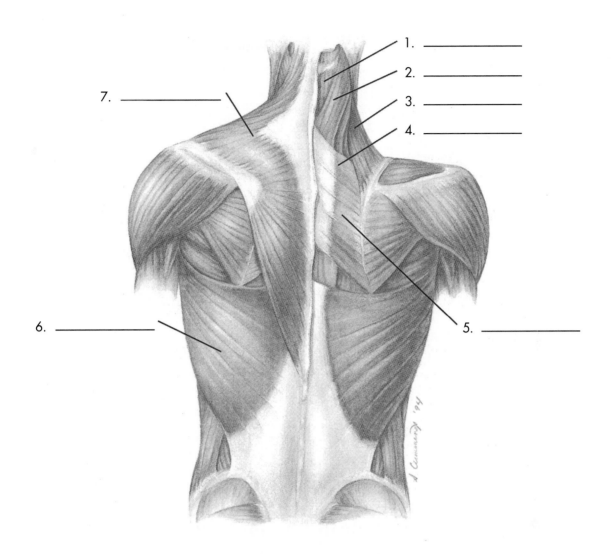

1. _____
2. _____
3. _____
4. _____
5. _____
6. _____
7. _____

Labeling Exercise 37
Back Muscles: First (Left) and Second (Right) Layers

Choices

Latissimus dorsi muscle   Semispinalis capitis muscle
Levator scapulae muscle   Splenius capitis muscle
Rhomboid major muscle   Trapezius muscle
Rhomboid minor muscle

Answers are on pages 297-306.

Anterior   **Posterior**

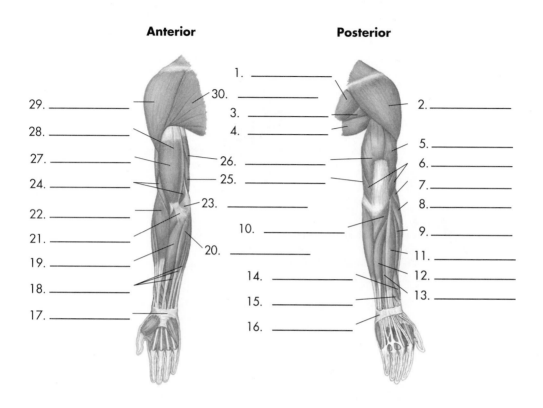

Labeling Exercise 38
Muscles of Arm

Choices

Abductor pollicis brevis
Abductor pollicis longus
Anconeus
Biceps brachii, long head
Biceps brachii, short head
Bicipital aponeurosis
Brachialis
Brachioradialis (2 times)
Deltoid (2 times)

Extensor carpi radialis brevis
Extensor carpi radialis longus
Extensor carpi ulnaris
Extensor digiti minimi
Extensor digitorum communis
Extensor retinaculum
Flexor carpi radialis
Flexor digitorum superficialis
Flexor retinaculum

Infraspinatus
Palmaris longus
Pectoralis major
Pronator teres
Teres major
Teres minor
Triceps, lateral head
Triceps, long head
Triceps, medial head (2 times)

Answers are on pages 297-306.

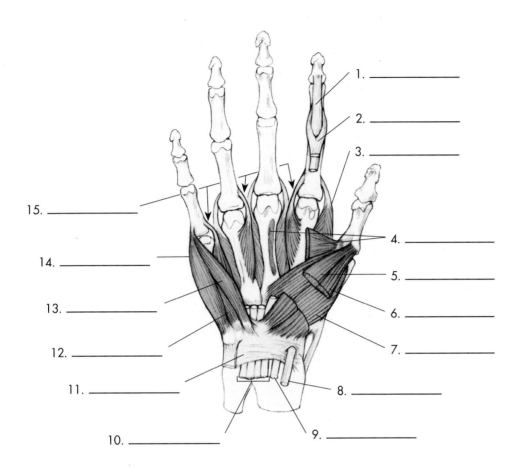

Labeling Exercise 39
Deeper Muscles of Palm: Anterior View

Choices

Abductor digiti minimi muscle
Abductor pollicis brevis muscle
Adductor pollicis muscle
First dorsal interosseous muscle
Flexor digiti minimi muscle
Flexor pollicis brevis muscle
Flexor retinaculum

Opponens digiti minimi muscle
Opponens pollicis muscle
Palmar interossei
Tendon of flexor carpi radialis
  muscle
Tendon of flexor digitorum
  profundus

Tendon of flexor digitorum
  superficialis
Tendon of pollicis longus muscle
Tendons of flexor digitorum
  superficialis muscle

Answers are on pages 297-306.

Anterior **Posterior**

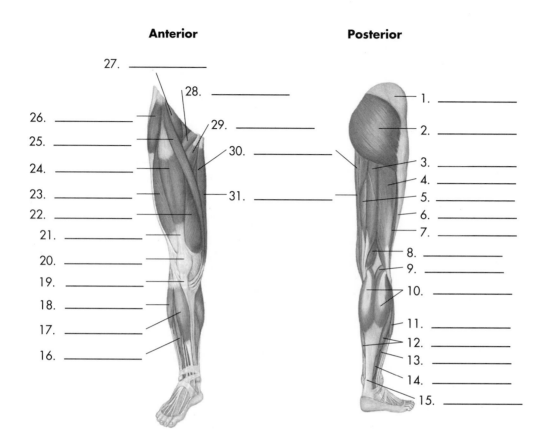

27. _____

28. _____

26. _____

29. _____

25. _____

30. _____

24. _____

23. _____   31. _____

22. _____

21. _____

20. _____

19. _____

18. _____

17. _____

16. _____

1. _____

2. _____

3. _____

4. _____

5. _____

6. _____

7. _____

8. _____

9. _____

10. _____

11. _____

12. _____

13. _____

14. _____

15. _____

Labeling Exercise 40
Muscles of Leg

Choices

Adductor longus
Adductor magnus
Biceps femoris long head
Biceps femoris short head
Calcaneal tendon (Achilles
    tendon)
Extensor digitorum longus
Fascia over gluteus medius
Flexor hallucis longus
Gastrocnemius

Gluteus maximus
Gracilis
Iliopsoas
Iliotibial tract
Patella
Patellar ligament
Pectineus
Peroneus brevis
Peroneus longus (2 times)
Plantaris

Rectus femoris
Sartorius
Semimembranosus (2 times)
Semitendinosus
Soleus
Tendon of rectus femoris
Tensor of fasciae latae
Tibialis anterior
Vastus lateralis
Vastus medialis

Modified from Mourad LA: *Orthopedic disorders,* St. Louis, 1991, Mosby.

Answers are on pages 297-306.

Answer Key for Labeling Exercises

Labeling Exercise 1

1. Rough endoplasmic reticulum
2. Lysosome
3. Golgi apparatus
4. Nucleolus
5. Smooth endoplasmic reticulum
6. Ribosomes
7. Cytoplasm
8. Nucleus
9. Mitochondrion
10. Cell (plasma) membrane

Labeling Exercise 2

1. Spinal cord
2. Spinal ganglion
3. Epineurium
4. Perineurium
5. Endoneurium
6. Axon
7. Motor end plate
8. Skin
9. Pain receptors
10. Muscle
11. Myelin sheath
12. Node of Ranvier
13. Nerve bundle (fasciculus)
14. Blood vessels

Labeling Exercise 3

1. Frontal bone
2. Nasal bone
3. Zygomatic bone
4. Sternum
5. Ribs
6. Vertebral column
7. Coxal (hip) bone
8. Ilium
9. Sacrum
10. Coccyx
11. Greater trochanter
12. Pubis
13. Ischium
14. Phalanges
15. Metatarsals
16. Tarsals
17. Fibula
18. Tibia
19. Patella
20. Femur
21. Phalanges
22. Metacarpals
23. Carpals
24. Ulna
25. Radius
26. Humerus
27. Xiphoid process
28. Costal cartilage
29. Scapula
30. Manubrium
31. Clavicle
32. Mandible
33. Maxilla
34. Orbit
35. Clavicle
36. Acromion process
37. Scapula
38. Ribs
39. Humerus
40. Ulna
41. Radius
42. Coxal (hip) bone
43. Sacrum
44. Calcaneus
45. Metatarsals
46. Phalanges
47. Tarsals
48. Fibula
49. Tibia
50. Femur
51. Phalanges
52. Metacarpals
53. Carpals
54. Lumbar vertebrae(5)
55. Thoracic vertebrae(12)
56. Cervical vertebrae(7)
57. Occipital bone
58. Parietal bone
59. Ischium
60. Coccyx

Labeling Exercise 4
1. Cervical curve
2. Thoracic curve
3. Lumbar curve
4. Sacral curve
5. First cervical vertebra (atlas)
6. Second cervical vertebra (axis)
7. Seventh cervical vertebra
8. First thoracic vertebra
9. Intervertebral disk
10. Intervertebral foramina
11. First lumbar vertebra
12. Body
13. Transverse process
14. Spinous process

Labeling Exercise 5
1. Jugular notch
2. Seventh cervical vertebra
3. First thoracic vertebra
4. Manubrium
5. Sternal angle
6. Body
7. Xiphoid process
8. Sternum
9. Floating ribs
10. False ribs
11. Costal cartilage
12. True ribs
13. Clavicle
14. Sternal end
15. Body
16. Head
17. Articular facets for body of vertebrae
18. Neck
19. Articular facet for transverse process of vertebra
20. Tubercle
21. Angle
22. Xiphoid process
23. Facets for attachment of costal cartilages 1 to 7
24. Jugular notch
25. Clavicular notch
26. Manubrium
27. Sternal angle
28. Body

Labeling Exercise 6
1. Sternal end
2. Body
3. Acromial end

Labeling Exercise 7
1. Scapular spine
2. Supraspinous fossa
3. Suprascapular notch
4. Infraspinous fossa
5. Infraglenoid tubercle
6. Glenoid fossa
7. Supraglenoid tubercle
8. Acromion
9. Coracoid process
10. Vertebral border
11. Lateral border
12. Scapular spine
13. Coracoid fossa
14. Glenoid fossa

Labeling Exercise 8
1. Greater tubercle
2. Head
3. Greater tubercle
4. Lesser tubercle
5. Surgical neck
6. Deltoid tuberosity
7. Radial fossa
8. Lateral epicondyle
9. Capitulum
10. Trochlea
11. Coronoid fossa
12. Medial epicondyle
13. Olecranon fossa

Labeling Exercise 9

1. Radial head
2. Radial tuberosity
3. Radius
4. Radial styloid
5. Ulnar styloid
6. Ulna
7. Interosseous membrane
8. Trochlear notch
9. Olecranon process of ulna

Labeling Exercise 10

1. Phalanges
2. Metacarpus
3. Carpus
4. Hamate
5. Pisiform
6. Triquetrum
7. Lunate
8. Styloid process
9. Ulnar head
10. Ulna
11. Radius
12. Ulnar notch of radius
13. Styloid process
14. Scaphoid
15. Capitate
16. Trapezium
17. Trapezoid
18. Sesamoids
19. Proximal
20. Middle
21. Distal

Labeling Exercise 11

1. Sacroiliac joint
2. Sacrum
3. Ilium
4. Pubis
5. Ischium
6. Symphysis pubis
7. Obturator foramen
8. Anterior superior iliac spine
9. Sacral promontory
10. Iliac crest
11. Ilium
12. Anterior superior iliac spine
13. Anterior inferior iliac spine
14. Lunate surface
15. Acetabulum
16. Acetabular notch
17. Inferior pubic ramus
18. Ischial ramus
19. Obturator foramen
20. Ischial tuberosity
21. Lesser sciatic notch
22. Ischial spine
23. Greater sciatic notch
24. Posterior inferior iliac spine
25. Posterior superior iliac spine
26. Iliac crest
27. Auricular surface
28. Posterior superior iliac spine
29. Posterior inferior iliac spine
30. Greater sciatic notch
31. Body of ischium
32. Ischial spine
33. Lesser sciatic notch
34. Ischial ramus
35. Inferior pubic ramus
36. Obturator foramen
37. Symphysis pubis
38. Pubic crest
39. Superior pubic ramus
40. Iliopectineal line
41. Anterior inferior iliac spine
42. Anterior superior iliac spine
43. Iliac fossa
44. Ilium

Labeling Exercise 12

1. Greater trochanter
2. Fovea capitis
3. Head of femur
4. Greater trochanter
5. Neck
6. Intertrochanteric fossa
7. Gluteal tuberosity
8. Lesser trochanter
9. Intertrochanteric line
10. Intertrochanteric crest
11. Pectineal line
12. Linea aspera
13. Lateral and medial supracondylar ridges
14. Medial and lateral supracondylar lines
15. Patellar groove
16. Adductor tubercle
17. Lateral epicondyle
18. Medial epicondyle
19. Lateral condyle
20. Medial condyle
21. Intercondylar fossa

Labeling Exercise 13

1. Intercondylar eminence
2. Medial condyle
3. Tibial tuberosity
4. Tibia
5. Medial malleolus
6. Lateral malleolus
7. Fibula
8. Neck of fibula
9. Head
10. Lateral condyle

Labeling Exercise 14

1. Tarsals
2. Lateral cuneiform
3. Cuboid
4. Calcaneus
5. Talus
6. Navicular
7. Tarsals
8. Intermediate cuneiform
9. Medial cuneiform
10. Metatarsals
11. Phalanges
12. Proximal phalanx
13. Middle phalanx
14. Distal phalanx
15. Distal phalanx of great toe
16. Proximal phalanx of great toe
17. Phalanges
18. Metatarsals
19. Tarsals
20. Calcaneus
21. Cuboid
22. Talus
23. Fibula
24. Tibia
25. Talus
26. Navicular
27. Cuneiforms

Labeling Exercise 15

1. Bone
2. Periosteum
3. Blood vessel
4. Nerve
5. Articular Cartilage
6. Joint cavity
7. Joint capsule
8. Articular Cartilage
9. Synovial membrane

Labeling Exercise 16
1. Coronal suture
2. Sagittal suture
3. Occipital bone
4. Parietal bone
5. Frontal bone

Labeling Exercise 17
1. Condylar process of mandible
2. Articular disk
3. Anterior tubercle, zygoma
4. Lateral temporomandibular ligament
5. Temporal bone, squamous part
6. Sphenoid, greater wing
7. Zygoma
8. Maxilla
9. Mandible
10. Pterygomandibular septa
11. Two heads of lateral pterygoid muscle
12. Stylomandibular ligament
13. External auditory meatus

Labeling Exercise 18
1. Humerus
2. Long head of biceps muscle
3. Transverse humeral ligament
4. Acromioclavicular ligament
5. Coracoclavicular ligament
6. Conoid ligament
7. Trapezoid ligament
8. Clavicle
9. Transverse scapular ligament
10. Suprascapular notch
11. Glenohumeral ligament
12. Scapula
13. Acromioclavicular ligament
14. Scapular spine and acromion

Labeling Exercise 19
1. Manubrium of sternum
2. Sternoclavicular ligament
3. Clavicle
4. First rib
5. Costoclavicular ligament
6. Second rib
7. Costal cartilages
8. Body of sternum
9. Synovial chondrosternal joint
10. Articular disk
11. Sternoclavicular joint

Labeling Exercise 20
1. Sternum
2. Clavicle
3. Coracoclavicular ligament
4. Acromioclavicular ligament
5. Coracoid process
6. Clavicle
7. Inferior border of scapula
8. Infraspinous fossa
9. Acromion
10. Scapular spine
11. Subscapular fossa
12. Acromioclavicular joint

Labeling Exercise 21
1. Lateral epicondyle
2. Medial epicondyle
3. Elbow joint capsule
4. Ulnar collateral ligament
5. Ulna
6. Radius
7. Annular ligament of radius
8. Radial collateral ligament
9. Radial tuberosity
10. Annular ligament
11. Anterior elbow capsule
12. Medial (ulnar) collateral ligament
13. Anterior band
14. Oblique band
15. Posterior band
16. Olecranon of ulna
17. Ulna
18. Radius

Labeling Exercise 22
1. Distal phalanges
2. Middle phalanges
3. Proximal phalanges
4. Metacarpals
5. Hamate
6. Pisiform
7. Triquetrum
8. Capitate
9. Lunate
10. Scaphoid
11. Trapezium
12. Trapezoid
13. Carpometacarpal
14. Metacarpophalangeal
15. Interphalangeal
16. Metacarpophalangeal (MCP)
17. Proximal interphalangeal (PIP)
18. Distal interphalangeal (DIP)

Labeling Exercise 23
1. Iliolumbar ligament
2. Sacroiliac joint
3. Greater sciatic foramen
4. Arcuate line
5. Inguinal ligament
6. Lesser sciatic foramen
7. Acetabulum
8. Coccyx
9. Pubic symphysis
10. Pubic tubercle
11. Pectineal line
12. Sacrotuberous ligament
13. Sacrospinous ligament
14. Sacroiliac ligament
15. Ischium

Labeling Exercise 24
1. Ilium
2. Ischiofemoral ligament
3. Greater trochanter
4. Lesser trochanter
5. Ischial tuberosity
6. Inferior pubic ramus
7. Pubofemoral ligament
8. Lesser trochanter
9. Greater trochanter
10. Iliofemoral ligament

Labeling Exercise 25
1. Anterior cruciate ligament
2. Fibular (lateral) collateral ligament
3. Tendon of popliteus muscle
4. Lateral meniscus
5. Transverse ligament
6. Fibular head
7. Patella
8. Patellar ligament
9. Medial meniscus
10. Tibial (medial) collateral ligament
11. Medial condyle
12. Posterior cruciate ligament
13. Posterior meniscus femoral ligament
14. Fibular (lateral) collateral ligament
15. Lateral condyle
16. Lateral meniscus
17. Popliteus tendon
18. Fibular head
19. Oblique popliteal ligament
20. Tibia
21. Popliteus muscle
22. Semimembranous tendon
23. Patellar tendon
24. Anterior cruciate ligament

Labeling Exercise 26
1. Medial malleolus
2. Anterior tibiotalar
3. Tibionavicular
4. Tibiocalcaneal
5. Posterior tibiotalar
6. Calcaneus
7. Navicular
8. Medial cuneiform

Labeling Exercise 27

1. Fascicle
2. Muscle fiber
3. Myofibril
4. Sarcolemma
5. Nucleus
6. Endomysium
7. Perimysium
8. Epimysium

Labeling Exercise 28

1. Superficial temporal artery
2. Facial artery
3. Carotid artery
4. Axillary artery
5. Brachial artery
6. Radial artery
7. Femoral artery
8. Popliteal (posterior to patella)
9. Dorsalis pedis

Labeling Exercise 29

1. Tonsils
2. Cervical lymph node
3. Right lymphatic duct
4. Peyer's patches
5. Red bone marrow
6. Inguinal lymph node
7. Spleen
8. Thoracic duct
9. Axillary lymph node
10. Thymus gland
11. Entrance of thoracic duct into subclavian vein

Labeling Exercise 30

1. Upper respiratory tract
2. Left and right primary bronchii
3. Lower respiratory tract
4. Bronchioles
5. Nasal cavity
6. Nasopharynx
7. Oropharynx
8. Laryngopharynx
9. Larynx
10. Pharynx
11. Trachea
12. Alveolar duct
13. Alveoli
14. Capillary
15. Alveolar sac

Labeling Exercise 31

1. Urinary bladder
2. Symphysis pubis
3. Prostate gland
4. Corpus cavernosum
5. Corpus spongiosum
6. Urethra
7. Testis
8. Glans
9. Bulbocavernosus muscle
10. Anus
11. Ejaculatory duct
12. Levator ani muscle
13. Seminal vesicle
14. Rectum
15. Epididymis
16. Penis

Labeling Exercise 32

1. Rectouterine fossa
2. Oviduct
3. Ovary
4. Uterus
5. Vesicouterine fossa
6. Bladder
7. Pubic symphysis
8. Clitoris
9. Urethral orifice
10. Vagina
11. Vaginal introitus
12. Labium minus
13. Urogenital diaphragm
14. Perineal body
15. Anal orifice
16. Anococcygeal raphe
17. Coccyx

Labeling Exercise 33
1. Cerebrum
2. Cerebellum
3. Brachial plexus
4. Musculocutaneous nerve
5. Spinal cord
6. Saphenous nerve
7. Digital nerves
8. Perineal nerve
9. Tibial nerve
10. Femoral cutaneous nerve
11. Ischial nerve
12. Femoral nerve
13. Cauda equina
14. Intercostal nerves

Labeling Exercise 34
1. Facial muscles
2. Cranial muscles
3. Sternocleidomastoideus
4. Trapezius
5. Pectoralis major
6. Serratus anterior
7. Rectus abdominis
8. Flexors of wrist and fingers
9. Obliquus externus
10. Tensor fasciae latae
11. Vastus lateralis
12. Rectus femoris
13. Patella
14. Tibialis anterior
15. Extensor digitorum longus
16. Peroneus longus
17. Peroneus brevis
18. Extensor hallucis longus tendon
19. Superior extensor retinaculum
20. Soleus
21. Gastrocnemius
22. Patellar tendon
23. Vastus medialis
24. Sartorius
25. Flexor retinaculum
26. Adductors of thigh
27. Extensors of wrist and fingers
28. Linea alba
29. Biceps brachii
30. Deltoideus

Labeling Exercise 35
1. Splenius capitis
2. Trapezius
3. Infraspinatus
4. Portion of rhomboideus
5. Obliquus externus
6. Gluteus maximus
7. Adductor magnus
8. Gracilis
9. Iliotibial tract
10. Plantaris
11. Gastrocnemius tendon (Achilles tendon)
12. Soleus
13. Superior peroneal retinaculum
14. Peroneus brevis
15. Peroneus longus
16. Gastrocnemius
17. Semimembranosus
18. Biceps femoris
19. Semitendinosus
20. Extensors of the wrist and fingers
21. Latissimus dorsi
22. Triceps
23. Teres major
24. Teres minor
25. Deltoideus
26. Seventh cervical vertebra
27. Sternocleidomastoideus

Labeling Exercise 36
1. Frontalis muscle
2. Temporalis muscle
3. Procerus muscle
4. Orbicularis oculi muscle (palpebral part)
5. Levator labii superioris
6. Zygomaticus major and minor muscles
7. Levator anguli oris
8. Parotid gland and duct
9. Buccinator muscle
10. Masseter muscle
11. Orbicularis oris muscle
12. Depressor labii inferioris
13. Mentalis
14. Depressor anguli oris
15. Platysma
16. Risorius
17. Nasalis
18. Zygomaticus major muscle
19. Zygomaticus minor muscle
20. Levator labii superioris alaeque nasi muscle
21. Orbicularis oculi (orbital part)
22. Frontalis muscle
23. Temporalis muscle
24. Procerus muscle
25. Orbicularis oculi muscle
26. Levator labii superioris alaeque nasi muscle
27. Nasalis muscle
28. Zygomaticus minor muscle
29. Zygomaticus major muscle
30. Orbicularis oris muscle
31. Depressor labii inferioris
32. Depressor anguli oris muscle
33. Mentalis muscle
34. Platysma muscle
35. Buccinator muscle
36. Masseter muscle
37. Parotid gland and duct
38. Auricular muscles
39. Superior
40. Posterior
41. Anterior
42. Occipitalis muscle
43. Galea aponeurotica

Labeling Exercise 37
1. Semispinalis capitis muscle
2. Splenius capitis muscle
3. Levator scapulae muscle
4. Rhomboid minor muscle
5. Rhomboid major muscle
6. Latissimus dorsi muscle
7. Trapezius muscle

Labeling Exercise 38
1. Infraspinatus
2. Deltoid
3. Teres minor
4. Teres major
5. Triceps, long head
6. Triceps, medial head
7. Brachioradialis
8. Extensor carpi radialis longus
9. Extensor carpi radialis brevis
10. Anconeus
11. Extensor digitorum communis
12. Extensor carpi ulnaris
13. Extensor digiti minimi
14. Abductor pollicis brevis
15. Abductor pollicis longus
16. Extensor retinaculum
17. Flexor retinaculum
18. Flexor digitorum superficialis
19. Flexor carpi radialis
20. Palmaris longus
21. Bicipital aponeurosis
22. Brachioradialis
23. Pronator teres
24. Brachialis
25. Triceps, medial head
26. Triceps, lateral head
27. Biceps brachii, long head
28. Biceps brachii, short head
29. Deltoid
30. Pectoralis major

Labeling Exercise 39

1. Tendon of flexor digitorum profundus
2. Tendon of flexor digitorum superficialis
3. First dorsal interosseous muscle
4. Adductor pollicis muscle
5. Flexor pollicis brevis muscle
6. Abductor pollicis brevis muscle
7. Opponens pollicis muscle
8. Tendon of flexor carpi radialis muscle
9. Tendon of pollicis longus muscle
10. Tendons of flexor digitorum superficialis muscle
11. Flexor retinaculum
12. Opponens digiti minimi muscle
13. Flexor digiti minimi muscle
14. Abductor digiti minimi muscle
15. Palmar interossei

Labeling Exercise 40

1. Fascia over gluteus medius
2. Gluteus maximus
3. Semitendinosus
4. Biceps femoris long head
5. Semimembranosus
6. Iliotibial tract
7. Biceps femoris short head
8. Semimembranosus
9. Plantaris
10. Gastrocnemius
11. Peroneus longus
12. Soleus
13. Peroneus brevis
14. Flexor hallucis longus
15. Calcaneal tendon (Achilles tendon)
16. Extensor digitorum longus
17. Tibialis anterior
18. Peroneus longus
19. Patellar ligament
20. Patella
21. Tendon of rectus femoris
22. Vastus medialis
23. Vastus lateralis
24. Rectus femoris
25. Sartorius
26. Tensor of fasciae latae
27. Iliopsoas
28. Pectineus
29. Adductor longus
30. Adductor magnus
31. Gracilis

CHAPTER

29
Muscle Quick Reference Guide

This chart is an abbreviated, simplified description of the main muscles and referred pain patterns encountered during massage application.

Muscle Name	Function	Trigger Point Referred Pain Pattern*
MUSCLES OF THE FACE AND HEAD		
Muscles of Facial Expression		
	Move scalp forward and backward; assist in raising the eyebrows and wrinkling the forehead; draw the eyebrows downward and medially; and create transverse wrinkles over the bridge of the nose.	Galea aponeurotica, muscles over the eyebrows, eyes, ears, nose, and scalp above the ears
Auricular (ear) muscles	Move the ear.	None identified
Eye muscles	Open and close the eyelids; provide intrinsic movement of the eyeball.	Superior orbital area above the eyelid
Muscles That Move the Mouth		
	Move lips; aid in mastication; force air out between the lips; and compress the cheek against the teeth.	
Muscles of Mastication (Chewing)		
	Move the mouth; close the jaw; provide side-to-side movement and biting; and elevate the mandible.	Near and in the zygomatic arch; anterior, medial, and posterior along the inferior aspect of the muscles near the tendinous junction at the coronoid process of the mandible; temporal region, eyebrow, upper teeth, cheek, and temporomandibular joint; back of the throat, into the ear; upper and lower jaw, the ear, and the eyebrow
MUSCLES OF THE NECK		
Anterior Triangle of the Neck		
Suprahyoid muscles	Affect movement of the tongue; elevate the hyoid bone;	Neck and throat

(Continued)

Muscle Name	Function	Trigger Point Referred Pain Pattern*
MUSCLES OF THE NECK—CONT'D	help produce sound and speech; draw the larynx and thyroid cartilage downward; depress the larynx; and elevate the thyroid cartilage.	
Infrahyoid muscles	Depress the hyoid bone; influence swallowing; and help produce sound.	Neck and throat
Sternocleidomastoideus	Assists in flexing the cervical portion of the vertebral column forward, elevating the thorax, and extending the head at the atlantooccipital joint; stabilizes the head; and resists forceful backward movement of the head, tilts head, rotates the head, and simultaneously acts to control rotation.	Several trigger points are located at the entire length of both divisions of the muscle. Head and face, particularly the occipital region, ear, and forehead. Autonomic nervous system phenomena and proprioceptive disturbances are common.
Posterior Triangle of the Neck		
Longus colli and capitus	Bend the neck forward (flexion); oblique portion bends neck laterally; inferior portion rotates neck to the opposite side; control acceleration of cervical extension, lateral extension, and contralateral rotation; and provide dynamic stabilization of cervical spine.	These muscles are difficult to palpate, and so no specific trigger point locations have been identified.
SCALENE GROUP		
Scalenus anterior	Bends the cervical portion of the vertebral column forward (flexion) and laterally; also rotates to the opposite side and assists in elevation of the first rib, thus functioning as an accessory muscle of respiration; checks (decelerates) cervical lateral flexion and rotation; and stabilizes cervical spine.	Pectoral region, rhomboid region, and the entire length of the arm into the hand
Scalenus medius	Acting from above, helps to raise the first rib, thus functioning as an accessory muscle of respiration; acting from below, bends the cervical part of the vertebral column to the same side; assists flexion of the neck; checks (decelerates) cervical lateral flexion and rotation; and stabilizes the cervical spine.	Pectoral region, rhomboid region, and the entire length of the arm into the hand
Scalenus posterior	When the second rib is fixed, bends the lower end of the cervical portion of the vertebral column to the same side	Pectoral region, rhomboid region, and the entire length of the arm into the hand

Muscle Name	Function	Trigger Point Referred Pain Pattern*
SCALENE GROUP—CONT'D	(lateral flexion); when the upper attachment is fixed, helps to elevate the second rib, thus functioning as an accessory muscle of respiration; checks (decelerates) cervical lateral flexion and rotation; and stabilizes the cervical spine.	
Deep Posterior Cervical Muscles Splenius capitis and cervicis	Extend the head and neck, draw the head dorsally and laterally and rotate the head to the same side; check and control cervical flexion and contralateral rotation; and stabilize the cervical spine.	Belly of the muscles closer to the head; to the top of the skull (the pain often feels as if it is inside the head), to the eye, and into the shoulder
Erector Spinae Group Spinalis thoracis, cervicis, and capitis Longissimus thoracis, cervicis, and capitis Iliocostalis lumborum, thoracis, and cervicis	Extend, rotate, and laterally flex the vertebral column and head; assist with anterior tilt elevation and rotation of the pelvis and spinal stabilization; control and decelerate vertebral flexor rotation and lateral flexion; and stabilize lumbar spine primarily.	Scapular, lumbar, abdominal, and gluteal areas, bandlike headache into the eyes, stiff neck
Oblique muscles, transversospinalis group: Semispinalis thoracis, cervicis, and capitis Multifidus Rotatores Intertransversarii lumborum, thoracis, and cervicis Interspinales	This group of muscles extends the motion segments of the back; rotates the thoracic, cervical, and lumbar vertebral joints; and stabilizes the vertebral column.	Scapular, lumbar, abdominal, and gluteal areas, bandlike headache into the eyes, stiff neck
Suboccipital muscles Rectus capitis posterior major and minor Oblique capitis superior and inferior	As a group these muscles extend and rotate the head in small, precise movements. More often these muscles isometrically function as stabilizers of the head and provide proprioceptive input about head position. These muscles are also important postural muscles and are neuro-reporting stations on balance and proprioceptive monitors of cervical spine and neck position.	Belly of the muscle, located with deep palpation at the base of the skull, around the ear on the same side; sensation of compressed junction of skull and neck, bandlike headache
MUSCLES OF THE TORSO **Muscles of the Thorax and Posterior Abdominal Wall** Diaphragm	Participates in respiration; during inspiration (breathing in),	None identified

(Continued)

Muscle Name	Function	Trigger Point Referred Pain Pattern*
MUSCLES OF THE TORSO—CONT'D		
	diaphragmatic contractions increase the capacity of the thoracic cavity; controls expiration as the diaphragm relaxes; and during breath holding, assists in stabilizing the lumbar and pelvic floor.	
Serratus posterior superior	Assists in lifting the ribs during inspiration.	Under the scapula near the insertion of the muscle on the ribs and under the upper portion of the scapula
Serratus posterior inferior	Depresses last four ribs (9-12). Some studies disagree that this is the function, finding no electromyographic activity of this muscle during respiration. Seems to act as a stabilizer during forced expirations such as coughing.	Nagging ache in the area of the muscle
External intercostals	Elevate ribs and draw adjacent ribs together; lift ribs, increasing the volume of the thoracic cavity—contralateral torso rotation; and stabilize the thorax.	The intercostals can develop trigger points, which are located by palpating the muscles between the ribs. Pain spans the intercostal segment, especially noticed with deep breathing or rotational movement.
Internal intercostals	Depress ribs and draw adjacent ribs together, decreasing volume of thoracic cavity—ipsilateral torso rotation; stabilize the thorax.	The intercostals can develop trigger points, which are located by palpating the muscles between the ribs. Pain spans the intercostal segment, especially noticed with deep breathing or rotational movement.
Innermost intercostals	The muscles of this small group attach to the internal aspects of two adjoining ribs. They are believed to act with the internal intercostals.	The intercostals can develop trigger points, which are located by palpating the muscles between the ribs. Pain spans the intercostal segment, especially noticed with deep breathing or rotational movement.
Transversus thoracis	Draws anterior portion of the ribs caudally (reduces thoracic cavity); stabilizes the ribcage.	None identified
Quadratus lumborum	Draws last rib downward; flexes lumbar vertebral column laterally to the same side; acts to elevate and anteriorly tilt pelvis; acting bilaterally, extends the lumbar spine and assists forced exhalation, as when coughing; restrains and checks lateral flexion; and assists normal inhalation by	Gluteal and groin area, sacroiliac joint and greater trochanter: these points are implicated in most low back pain. The dual function of lumbar stabilization (isometric function) and respiration (concentric function) can cause severe pain in the low back with a cough or sneeze if these

Muscle Name	Function	Trigger Point Referred Pain Pattern*
MUSCLES OF THE TORSO—CONT'D		
	stabilizing the diaphragm and the twelfth rib and stabilizing the lumbar area.	trigger points are active. Low back pain often is related more to maintenance of posture than trigger point activity; therefore one commonly finds corresponding pain patterns in the muscles that laterally flex the head and neck, such as the scalene muscles.
Psoas major and minor	With origin fixed, flex the hip joint by flexing the femur on the pelvis; may assist in lateral rotation of the hip joint; acting bilaterally, flex the hip joint by flexing the trunk on the pelvis; can assist extension of the lumbar spine, increasing lumbar lordosis; acting unilaterally, may assist in lateral flexion of the trunk toward the same side; restrain and check trunk and hip extension and contralateral flexion of the trunk; control tendency of lordosis; and stabilize lumbar spine and help to maintain upright posture.	Entire lumbar area into the superior gluteal region; front of the thigh; menstrual aching; and can mimic appendicitis. Shortening is a major cause of low back pain. If tension or trigger point activity is located at insertion, pain can mimic a groin pull. Because of postural reflexes, muscles that flex the head and neck are facilitated with psoas activation. A common correlation exists between neck pain and stiffness and psoas pain and low back stiffness. Massage often must address both areas in sequence to be effective.
Iliacus	Flexes the hip joint; may assist in lateral rotation and abduction of the hip joint; with insertion fixed and acting bilaterally, flexes the hip joint by flexing the trunk on the femur; tilts pelvis forward (anterior) when legs are fixed; decelerates hip extension; and stabilizes the pelvis.	Inner border of the ilium behind the anterior superior iliac spine
Muscles of the Anterior Abdominal Wall		
Transversus abdominis	Constricts and compresses the abdomen, increasing intraabdominal pressure, and supports the abdominal viscera; assists in forced expiration.	Pain located throughout the area but concentrated more in the external circle of the abdominal wall rather than toward the middle near the umbilicus
Obliquus internus abdominis	Compresses the abdominal cavity (some isometric activity); assists with posterior tilt of the pelvis; flexes the vertebral column, bringing the costal cartilage toward the pubis; laterally bends and ipsilaterally rotates the vertebral column (brings the shoulder of the opposite side	Pain located throughout the area but concentrated more in the external circle of the abdominal wall rather than toward the middle near the umbilicus

(Continued)

Muscle Name	Function	Trigger Point Referred Pain Pattern*
MUSCLES OF THE TORSO—CONT'D		
	forward); and restrains trunk extension.	
Obliquus externus abdominis	Compresses the abdominal cavity (some isometric activity); assists in forced expiration; with both sides acting, flexes the vertebral column, bringing the pubis toward the xiphoid process of sternum; supports posterior pelvic rotation; laterally bends and brings the shoulder of the same side forward; and restrains trunk extension.	Pain located throughout the area but concentrated more in the external circle of the abdominal wall rather than toward the middle near the umbilicus
Rectus abdominis	Flexes the vertebral column, bringing the sternum toward the pelvis; compresses the abdominal cavity; assists with posterior tilt of the pelvis (some isometric activity); assists in forced expiration; and restrains trunk extension.	Trigger points often found in the rectus abdominis just below the umbilicus on either side of the linea alba and near the attachment on the ribs. Pain is referred in local area or to groin.
MUSCLES OF SCAPULAR STABILIZATION		
Trapezius	Upper trapezius elevates the shoulder and, with the shoulder fixed, can assist in drawing the head backward and laterally to tilt chin; the middle portion adducts (retracts) the scapula, draws back the acromion process, and rotates the scapula; lower fibers depress the scapula; the entire muscle, acting bilaterally, assists extension of the cervical and thoracic spine; upper trapezius restrains and controls flexion, lateral flexion, and rotation of the neck and head. Middle trapezius controls and restrains scapular abduction (protraction). Lower trapezius restrains scapular elevation. Trapezius stabilizes scapula and cervical spine.	Neck behind the ear and to the temple; subscapular area; acromial pain
Rhomboideus major and minor	Adduct (retract) and elevate the scapula and also rotate it downward so that the glenoid cavity faces down toward feet; restrain protraction and upward rotation of scapula; stabilize the scapula.	At the attachment point near the scapular border; scapular region
Levator scapulae	Raises the scapula and draws it medially; with the scapula fixed, extends the neck laterally	Belly of the muscle just as it begins the rotation and at the attachment near the scapula;

Muscle Name	Function	Trigger Point Referred Pain Pattern*
MUSCLES OF SCAPULAR STABILIZATION—CONT'D		
	and rotates it to the same side; bilaterally extends the neck; restrains and controls head and neck flexion, scapular depression, and lateral flexion of cervical spine; and stabilizes cervical/scapular function.	angle of the neck and along the vertebral border of the scapula; stiff neck in rotation
Pectoralis minor	Assists in drawing the scapula forward (protraction) around the chest wall; rotates the scapula to depress the point of the shoulder; assists in forced inspiration; restrains the scapula retraction; and stabilizes the scapula during movement.	Near the attachment at the coracoid process and at the belly of the muscle. May mimic angina with pain in front of the chest from the shoulder and down the ulnar side of the arm into the fingers.
Serratus anterior	Abducts (protracts) the scapula; rotates the scapula so that the glenoid cavity faces cranially (toward the head); raises the ribs with the scapula fixed and therefore is an accessory muscle of respiration; controls scapular retraction; and holds the medial border of the scapula firmly against the thorax and prevents winging of the scapula.	Along the midaxillary line near the ribs; side and back of the chest and down the ulnar aspect of the arm into the hand. May result in shortness of breath and pain during inhalation.
MUSCLES OF THE MUSCULOTENDINOUS (ROTATOR) CUFF		
Supraspinatus	Abducts the arm; restrains adduction of the arm; and acts to stabilize the humeral head in the glenoid cavity during movements of the shoulder joint.	Shoulder, deltoid, and down the arm to the elbow, often experienced as a dull ache
Infraspinatus	Provides lateral or external rotation of the arm at the shoulder; restrains and controls internal (medial) rotation of the arm at the shoulder; and acts to stabilize the humeral head in the glenoid cavity during movements of the shoulder joint.	Deep into the shoulder and deltoid area, down the arm, suboccipital area, medial border of the scapula, with limits reaching behind back
Teres minor	Provides adduction and lateral (external) rotation of the arm; restrains internal (medial) rotation of arm; and acts to stabilize the humeral head in the glenoid cavity during movements of the shoulder joint.	Posterior deltoid region; client often experiences limited range of motion when reaching behind the back, such as putting hands in back pocket of pants.
Subscapularis	Rotates humerus medially (internal rotation) and draws it	Access is through the axilla near the attachment at the

(Continued)

Muscle Name	Function	Trigger Point Referred Pain Pattern*
MUSCLES OF THE MUSCULOTENDINOUS (ROTATOR) CUFF—CONT'D	forward and down when the arm is raised; restrains lateral (external) rotation of the arm; and stabilizes humeral head in the glenoid fascia during movement of the shoulder.	humerus and in the belly of the muscle. Pain in posterior deltoid, scapular region, triceps area and into the wrist often is mistaken for bursitis because pain often refers to the insertion at the shoulder.
MUSCLES OF THE SHOULDER JOINT		
Deltoideus	Provides flexion and medial and lateral rotation of the arm and abduction of the arm. Anterior deltoid restrains and controls extensor and external rotator of the arm. Middle deltoid restrains arm adduction. Posterior deltoid restrains flexion and internal rotators and horizontal adduction of the arm. Deltoid stabilizes glenohumeral joint during arm movement.	Deltoid region and down the lateral side of the arm
Pectoralis major	With proximal attachment (origin) fixed, adducts and draws the humerus forward (flexion) and horizontal and medially (internally) rotates it; with insertion fixed and arm abducted, assists in elevating the thorax (as in forced inspiration); controls arm extension, horizontal abduction, and external rotation; and stabilizes the shoulder during overhead activity.	Chest and breast and down the ulnar aspect of the arm to the fourth and fifth fingers
Subclavius	Draws the clavicle forward and down; stabilizes the clavicle.	Chest and breast and down the ulnar aspect of the arm to the fourth and fifth fingers
Latissimus dorsi	With proximal attachment (origin) fixed, medially or internally rotates, adducts, and extends the humerus; depresses the shoulder girdle and assists in lateral flexion of the trunk; with insertion fixed, assists in tilting the pelvis anteriorly and laterally; acting bilaterally, assists in hyperextending the spine and tilting the pelvis anteriorly; controls abduction, flexion, and external (lateral) rotation of humerus; and stabilizes the lumbar and pelvic area by maintaining tension on the thoracolumbar fascia.	Posterior axillary area just as the muscle begins to twist around the teres major; belly of the muscle near the rib attachments; just below the scapula and into the ulnar side of the arm; anterior deltoid region and abdominal oblique area.

Muscle Name	Function	Trigger Point Referred Pain Pattern*
MUSCLES OF THE SHOULDER JOINT—CONT'D		
Teres major	Medially or internally rotates, adducts, and extends the arm; upwardly rotates the scapula; controls and restrains flexion, abduction, and external rotation of the arm; and stabilizes the glenohumeral joint.	Near the musculotendinous junction at both attachments; posterior deltoid region and down the dorsal portion of the arm
Coracobrachialis	Flexes and adducts the humerus; controls extension and abduction of the humerus; stabilizes the shoulder and scapula.	Front of shoulder, posterior aspect of the arm down the triceps and dorsal forearm into the dorsal hand
MUSCLES OF THE ELBOW AND RADIOULNAR JOINTS		
Biceps brachii	Provides flexion of the humerus. The long head may assist with abduction if the humerus is laterally rotated. The short head assists arm adduction. With proximal attachment (origin) fixed, flexes the forearm toward the humerus and supinates the forearm; with insertion fixed, flexes the elbow joint, moving the humerus toward the forearm, as in a pull-up or chin-up; restrains and controls elbow extension and extension of the humerus; stabilizes the humerus at the shoulder and the elbow joint during full extension; and stabilizes the elbow when flexed and holding a weight.	Front of the shoulder at the anterior deltoid region and into the scapular region; also into the antecubital space or the front of the elbow
Brachialis	Flexes the elbow joint; restrains and controls elbow extension; stabilizes the elbow in full extension and fixed flexion.	Primarily to the thumb, with some pain in the anterior deltoid area and at the elbow
Brachioradialis	Flexes the elbow joint after brachialis and biceps initiate movement; assists in pronation and supination of the forearm to midposition; restrains and controls elbow extension; and stabilizes the elbow in full extension and fixed flexion.	Wrist and base of the thumb in the web space between the thumb and index finger and to the lateral epicondyle at the elbow
Pronator teres	Pronates the forearm; assists in flexing the elbow joint; controls supination of the forearm; and stabilizes the elbow joint and radioulnar joint.	Radial side of the forearm into the wrist and thumb. Pain may mimic carpal tunnel syndrome.
Supinator	Supinates the forearm; assists with flexion of the forearm at the elbow when the hand is held half way between supination and pronation;	Lateral epicondyle and dorsal aspect of the arm (pain mimics tennis elbow); near the radius in the antecubital space

(Continued)

Muscle Name	Function	Trigger Point Referred Pain Pattern*
MUSCLES OF THE ELBOW AND RADIOULNAR JOINTS—CONT'D		
	restrains and controls pronation of the forearm; and stabilizes the elbow and radioulnar joint.	
Pronator quadratus	Provides pronation of the forearm; restrains and controls supination of the forearm.	Belly of the muscle; active supination
Triceps brachii	Extension of the forearm; in addition, the long head adducts and assists in extension of the humerus; restrains elbow flexion and arm abduction and flexion; stabilizes the elbow in extension and fixed flexion to allow carrying weight in the hands; and assists in stabilizing the glenohumeral joint.	Length of posterior arm
Anconeus (elbow)	Assists the triceps in extension of the elbow joint; balances elbow flexion; and stabilizes the joint capsule of the elbow.	Elbow at lateral epicondyle
MUSCLES OF THE WRIST AND HAND JOINTS **Anterior Flexor Group:** **Superficial Layer**		
Flexor carpi radialis	Flexes and abducts the wrist (radial deviation); may assist in pronation of the forearm and flexion of the elbow; restrains and controls extension and adduction of the wrist; and stabilizes the wrist.	Into the wrist and fingers; occasionally into the elbow
Palmaris longus	Flexes the wrist; may assist in flexion of the elbow and pronation of the forearm; restrains wrist extension; and tenses the palmar fascia.	Into the wrist and fingers; occasionally into the elbow
Flexor carpi ulnaris	Flexes and adducts (ulnar deviation) the wrist; may assist in elbow flexion; controls and restrains wrist extension and abduction; and stabilizes wrist.	Into the wrist and fingers; occasionally into the elbow
Flexor digitorum superficialis	Flexes the proximal interphalangeal joints of the second through fifth digits; assists in flexion of the wrist; restrains and controls finger extension; and stabilizes wrist and hand joints.	Into the wrist and fingers; occasionally into the elbow
Flexor digitorum profundus	Flexes the distal interphalangeal joints of the second through fifth digits; assists in flexion of the proximal interphalangeal and metacarpophalangeal joints;	Into the wrist and fingers; occasionally into the elbow

Muscle Name	Function	Trigger Point Referred Pain Pattern*
MUSCLES OF THE WRIST AND HAND JOINTS—CONT'D		
	assists in adduction of the index, ring, and little fingers and in flexion of the wrist; restrains and controls extension of the fingers; and stabilizes the fingers.	
Flexor pollicis longus	Flexes interphalangeal joint of the thumb; assists in flexion of the metacarpophalangeal and carpometacarpal joints; restrains thumb; and stabilizes the thumb.	Thumb
Posterior Extensor Group: Superficial Layer		
Extensor carpi radialis longus	Extends and abducts (ulnar deviation) the wrist; may assist in flexion of the elbow and pronation of the forearm; restrains and controls wrist flexion and adduction; and stabilizes the wrist and elbow joints.	From the lateral epicondyle at the elbow down the dorsum of the forearm to various parts of the hand, especially to the web of the thumb
Extensor carpi radialis brevis	Extends the wrist and assists in abduction (radial deviation) of wrist and weak flexion of the forearm; restrains and controls wrist flexion and adduction; and stabilizes the wrist.	From the lateral epicondyle at the elbow down the dorsum of the forearm to various parts of the hand, especially to the web of the thumb
Extensor digitorum	Extends the metacarpophalangeal joints; extends the interphalangeal joint of the second through fifth digits (with the lumbricales and interosseous muscles); assists in extension of the wrist; restrains and controls wrist and finger flexion; and stabilizes the wrist.	From the lateral epicondyle at the elbow down the dorsum of the forearm to various parts of the hand, especially to the web of the thumb
Extensor digiti minimi	Extends the metacarpophalangeal and (with the interosseous and lumbrical muscles) the interphalangeal joints of the little finger; assists in abduction of the little finger; controls and restrains flexion and adduction of the little finger; and stabilizes the joints of the little finger.	From the lateral epicondyle at the elbow down the dorsum of the forearm to various parts of the hand, especially to the web of the thumb
Extensor carpi ulnaris	Extends and abducts (ulnar deviation) the wrist; controls wrist flexion and adduction; and stabilizes the wrist.	From the lateral epicondyle at the elbow down the dorsum of the forearm to various parts of the hand, especially to the web of the thumb
Extensor pollicis brevis	Extends and abducts the carpometacarpal joint of the	From the lateral epicondyle at the elbow down the dorsum of

(Continued)

Muscle Name	Function	Trigger Point Referred Pain Pattern*
MUSCLES OF THE WRIST AND HAND JOINTS—CONT'D	thumb; extends the metacarpophalangeal joint; assists in abduction (radial deviation) of the wrist; assists supination of the forearm; restrains flexion of the thumb and adduction of the wrist; and stabilizes the thumb.	the forearm to various parts of the hand, especially to the web of the thumb
Posterior Extensor Group: Deep Layer		
Abductor pollicis longus	Abducts and extends the carpometacarpal joint of the thumb; abducts (radial deviation) and assists in wrist flexion and supination of the forearm; controls thumb adduction; and stabilizes thumb and wrist.	To the web of the thumb
Extensor pollicis longus	Extends the interphalangeal joint and assists in extension of the metacarpophalangeal and carpometacarpal joints of the thumb; assists in abduction (radial deviation) and extension of the wrist; restrains thumb and wrist flexion; and stabilizes thumb and wrist.	To the web of the thumb
Extensor indicis	Extends the metacarpophalangeal joint and, with the lumbrical and interosseous muscles, extends the interphalangeal joints of the index finger; may assist in adduction of the index finger and supination of the forearm; and restrains, stabilizes, and controls flexion of the index finger.	Dorsum of the forearm to various parts of the hand
INTRINSIC MUSCLES OF THE HAND **Thenar Eminence Muscles**		
Opponens pollicis	Adducts the carpometacarpal joint of the thumb; adducts and assists in flexion of the metacarpophalangeal joint; aids in opposition of the thumb to each of the other digits; controls and restrains abduction of the thumb; and stabilizes the thumb.	Into the thumb and the wrist
Abductor pollicis brevis	Abducts and aids in opposition of the thumb; controls and restrains abduction of the thumb; and stabilizes thumb.	Into the thumb and the wrist

Muscle Name	Function	Trigger Point Referred Pain Pattern*
INTRINSIC MUSCLES OF THE HAND—CONT'D		
Flexor pollicis brevis	Flexes the proximal phalanx of the thumb; assists in opposition of the thumb; restrains and controls flexion of the thumb; and stabilizes the thumb.	Into the thumb and the wrist
Hypothenar Muscles		
Opponens digiti minimi	Provides flexion and slight rotation of the carpometacarpal joint of the little finger; helps to cup the palm of the hand; and stabilizes the little finger.	The little finger and wrist
Abductor digiti minimi	Abducts and assists in extension of the metacarpophalangeal joint of the little finger; controls and restrains abduction and extension of the little finger; and stabilizes the little finger.	The little finger and wrist
Flexor digiti minimi (brevis)	Flexes the metacarpophalangeal joint of the little finger; assists in opposition of the little finger to the thumb; controls extension of the little finger; and stabilizes the little finger.	The little finger and wrist
Deep Muscles of the Hand		
Adductor pollicis	Adducts the thumb and aids in opposition; restrains thumb abduction; and stabilizes the thumb.	The thumb
Interossei palmares	Adducts the index, ring, and little fingers toward the middle digit; assists in restraining abduction of the fingers; and stabilizes the hand.	Into the associated finger
Interossei dorsales	Abducts the index, middle, and ring fingers from the midline of the hand.	Into the associated finger
Lumbricales	Extends the interphalangeal joints and simultaneously flexes the metacarpophalangeal joint of the second through fifth digits.	Into the associated finger
MUSCLES OF THE GLUTEAL REGION		
Gluteus maximus	Extends and laterally rotates the hip joint; upper fibers assist abduction of the hip; lower fibers assist in adduction of the hip joint; with femur fixed, assists in extension of the trunk and posterior tilt of the pelvis; the gluteus maximus is active primarily during strenuous	Regionally into the gluteal region, especially to the ischial tuberosity, the tip of the greater trochanter, and the sacrum

(Continued)

Muscle Name	Function	Trigger Point Referred Pain Pattern*
MUSCLES OF THE GLUTEAL REGION—CONT'D		
	activity, such as running, jumping, and climbing stairs; and restrains and controls hip and trunk flexion and medial rotation and abduction of the hip. These muscles are important postural muscles that help maintain the upright posture, stabilize the pelvis, and provide tension to the iliotibial tract to keep the fascial band taut.	
Gluteus medius	Abducts the hip joint; anterior fibers medially rotate and assist in flexion of the hip joint and anterior tilt of the pelvis; posterior fibers laterally rotate and assist in extension of the hip joint and posterior tilt of the pelvis; restrains lateral rotation and extension of the hip; and stabilizes the pelvis when a person is standing on one foot.	Along the musculotendinous junction at the iliac crest; low back, posterior crest of the ilium to the sacrum, and to the posterior and lateral areas of the buttock into the upper thigh
Gluteus minimus	Abducts the hip joint and medially rotates the thigh when the limb is extended; restrains and controls hip adductors and lateral rotation; and keeps the pelvis level when a person is standing on one foot.	Lower lateral buttock and down the lateral to posterior aspect of the thigh, knee, and leg to the ankle
Tensor fasciae latae	Flexes, medially rotates, and may assist in abduction of the hip joint; assists in anterior pelvic tilt; extends the knee; restrains hip extension and lateral rotation; tenses the iliotibial tract, counterbalancing the backward pull of the gluteus maximus on the iliotibial tract; and stabilizes the pelvis and knee.	Localized in the hip and down the lateral side of the leg to the knee
Deep Lateral Rotators		
Piriformis Obturator internus and externus Gemellus superior and inferior	Provide lateral rotation and abduction of the hip joint when the thigh is flexed and posterior pelvic tilt; restrain medial rotation and adduction of the hip; and stabilize the hip joint.	The belly of each muscle can house trigger points. Sacroiliac region, entire buttock, and down the posterior thigh to just above the knee
Quadratus femoris	Laterally rotates the hip joint and adducts the thigh; restrains internal rotation and abduction of the hip joint; and stabilizes the hip joint.	The main trigger points are near the attachments and the insertion. Tension in this muscle may cause deep hip and groin pain.

Muscle Name	Function	Trigger Point Referred Pain Pattern*
MUSCLES OF THE POSTERIOR THIGH		
Semimembranosus	Flexes the knee and medially rotates the knee joint when the knee is semiflexed; moves the medial meniscus posteriorly during knee flexion; extends and assists in medial rotation and adduction of the hip joint; posteriorly tilts the pelvis; restrains and controls knee extension and lateral rotation; assists in controlling lateral rotation of the hip and flexors; and stabilizes the knee and hip complex.	Several areas in the belly of each muscle and at the musculotendinous junction nearer the knee; ischial tuberosity, back of the knee, and the entire posterior leg to midcalf
Semitendinosus	Flexes the knee and medially rotates the knee joint when the knee is semiflexed; extends and assists in medial rotation and adduction of the hip joint; restrains and controls knee extension and lateral rotation; assists in controlling lateral rotation of the hip and flexors; and stabilizes the knee and hip complex.	Several areas in the belly of each muscle and at the musculotendinous junction nearer the knee; ischial tuberosity, back of the knee, and the entire posterior leg to midcalf
Biceps femoris	Flexes and laterally rotates the knee joint when the knee is semiflexed; long head also extends and assists in lateral rotation of the hip joint and posteriorly tilts the pelvis; restrains and controls knee extension and medial rotation; also restrains hip flexion and medial rotation; and stabilizes the hip and knee complex.	Several areas in the belly of each muscle and at the musculotendinous junction nearer the knee; ischial tuberosity, back of the knee, and the entire posterior leg to midcalf
MUSCLES OF THE MEDIAL THIGH		
Pectineus	Adducts, flexes, and assists in medial rotation of the hip joint and anterior tilt of the pelvis; restrains abduction, extension, and lateral rotation of hip; and stabilizes the hip.	Deep in the groin into the medial thigh and downward to the knee and shin. Pain may mimic hamstring tension.
Adductor brevis	Adducts and assists in flexing the hip joint anteriorly and tilts the pelvis; restrains and controls abduction and extension of the hip; and stabilizes the hip and trunk in the standing position.	Deep in the groin into the medial thigh and downward to the knee and shin. Pain may mimic hamstring tension.

(Continued)

Muscle Name	Function	Trigger Point Referred Pain Pattern*
MUSCLES OF THE MEDIAL THIGH—CONT'D		
Adductor longus	Adducts and assists in flexing the hip joint and anteriorly tilts the pelvis; restrains and controls abduction and extension of the hip; and stabilizes the hip and trunk in the standing position.	Deep in the groin into the medial thigh and downward to the knee and shin. Pain may mimic hamstring tension.
Adductor magnus	Adducts the hip joint and posteriorly tilts the pelvis; upper portion medially rotates and flexes, whereas the lower portion laterally rotates and extends the hip joint; restrains and controls hip abduction; and stabilizes the trunk, pelvis, and hip.	Deep in the groin into the medial thigh and downward to the knee and shin. Pain may mimic hamstring tension.
Gracilis	Adducts and flexes the hip joint; assists with anterior tilt of the pelvis; flexes the knee and medially rotates the knee joint when the knee is semiflexed; controls and restrains hip abduction and extension and knee extension and lateral rotation; and assists in controlling and stabilizing the valgus angulation of the knee and stabilizing the pelvic and knee complex.	Deep in the groin into the medial thigh and downward to the knee and shin. Pain may mimic hamstring tension.
MUSCLES OF THE ANTERIOR THIGH		
Sartorius	Flexes, laterally rotates, and abducts the hip joint; also weakly flexes the torso toward the pelvis when the leg is fixed and anteriorly and laterally tilts the pelvis; flexes and assists in medial rotation of the knee joint; controls and restrains extension, medial rotation, and adduction of the hip and assists in restraining trunk extension; at the knee, restrains and controls extension and lateral rotation of the knee; and stabilizes the knee and hip complex.	Into hip and medial knee
Quadriceps Femoris Group		
Rectus femoris	Extends the knee joint; flexes the hip joint; anteriorly tilts the pelvis; restrains and controls knee flexion and hip extension; and stabilizes the knee and hip complex.	Into hip and knee
Vastus lateralis	Extends the knee joint and exerts a lateral pull on the	Into hip and lateral knee

Muscle Name	Function	Trigger Point Referred Pain Pattern*
MUSCLES OF THE ANTERIOR THIGH—CONT'D		
	patella; controls and restrains knee flexion and medial pull of patella; and stabilizes iliotibial tract and knee.	
Vastus medialis	Extends the leg and draws the patella medially, particularly the lower oblique aspect of the muscle (vastus medialis oblique) with attachment into the adductor magnus; controls and restrains knee flexion and lateral movement of patella; and stabilizes the knee and patella.	Entire anterior thigh, with concentration at the knee
Vastus intermedius	Extends the knee joint; restrains and controls knee flexion; and stabilizes the knee and patella.	Into the knee
MUSCLES OF THE ANTERIOR AND LATERAL LEG **Anterior Muscles**		
Tibialis anterior	Provides dorsiflexion of the ankle joint; assists in inversion and adduction of the foot. Note: Combined action of eversion and adduction results in supination. Eccentric function: Restrains and controls plantar flexion and eversion of the foot. Isometric function: Stabilizes the ankle.	Down the leg to the ankle and into the toes
Extensor digitorum longus	Extends the phalanges of the second through fifth digits; assists in dorsiflexion of the ankle joint and eversion and abduction of the foot; restrains and controls flexion of the toes, plantar flexion, and invasion of the ankle and foot; and stabilizes the ankle and foot.	Down the leg to the ankle and into the toes
Extensor hallucis longus	Extends the metatarsophalangeal joint of the great toe; also assists in inverting and adducting (supination) the foot and dorsiflexing the ankle joint; restrains and controls flexion of the great toes, eversion of the foot, and plantar flexion of the ankle; and stabilizes the great toe and assists in stabilizing the ankle.	Down the leg to the ankle and into the toes
Fibularis (peroneus) tertius	Dorsiflexes the ankle joint; everts and abducts (pronates) the foot; assists in controlling	Down the leg to the ankle

(Continued)

Muscle Name	Function	Trigger Point Referred Pain Pattern*
MUSCLES OF THE ANTERIOR AND LATERAL LEG—CONT'D	and restraining plantar flexion of the ankle and inversion of the foot; and assists in stabilizing the ankle.	
Lateral Muscles		
Fibularis (peroneus) longus and brevis	Everts and abducts (pronates) the foot; assists in plantar flexion of the ankle joint; restrains and controls dorsiflexion of the ankle and inversion of the foot; and stabilizes the ankle.	To the malleolus lateralis and the heel
POSTERIOR LEG MUSCLES		
Popliteus	Assists in restraining knee extension; stabilizes the knee.	To the back of the knee
Tibialis posterior	Inverts the foot; assists in plantar flexion of the ankle joint; restrains and controls eversion of the foot and dorsiflexion of the ankle; and stabilizes the ankle.	Down the posterior leg to the heel and the sole of the foot into the plantar surface of the toes. Can be a factor in knee pain and restricted mobility of the knee and ankle.
Flexor digitorum longus	Flexes the joints of the second through fifth digits; assists in plantar flexion of the ankle joint and inversion and adduction (supination) of the foot; restrains and controls extension of the toes and assists in controlling dorsiflexion of the ankle and eversion of the foot; and stabilizes the ankle and toes.	Down the posterior leg to the heel and the sole of the foot into the plantar surface of the toes. Can be a factor in knee pain and restricted mobility of the knee and ankle.
Flexor hallucis longus	Flexes the joints of the great toe; provides plantar flexion of the ankle joint and inverts the foot; restrains extension of the great toe and assists in controlling dorsiflexion of the ankle and eversion of the foot; and stabilizes the great toe, ankle, and foot.	Down the posterior leg to the heel and the sole of the foot into the plantar surface of the great toe
Plantaris	Provides plantar flexion of the ankle joint; assists in flexion of the knee joint; restrains dorsiflexion of the ankle and assists in controlling extension of the knee; and assists in stabilizing the ankle/knee complex.	Can be a factor in knee pain and restricted mobility of the knee and ankle.
Soleus	Provides plantar flexion of the ankle joint and assists inversion of the foot at the ankle; restrains and controls	Down the posterior leg to the heel and the sole of the foot into the plantar surface of the toes. Can restrict mobility of the ankle.

Muscle Name	Function	Trigger Point Referred Pain Pattern*
POSTERIOR LEG MUSCLES—CONT'D		
	dorsiflexion and eversion of the ankle; and stabilizes the leg over the foot and ankle.	
Gastrocnemius	Provides plantar flexion of the ankle joint; assists in flexion of the knee joint and inversion of the foot; restrains and controls dorsiflexion of the ankle and extension of the knee; and stabilizes the knee and ankle complex and is involved in maintaining balance in static standing.	Down the posterior leg to the heel and the sole of the foot into the plantar surface of the toes. Can be a factor in knee pain and restricted mobility of the knee and ankle.
MUSCLES OF THE FOOT		
Dorsal Aspect		
Extensor digitorum brevis	Extends metatarsophalangeal joint of the first toe and extends the interphalangeal and metatarsophalangeal joints of the second through fourth toes.	The entire foot with areas concentrated at the toes, the ball of the foot, and the heel
Plantar Aspect: Superficial Layer		
Abductor hallucis	Abducts and assists in flexion of the metatarsophalangeal joint of the large toe.	The entire foot with areas concentrated at the large toe, the ball of the foot, and the heel
Flexor digitorum brevis	Flexes the proximal interphalangeal joints and assists in flexion of the metatarsophalangeal joints of the second through fifth toes.	The entire foot with areas concentrated at the toes, the ball of the foot, and the heel
Abductor digiti minimi	Abducts and assists in flexing the metatarsophalangeal joint of the fifth toe.	The entire foot with areas concentrated at the small toe
Plantar Aspect: Second Layer		
Quadratus plantae	Modifies the line of pull of the flexor digitorum longus and assists in flexion of the second through the fifth digits.	The entire foot
Lumbricales	These muscles flex the metatarsophalangeal joints and extend the interphalangeal joints of the second through the fifth digits.	Several areas concentrated in the belly of each muscle; the entire foot with areas concentrated at the large toe, the ball of the foot, and the heel
Plantar Aspect: Third Layer		
Flexor hallucis brevis	Flexes the metatarsophalangeal joint of the large toe.	The entire foot with areas concentrated at the large toe
Adductor hallucis	Adducts and assists in flexion of the metatarsophalangeal joint of the large toe.	The entire foot with areas concentrated at the large toe
Flexor digiti minimi brevis	Flexes the metatarsophalangeal joint of the fifth toe.	The entire foot with areas concentrated at the toes

(Continued)

Muscle Name	Function	Trigger Point Referred Pain Pattern*
MUSCLES OF THE FOOT—CONT'D		
Plantar Aspect: Fourth Layer		
Interossei plantares	These muscles adduct the third, fourth, and fifth toes toward an axis through the second toe; assist in flexion of the metatarsophalangeal joints of the third through fifth toes.	The entire foot
Interossei dorsales	These muscles abduct the second, third, and fourth toes from a longitudinal axis through the second toe; also assist in flexion of the metatarsophalangeal joints of the second through the fourth digits and extension of interphalangeal joint of the second through fourth digits.	The entire foot

From Fritz S: *Mosby's essential sciences for therapeutic massage,* ed 2, St Louis, 2004, Mosby.
* The most common location of trigger points is in the belly of the muscles or at the attachments.

CHAPTER

30

Diseases and Indications/Contraindications to Massage Therapy

Disease	Indications/Contraindications of Massage Therapy	Mosby's Essential Sciences for Therapeutic Massage
Alzheimer's disease	The degeneration of Alzheimer's disease may be slowed with therapeutic intervention and medication. Studies indicate that sensory stimulation modalities such as rhythmic massage and movement may provide calming and orienting influences.	4
Amyotrophic lateral sclerosis Also known as Lou Gehrig disease, ALS is a progressive disease beginning in the central nervous system that involves the degeneration of motor neurons and eventually results in the atrophy of voluntary muscle.	Massage is indicated for ALS, with caution and under a doctor's supervision. The degrees of pressure and intensity need to be adjusted as the disease progresses. General constitutional methods are indicated. The practitioner should avoid stressing the system and should work toward general restorative processes that reduce pain, support sleep, and create an overall sense of well-being.	4
Aneurysm An aneurysm is a weakening and bulging of any artery, including those in the brain.	Contraindicated. Refer client immediately to a physician.	4
Ankylosing spondylitis Also called rheumatoid inflammatory disorder, this disease destroys the articular hyaline cartilage, causing the bones to fuse and spinal ligaments to ossify, and tends to begin in the sacroiliac joints and progress up the spine.	Massage therapy modalities are effective in managing backache. The benefits derived are from reduction in protective muscle spasm compensation (guarding) and generalized pain-modulating effects. Be aware that protective spasm provides stabilization. The goal is not to eliminate protective spasm but to support the body in managing dysfunctional patterns. Complex backache involving the joint structures requires the practitioner to incorporate therapeutic massage into a total treatment program supervised by the appropriate health care professional.	8
Anterior compartment syndrome This syndrome covers any condition that increases pressure in the anterior compartment of the leg, interfering with blood flow and compressing the nerves.	Treatment is contraindicated regionally unless supervised by the diagnosing or treating health care provider. Massage methods may soften the connective tissue sheath, relieving some of the pressure, but could aggravate the flow to the area, thus increasing the pressure. Elevation and ice may help.	9

(Continued)

327

Disease	Indications/Contraindications of Massage Therapy	*Mosby's Essential Sciences for Therapeutic Massage*
Anxiety Endogenous anxiety is a biochemical phenomenon usually unrelated to environmental stimuli. Reactive, or exogenous, anxiety is prompted by an anxiety-provoking stimulus such as specific events, situations, relationships, or conflicts.	Massage and exercise often are effective as part of a comprehensive management strategy dealing with anxiety symptoms.	5
Bartholin's cyst The cyst occurs in the Bartholin's glands located on each side of the vaginal opening.	Most reproductive system conditions present regional contraindications. As with most chronic illness and pain, therapeutic massage offers generalized support for homeostasis and can offer palliative or comfort care for the maintenance of these conditions.	12
Bell's palsy This palsy causes partial or total paralysis of the facial muscles on one side as the result of inflammation or injury to the seventh cranial nerve.	Massage approaches for infectious disease can be supportive and can reduce stress. The practitioner must gauge the intensity and duration of any therapeutic intervention so that the demand to adapt does not overtax an already stressed system, aggravating the condition. The less-is-more philosophy of intervention, which calls for shorter, more frequent interventions, often is indicated.	5
Bladder infection (cystitis) The bacteria in the bladder spread from the perineal region.	Therapeutic massage modalities may be useful for pain and stress management, but only with the careful supervision of the treating physician. Acute infectious processes contraindicate massage until the infection has run its course. Therapeutic massage may support chronic infection treatment as part of a supervised treatment plan. Stress is a contributing factor to incontinence. Any form of stress management helps somewhat with stress and urge incontinence. The practitioner needs to consider that incontinent clients require frequent and easy access to the restroom.	12
Breathing pattern disorder This is a complex, altered breathing function.	Therapeutic massage approaches and moderate application of movement therapies such as tai chi, yoga, or aerobic exercise assist with breathing. Almost every meditation or relaxation system uses breathing patterns because they are a direct link to altering autonomic nervous system patterns, which in turn alter mood, feelings, and behavior.	12
Bursitis The inflammation of the bursae, especially those located between the bony prominences and a muscle or tendon such as in the shoulder, elbow, hip, or knee, usually results from trauma and repetitive use.	Therapeutic massage can be a beneficial adjunct treatment, especially with the symptomatic management of pain in supporting increase in range of motion. Massage directly over the bursas is contraindicated.	8
Carpal tunnel syndrome This syndrome results from irritation of the meridian nerve as it passes under the transverse carpal ligament into the wrist.	Various forms of massage application reduce muscle spasm, lengthen shortened muscles, and soften and stretch connective tissue, restoring a more normal space around the nerve and alleviating impingement. When massage is combined with other appropriate methods, surgery is seldom necessary. If surgery is	5

Disease	Indications/Contraindications of Massage Therapy	*Mosby's Essential Sciences for Therapeutic Massage*
	performed, the practitioner must manage adhesions appropriately to prevent reentrapment of the nerve by maintaining soft tissue suppleness around the healing surgical area and, as healing progresses, extending the soft tissue methods to deal with the forming scar more directly. Before doing any work near the site of a recent incision, one must obtain physician's approval. In general, work close to the surgical area can begin after the stitches have been removed and all inflammation is gone. Direct work on a new scar usually is safe 8 to 12 weeks into the healing period.	
Cervical cancer Cervical dysplasia is a change in the cells of the cervix. Some of these abnormal cells can develop into cancerous cells.	Massage for clients with malignancies is contraindicated unless the appropriate health care professional gives approval and supervision. As with most chronic illness and pain, therapeutic massage offers generalized support for homeostasis and can offer palliative or comfort care for the maintenance of these conditions.	12
Cervicitis Cervicitis is inflammation of the cervix.	Most reproductive system conditions present regional contraindications. As with most chronic illness and pain, therapeutic massage offers generalized support for homeostasis and can offer palliative or comfort care for the maintenance of these conditions.	12
Chorea Chorea results from the degeneration of neurons in the basal ganglia.	Therapeutic massage is supportive in a multidisciplinary treatment. The practitioner can manage secondary muscle tension effectively with massage therapy and other forms of soft tissue manipulation.	4
Cirrhosis Cirrhosis is infiltration of connective tissue into the functioning cells of the liver, causing slow deterioration of the liver.	Caution is indicated depending on degree of liver function. Nonstressful general massage may be beneficial in stress management.	12
Club foot This deformity is evident in most cases when a child is born with one or both feet bent downward and adducted; in other cases the feet are pointed upward and abducted.	If skeletal problems create or are part of a permanent condition, supportive care is required. Massage methods are helpful in managing compensatory muscle spasms and connective tissue changes. Light, superficial methods, such as the gentle laying on of hands, are helpful.	8
Colon cancer This cancer usually affects the lowest part of the rectum.	Comprehensive stress management programs with medical supervision, including therapeutic massage methods, are often effective in managing these conditions.	12
Concussion A concussion is a brain trauma that may be mild, moderate, or severe.	Massage and bodywork is an effective part of a supervised comprehensive care program. Massage and other forms of bodywork can help manage secondary muscle tension.	4
Conn's syndrome If caused by an adrenal tumor, the disease is primary hyperaldosteronism. In rare cases, if caused by a nonspecific enlargement of the adrenal glands, the disease is called aldosteronism.	After these conditions are diagnosed, stress management can be an important part of ongoing therapeutic management.	6

(Continued)

Disease	Indications/Contraindications of Massage Therapy	*Mosby's Essential Sciences for Therapeutic Massage*
Constipation Constipation is difficulty passing stools or an incomplete or infrequent passage of hard stools.	After this condition is diagnosed, stress management can be an important part of ongoing therapeutic management. A specific type of massage to the large intestine can assist in managing constipation. The practitioner can teach this method to the client for self-care. The method is contraindicated in inflammatory bowel disease, and one should obtain permission from the physician for any other conditions.	12
Contracture Contracture is the chronic shortening of a muscle, especially the connective tissue component.	Gentle, slow intervention using connective tissue methods and stretching may improve contractures. Applying massage may prevent or slow the development of a contracture. The practitioner must consider the reason for the contracture when developing a treatment plan.	9
Contusion A muscle bruise results from trauma to the muscles and involves local internal bleeding and inflammation.	Direct work over the area of injury is contraindicated regionally until all signs of inflammation have dissipated.	9
Cramps Cramps are painful muscle contractions, may result from mild myositis or fibromyositis, and can be a symptom of any irritation or of an electrolyte imbalance.	The practitioner can manage simple cramps or spasms by firmly pushing the belly of the muscle together or by initiating reciprocal inhibition, which involves placing the attachment and insertion of the cramping muscle close together and then contracting the antagonist. The muscle lengthens gently after the cramp or spasm subsides.	9
Cushing's syndrome This syndrome is caused by excessive production of adrenocorticotropic hormone in the body.	After diagnosis of these conditions, stress management can be an important part of ongoing therapeutic management.	6
Cystic fibrosis This genetic disease involves exocrine gland dysfunction.	Percussion helps loosen the phlegm but should not be attempted without medical supervision and training.	12
Depression Depression is associated with a decrease in the neurotransmitters norepinephrine, serotonin, and dopamine.	Therapeutic massage is supportive in a multidisciplinary treatment of depression because such methods influence serotonin, among other neurotransmitters. In addition, the practitioner can manage secondary muscle tension effectively with massage therapy and other forms of soft tissue manipulation.	4
Diabetes mellitus This disease results from the pancreas not producing enough insulin or not producing any insulin.	A general stress management program is supportive in managing diabetes. Therapeutic massage can be an integral part of such a program. An important part of working with the diabetic client is that massage be a part of an overall treatment program with medical supervision. Careful observation of the feet during massage supports a hygiene program. The practitioner should refer the client for immediate medical care for any noted tissue changes. In pain management of diabetic neuropathy, massage approaches used as part of a supervised program can prove beneficial for short-term reduction of pain symptoms.	6

Disease	Indications/Contraindications of Massage Therapy	Mosby's Essential Sciences for Therapeutic Massage
Disk degeneration Disk degeneration occurs when the fibrocartilage surrounding the intervertebral disk ruptures, releasing the nucleus pulposus, which cushions the vertebrae above and below.	Various forms of massage are important in managing the muscle spasm and pain. The muscle spasms serve a stabilizing and protective function called guarding. Without some protective spasm, the nerve could be damaged further, but too much muscle spasm increases the discomfort. Therapeutic intervention seeks to reduce pain and excessive tension and restore moderate mobility while allowing for the resourceful compensation produced by the muscle tension pattern.	5
Dislocation Dislocation is displacement of the bones of a joint; a subluxation is a partial dislocation.	Massage and bodywork are contraindicated locally over a trauma area until healing is complete. Light, subtle methods of touch therapies (e.g., a gentle laying on of hands) may be beneficial in diminishing pain. The process usually is calming and soothing, which encourages healing through stress management. Massage methods are beneficial in supporting the rest of the body during the healing process, especially in managing compensation patterns caused by immobilization of an area. Massage and other forms of bodywork can help manage secondary muscle tension.	8
Diverticula These small, saclike outpouchings of the intestinal wall occur in weak areas of the colon near where vessels are located.	Abdominal pain or referred back pain may indicate one of several gastrointestinal disorders. In such cases, referral is necessary for proper diagnosis.	12
Dupuytren's contracture This disorder is a thickened plaque overlying the tendon of the ring finger and occasionally the little finger at the level of the distal palmar crease.	Treatment is contraindicated regionally if methods increase symptoms.	9
Ectopic pregnancy Ectopic pregnancy occurs when the zygote fails to implant itself in the uterus and starts to develop in the fallopian tube.	Refer client immediately to a physician.	12
Edema Edema is a condition in which excess fluid accumulates within the interstitial spaces.	Therapeutic massage tends to increase blood volume through the kidneys via mechanical and reflexive processes. In the healthy individual, therapy supports the filtration process. For those with kidney disease the increased volume can strain the kidney function. General contraindications exist for anyone with kidney disease.	12
Emphysema This chronic pulmonary disease is marked by an abnormal increase in the size of air spaces distal to the terminal bronchiole, with destruction of the alveolar walls.	Simple palliative measures to provide comfort and encourage sleep are appropriate. In chronic conditions such as emphysema, general stress management and maintenance of normal function of the muscles of respiration are beneficial, again after one gauges the appropriate added stress levels caused by the massage stimulation.	12
Encephalitis Encephalitis is a bacterial or viral infection of the brain.	Infectious processes are contraindicated for massage intervention unless closely supervised by appropriate medical personnel. Refer a client with	4

(Continued)

Disease	Indications/Contraindications of Massage Therapy	*Mosby's Essential Sciences for Therapeutic Massage*
	unusual or unexplained stiff neck immediately for diagnosis.	
Endometriosis In this disease, endometrial tissue is present in nonuterine locations, such as the intestines, ovaries, or even in the fallopian tubes.	Most reproductive system conditions present regional contraindications. As with most chronic illness and pain, therapeutic massage offers generalized support for homeostasis and can offer palliative or comfort care for the maintenance of these conditions.	12
Epicondylitis Epicondylitis is inflammation of the epicondyle of the humerus and surrounding tissues.	Therapeutic massage can be a beneficial adjunct treatment, especially with the symptomatic management of pain supporting increase in range of motion.	8
Fibromyalgia This syndrome has symptoms of widespread pain or aching, persistent fatigue, generalized morning stiffness, nonrestorative sleep, and multiple tender points.	General constitutional approaches seem to work best to aid in symptomatic pain reduction and restoration of the sleep pattern. The client should avoid any form of therapy that causes therapeutic inflammation, including intense exercise and stretching programs, until healing mechanisms in the body are functioning. If tender points have been injected with antiinflammatory medications, anesthetics, or other substances, the practitioner should not massage over these areas.	9
Flaccid muscles Flaccid muscles have decreased tone.	Flaccid or spastic muscles often are associated with motor neuron disorders. The reason for the change in tone determines the appropriateness of therapeutic massage. These conditions differ from general muscle tension or weakness in that the dysfunction has a physical cause rather than a functional one.	9
Fracture Fractures are breaks or ruptures in a bone.	Massage and bodywork are contraindicated locally over a trauma area until healing is complete. Light, subtle methods of touch therapies (e.g., a gentle laying on of hands) may be beneficial in diminishing pain. Stress fractures may not be readily detectable. Referral is indicated if the history points toward a mechanical stress condition such as participation in a recent athletic event.	8
Gallbladder disease (cholelithiasis) The disease almost always results from a gallstone composed of bile salts and/or cholesterol lodged in the cystic duct.	Abdominal pain or referred back pain may indicate one of several gastrointestinal disorders. In such cases, referral is necessary for proper diagnosis. Many gastrointestinal diseases are bacterial or viral and are contagious. The practitioner should take appropriate precautions to maintain sanitary practice. Most chronic gastrointestinal diseases have a strong correlation to stress. The intestinal tract is highly responsive to changes in autonomic function and endocrine patterns. Sympathetic arousal changes peristaltic action and can send the intestinal tract into all kinds of dysfunction. Comprehensive stress management programs, including therapeutic massage methods, are often effective in managing these conditions.	12
Gibbus Gibbus is an angular deformity of a collapsed vertebra.	Most backaches are preventable. Massage therapy modalities are effective in managing backache. The benefits derived are from reduced protective muscle spasm compensation (guarding) and the generalized pain-modulating effects. Be aware that protective	8

Disease	Indications/Contraindications of Massage Therapy	*Mosby's Essential Sciences for Therapeutic Massage*
	spasm provides stabilization. The goal is not to eliminate protective spasm but to support the body in managing dysfunctional patterns. The joint structures require that therapeutic massage be incorporated into a total treatment program with supervision by the appropriate health care professional.	
Glomerulonephritis This group of diseases involves antigen-antibody reactions affecting the glomeruli.	Therapeutic massage tends to increase blood volume through the kidneys via mechanical and reflexive processes. In the healthy individual, therapy supports the filtration process. For those with kidney disease the increased volume can strain the kidney function. General contraindications exist for anyone with kidney disease. Therapeutic massage modalities may be useful for pain and stress management.	12
Gout Gout is a form of arthritis caused by a disturbance of metabolism.	Massage therapy is contraindicated regionally.	8
Growing pains These pains occur during growth spurts in children and adolescents when the bone grows faster than the attached muscles	Treatment of local areas may be contraindicated if inflammation is present. Methods that do not introduce any sort of therapeutic inflammation often soothe general growing pains. The practitioner should avoid intense stretching and frictioning methods. Methods that relax and lengthen the muscle and soften the connective tissue are appropriate.	7
Headache Pain occurs in the forehead, eyes, jaw, temples, scalp, skull, occiput, or neck.	Massage therapy is effective in treating muscle tension headache but much less so with migraine or cluster headaches and can relieve secondary muscle tension headache caused by the pain of the primary headache. Headache is often stress induced. Stress management in all forms usually is indicated in chronic headache conditions.	4
Hepatitis Hepatitis is an infection of the liver.	Abdominal pain or referred back pain may indicate one of several gastrointestinal disorders. In such cases, referral is necessary for proper diagnosis. Many gastrointestinal diseases are bacterial or viral and are contagious. The practitioner should take appropriate precautions to maintain sanitary practice.	12
Hernia Hernia usually is caused by the weakness of abdominal muscles or protrusion of an abdominal organ (commonly the small intestine) through an opening in the abdominal wall.	Treatment of a client with a hernia is contraindicated regionally, and referral is indicated for initial diagnosis or for any change in a hernia.	9
Hyperparathyroidism Primary hyperparathyroidism usually results from a benign tumor, and secondary hyperparathyroidism results mostly from kidney disease.	The symptoms of hyperparathyroidism include mild to severe skeletal pain. Osteoporosis may result as well. The client may seek therapeutic massage for these conditions, and massage practitioners must take care to provide the appropriate referral to determine the underlying cause of the problem.	6
Hyperthyroidism or thyrotoxicosis	Because thyroid conditions can go undiagnosed as a result of the symptoms being common to many	6

(Continued)

Disease	Indications/Contraindications of Massage Therapy	Mosby's Essential Sciences for Therapeutic Massage
These diseases result from overfunction of the thyroid.	stress-related conditions, referring clients for medical assessment to rule out thyroid dysfunction is important when they have any symptom of hyperthyroidism or hypothyroidism.	
Hypothyroidism This condition results from underfunction of the thyroid.	Some studies suggest that mild cases of hypothyroidism respond to cold water therapy and moderate aerobic exercise. Exposure to cold triggers release of thyroid-stimulating hormone. Therapeutic massage may be beneficial in managing symptoms of hyperthyroidism and hypothyroidism. Because thyroid conditions can go undiagnosed as a result of the symptoms being common to many stress-related conditions, referring clients for medical assessment to rule out thyroid dysfunction is important when they have any symptom of hyperthyroidism or hypothyroidism.	6
Immobilization External restraint mechanisms such as casts may cause reactions such as pain and inflammation or paralysis.	Dynamic movable splinting devices such as air casts and continuous passive motion devices that are capable of moving joints passively and repeatedly through a specified position of the physiologic range of motion have been beneficial in reducing immobilization in joints. Therapeutic massage can maintain pliability in accessible connective tissue structures. Therapeutic massage methods and movement approaches are beneficial in assisting a return to normal function after removal of the splinting.	8
Immune system	Therapeutic massage approaches support immune function by supporting balanced homeostatic functions. No specific methods are used for the immune system, yet any behavior that supports wellness, including regular massage, supports immunity. Any modality that normalizes autonomic nervous system functions supports immunity.	11
Infectious arthritis Infections such as rheumatic fever, gonorrhea, and tuberculosis can cause infectious arthritis.	Infectious disease is a contraindication of massage unless the appropriate health care professionals directly supervise the massage therapy.	8
Infertility Infertility is a decrease in the ability to conceive.	Most reproductive system conditions present regional contraindications. Therapeutic massage offers generalized support for homeostasis.	12
Irritable bowel syndrome Also called spastic, or irritable, colon.	Referral is necessary for proper diagnosis. Most chronic gastrointestinal diseases have a strong correlation to stress. The intestinal tract is highly responsive to changes in autonomic function and endocrine patterns. Sympathetic arousal changes peristaltic action and can send the intestinal tract into all kinds of dysfunction. Comprehensive stress management programs, including therapeutic massage methods, are often effective in managing these conditions.	12
Joint injuries	Pain and swelling of joint injury can be overcome with the judicious and short-term use of pain medication, antiinflammatory medications, and appropriate rehabilitation exercise. Massage, myofascial release, and trigger point work are often	8

Disease	Indications/Contraindications of Massage Therapy	*Mosby's Essential Sciences for Therapeutic Massage*
	effective after the acute phase (2-3 days). The application of ice along with rehabilitation exercise is beneficial. Management and rehabilitation of joint problems is a long-term process often requiring a multidisciplinary approach. Ice is contraindicated in some conditions and thus should be used with caution. Although direct work over an area that is actively healing is contraindicated unless supervised, massage and other forms of soft tissue work, coupled with movement therapies, can manage compensatory patterns that develop because of casting and other forms of immobilization.	
Kidney failure Also known as renal failure, the disease is the inability of the kidneys to excrete waste products and retain electrolytes.	Therapeutic massage tends to increase blood volume through the kidneys via mechanical and reflexive processes. In the healthy individual, therapy supports the filtration process. For those with kidney disease the increased volume can strain the kidney function. General contraindications exist for anyone with kidney disease.	12
Kidney stones These are small crystalline substances that develop in the kidney.	Therapeutic massage tends to increase blood volume through the kidneys via mechanical and reflexive processes. For those with kidney disease the increased volume can strain the kidney function. General contraindications exist for anyone with kidney disease. Therapeutic massage modalities may be useful for pain and stress management, but only with the careful supervision of the treating physician.	12
Kyphosis Kyphosis is a rounded thoracic convexity.	Massage therapy modalities are effective in managing backache. The benefits derived are from reduction in protective muscle spasm compensation (guarding) and generalized pain-modulating effects. Be aware that protective spasm provides stabilization. The goal is not to eliminate protective spasm but to support the body in managing dysfunctional patterns. Complex backache involving the joint structures requires the practitioner to incorporate therapeutic massage into a total treatment program supervised by the appropriate health care professional.	8
Legg-Calvé-Perthes disease This disease is the degeneration and necrosis at the head of the femur, followed by recalcification.	Necrosis usually is a localized condition that requires regional avoidance of the involved bone area. Because massage provides the generalized effect of enhanced circulation, indirect benefits might be realized with careful use of these methods. However, because these disorders are pathologic conditions, the primary health care provider must give permission for and supervise any massage.	7
List List is a lateral tilt of the spine	Massage therapy modalities are effective in managing backache. The benefits derived are from reduction in protective muscle spasm compensation (guarding), and generalized pain-modulating effects. Be aware that protective spasm provides stabilization. The goal is not to eliminate protective spasm but to support the body in managing dysfunctional patterns. Complex backache involving	8

(Continued)

Disease	Indications/Contraindications of Massage Therapy	Mosby's Essential Sciences for Therapeutic Massage
	the joint structures requires that therapeutic massage be incorporated into a total treatment program with supervision by the appropriate health care professional.	
Lordosis Lordosis is an accentuation of the normal lumbar curve that develops to compensate for the protuberant abdomen of pregnancy or great obesity.	Massage therapy modalities are effective in managing backache. The benefits derived are from reduction in protective muscle spasm compensation (guarding) and generalized pain-modulating effects. Be aware that protective spasm provides stabilization. The goal is not to eliminate protective spasm but to support the body in managing dysfunctional patterns. Complex backache involving the joint structures requires that therapeutic massage be incorporated into a total treatment program with supervision by the appropriate health care professional.	8
Lymphatic system disorders	Massage is contraindicated for malignant and infectious conditions until the client's health care professional gives approval. Modification of massage application is necessary depending on the type of treatment the client is receiving and the stress and fatigue levels. Massage that relaxes the client supports well-being and is helpful. The practitioner can manage simple edema with massage application focused to support the lymphatic system. More complicated lymphedema requires support of the appropriate health care professional concerning massage application.	11
Malabsorption syndromes These diseases involve poor absorption of nutrients.	The intestinal tract is highly responsive to changes in autonomic function and endocrine patterns. Sympathetic arousal changes peristaltic action and can send the intestinal tract into all kinds of dysfunction. Comprehensive stress management programs, including therapeutic massage methods, are often effective in managing these conditions.	12
Meningitis Meningitis is a bacterial or viral infection in the meninges, mainly in the subarachnoid fluid.	Infectious processes contraindicate massage intervention unless closely supervised by appropriate medical personnel. Immediately refer the client with unusual or unexplained stiff neck for diagnosis.	4
Miscarriage Miscarriage is termination of pregnancy.	Refer the client immediately to the appropriate physician or emergency room.	12
Multiple sclerosis Multiple sclerosis is a disease of autoimmune or viral cause (or both) in which myelin degenerates in random areas of the central nervous system.	Massage can be an effective part of a comprehensive, long-term care program. Stress management also is an important component of an overall care program for any chronic disease. Massage and other forms of bodywork can help manage secondary muscle tension caused by the alteration of posture and the use of equipment such as wheelchairs, braces, and crutches. Because therapeutic massage produces some stress, the practitioner must gauge the intensity and duration of any therapeutic intervention so as not to aggravate the condition.	5

Disease	Indications/Contraindications of Massage Therapy	*Mosby's Essential Sciences for Therapeutic Massage*
Muscle infection Infection of muscle is caused by several bacteria, viruses, and parasites, often producing local or widespread myositis (muscle inflammation).	Massage therapy is contraindicated until infection is no longer present.	9
Muscle strain Strain is an injury to skeletal muscles from overexertion or trauma and can range from mild to moderate to severe.	Direct work over the area of injury is contraindicated regionally until all signs of inflammation have dissipated. The use of ice and gentle range of motion can support healing. Methods to manage distortion in posture resulting from compensation in the rest of the body are helpful.	9
Muscle tension and headache The contracted muscles exert pressure on the nerves and blood vessels in the area, causing the pain, which is a dull, persistent ache with feelings of tightness around the head, temples, forehead, and occipital areas.	Various strategies are available to treat stress-induced muscle tension headaches, including massage. Chronic patterns often indicate connective tissue shortening. Headaches respond best to whole-body therapy, which not only addresses the immediate areas but also relaxes the entire body.	9
Muscular dystrophy This group of disorders is characterized by atrophy of skeletal muscles with no malfunction of the nervous system.	Careful intervention may slow the atrophy process. Passive and active range-of-motion methods not only directly affect the muscles and joints but also aid in the circulation and elimination processes. Abdominal massage may help with constipation. The practitioner should avoid methods that cause any inflammation.	9
Myasthenia gravis In this autoimmune disease the immune system attacks muscle cells at the neuromuscular junction and interferes with the action of acetylcholine.	General constitutional massage methods are indicated. The practitioner should avoid stressing the system and should work toward general restorative processes that reduce pain, support sleep, and create an overall sense of well-being.	5
Myelitis Myelitis is an infection of the spinal cord and/or brainstem.	Infectious processes are contraindicated for massage intervention unless closely supervised by the appropriate medical personnel. Immediately refer clients with unusual or unexplained stiff neck for diagnosis.	4
Myofascial system disorders	Intervention focuses on reversing nonproductive processes and supporting resourceful compensation patterns that develop in response to chronic problems. The goal is to support circulation, connective tissue strength and pliability, and nervous system interaction. The compression and stroking of massage support circulation. Connective tissue responds to methods that affect the viscoelastic, plastic, and colloid properties. Muscle tension patterns respond to compression and drag that stimulate proprioceptors. Muscle energy methods systematically use contraction and relaxing of muscles combined with lengthening to restore normal length of the muscles. Trigger points respond to methods that reduce hyperactivity, such as muscle energy methods and compression. Calming the sympathetic arousal is also necessary.	9

(Continued)

Disease	Indications/Contraindications of Massage Therapy	*Mosby's Essential Sciences for Therapeutic Massage*
Myoma Also called a fibroid, myoma is a benign tumor in the uterus that grows inside the uterine muscle wall or attaches to the wall.	Massage is contraindicated. Most reproductive system conditions present regional contraindications. As with most chronic illness and pain, therapeutic massage offers generalized support for homeostasis and can offer palliative or comfort care for the maintenance of these conditions.	12
Myopathies: metabolic and toxic	Treatment for these types of myopathy usually is not contraindicated, as long as the therapeutic approaches are general and focus on supporting body restoration and the healing processes. Massage can support detoxification efforts, because these methods enhance circulation. The practitioner must take care in toxic conditions not to tax an already overloaded system.	9
Myositis ossificans This disease involves an inflammatory process that stimulates the formation of osseous tissue in the fascial components of muscles.	Treatment is contraindicated regionally.	9
Neuropathy Neuropathy is the inflammation or degeneration of the peripheral nerves.	Nerve pain is difficult to manage, does not respond well to analgesics, and often is intractable. Massage, because of the interface with the nervous system, may provide short-term, symptomatic pain relief through shifts in neurotransmitters and stimulation of alternate nerve pathways, resulting in hyperstimulation analgesia and counterirritation. Any therapy that increases mood-elevating and pain-modulating mechanisms makes coping with nerve pain somewhat easier for short periods.	5
Obstruction of the urethra causing retention of urine	Refer the client to a physician for diagnosis.	12
Osgood-Schlatter disease This disease occurs when the tubercle becomes inflamed or separates from the tibia because of irritation caused by the patellar tendon pulling on the tubercle during periods of rapid growth or overuse of the quadriceps.	Treatment of local areas may be contraindicated if inflammation or necrosis is present. Methods that relax and lengthen the muscle and soften the connective tissue are appropriate.	7
Osteitis fibrosa cystica In this disease, fibrous tissue and cysts replace bone tissue, making the bones weak and prone to fracture.	The practitioner must exercise caution before using any massage and bodywork requiring any amount of compressive force on a client with a condition that causes demineralization of bone or that results in brittle, fragile bones. A fragile skeletal structure, regardless of the cause, is a contraindication for any type of compressive force or joint movement methods unless the appropriate medical professionals carefully supervise these methods. Light, superficial methods, such as the gentle laying on of hands used in some forms of touch systems, might be indicated with supervision. One may use massage methods on the unaffected areas and avoid the involved area.	7
Osteoarthritis A degenerative joint disease, osteoarthritis is the breakdown of	Because the progression and flare-ups of the disease are often stress related, the generalized gentle stress-reduction methods provided by massage therapy	8

Disease	Indications/Contraindications of Massage Therapy	*Mosby's Essential Sciences for Therapeutic Massage*
joints caused by normal wear and tear.	may be beneficial in long-term management of the condition, if supervised as part of a total care program. The practitioner should avoid frictioning techniques or any other forms of bodywork that cause inflammation. General systemic changes in the neurotransmitters and hormones that accompany exercise and many forms of bodywork can elevate mood and thus reduce pain perception.	
Osteochondritis dissecans This condition affects a joint in which a fragment of cartilage and its underlying bone become detached from the articular surface.	Massage therapy is contraindicated regionally.	7
Osteogenesis imperfecta This group of hereditary disorders appears in newborns or young children. The bones are deformed and fragile as a result of demineralization and defective formation of connective tissue.	If skeletal problems create or are part of a permanent condition, supportive care is required. Massage methods are helpful in managing compensatory muscle spasms and connective tissue changes. Any type of compressive force or joint movement methods are contraindicated for a fragile skeletal structure, regardless of the cause, unless carefully supervised by the appropriate medical professionals. Light, superficial methods, such as the gentle laying on of hands used in some forms of touch systems, might be indicated, again with supervision.	7
Osteomyelitis Osteomyelitis is an inflammation in the bone, bone marrow, or periosteum, usually caused by pyogenic (pus-producing) bacteria.	Massage is contraindicated in infectious disease unless carefully supervised by medical personnel. The therapist always must refer clients with vague pain symptoms for proper diagnosis.	7
Osteonecrosis (ischemic necrosis) Osteonecrosis is the death of a segment of bone, usually caused by insufficient blood flow to a region of the skeleton.	Necrosis usually is a localized condition that requires regional avoidance of the involved bone area. Because massage provides the generalized effect of enhanced circulation, the practitioner might realize indirect benefits with careful use of these methods. However, because these disorders are pathologic conditions, one must give massage with the permission and supervision of the primary health care provider.	7
Osteoporosis In this disorder the bone lacks calcium and other minerals and bone protein.	The practitioner must exercise caution before using any massage and bodywork requiring any amount of compressive force on a client with a condition that causes demineralization of bone or that results in brittle, fragile bones. A fragile skeletal structure, regardless of the cause, is a contraindication for any type of compressive force or joint movement methods unless the appropriate medical professionals carefully supervise these methods. Light, superficial methods, such as the gentle laying on of hands used in some forms of touch systems, might be indicated with supervision. Bone involvement may be localized, such as with radiation treatment. In these cases, one can use bodywork methods on the unaffected areas and avoid the involved area.	7

(Continued)

Disease	Indications/Contraindications of Massage Therapy	*Mosby's Essential Sciences for Therapeutic Massage*
Paget's disease (osteitis deformans) This disease occurs when the bones undergo normal periods of calcium loss followed by periods of excessive new cell growth.	The practitioner must exercise caution before using any massage and bodywork requiring any amount of compressive force on a client with a condition that causes demineralization of bone or that results in brittle, fragile bones. A fragile skeletal structure, regardless of the cause, is a contraindication for any type of compressive force or joint movement methods unless the appropriate medical professionals carefully supervise these methods. Light, superficial methods, such as the gentle laying on of hands used in some forms of touch systems, might be indicated with supervision.	7
Pancreatitis Pancreatitis is the inflammation of the pancreas.	Abdominal pain or referred back pain may indicate one of several gastrointestinal disorders. In such cases, referral is necessary for proper diagnosis.	12
Parkinson's disease In this disease, neurons that release the neurotransmitter dopamine in the brain degenerate, thus slowing or stopping its release.	Because massage has been shown to increase dopamine activity, its use is indicated for managing Parkinson's disease and tremor. In addition, the practitioner can manage secondary muscle tension effectively with massage therapy and other forms of soft tissue manipulation.	4
Peptic ulcer A gastric or duodenal ulcer affects the lining of the esophagus, stomach, or duodenum.	Abdominal pain or referred back pain may indicate one of several gastrointestinal disorders. In such cases, referral is necessary for proper diagnosis. Most chronic gastrointestinal diseases have a strong correlation to stress. The intestinal tract is highly responsive to changes in autonomic function and endocrine patterns. Sympathetic arousal changes peristaltic action and can send the intestinal tract into all kinds of dysfunction. Comprehensive stress management programs, including therapeutic massage methods, are often effective in managing these conditions.	12
Plantar fasciitis This condition is an inflammation of the plantar fascia and surrounding myofascial structures.	Acute-phase plantar fasciitis responds to rest and ice. After the inflammation has diminished, soft tissue methods that address the connective tissue and judicial use of stretching are beneficial.	9
Poliomyelitis—postpolio syndrome Poliomyelitis is a viral infection of the nerves that control skeletal muscle movement. Years later, postpolio syndrome can cause fatigue and muscle aching and weakness.	For postpolio syndrome, general constitutional approaches seem to work best to aid in overall pain reduction and restoration of the sleep pattern. The practitioner should avoid any form of therapy that causes therapeutic inflammation, including intense exercise and stretching programs.	9
Preeclampsia Also termed pregnancy-induced hypertension or toxemia, the condition is a complication of pregnancy characterized by increasing hypertension, proteinuria, and edema.	Refer the client immediately for medical treatment.	12
Pregnancy abnormality and bleeding during pregnancy	Refer the client immediately to the appropriate physician or emergency room.	12
Prostatitis Infection of the prostate usually	Massage therapy is contraindicated until infection is no longer present.	12

Disease	Indications/Contraindications of Massage Therapy	*Mosby's Essential Sciences for Therapeutic Massage*
	results from a urinary tract infection.	
Pyelonephritis Infection of the kidney affects the nephrons, or filtering units.	Therapeutic massage tends to increase blood volume through the kidneys via mechanical and reflexive processes. Acute infectious processes contraindicate massage until the infection has run its course. The appropriate health care professional may support chronic infection treatment as part of a supervised treatment plan.	12
Radiation therapy disorders	The practitioner must exercise caution before using any massage and bodywork requiring any amount of compressive force on a client with a condition that causes demineralization of bone or that results in brittle, fragile bones. A fragile skeletal structure, regardless of the cause, is a contraindication for any type of compressive force or joint movement methods unless the appropriate medical professionals carefully supervise these methods. Light, superficial methods, such as the gentle laying on of hands used in some forms of touch systems, might be indicated with supervision. One can use massage methods on the unaffected areas and avoid the involved area.	7
Reflux esophagitis Regurgitation of gastric acid up through an open esophageal sphincter causes heartburn.	Abdominal pain or referred back pain may indicate one of several gastrointestinal disorders. In such cases, referral is necessary for proper diagnosis. Most chronic gastrointestinal diseases have a strong correlation to stress. The intestinal tract is highly responsive to changes in autonomic function and endocrine patterns. Sympathetic arousal changes peristaltic action and can send the intestinal tract into all kinds of dysfunction. Comprehensive stress management programs, including therapeutic massage methods, are often effective in managing these conditions.	12
Regional enteritis Also called Crohn's disease, enteritis is a chronic inflammation of the intestine, most commonly the ileum.	Abdominal pain or referred back pain may indicate one of several gastrointestinal disorders. In such cases, referral is necessary for proper diagnosis. Many gastrointestinal diseases are bacterial or viral and are contagious. The intestinal tract is highly responsive to changes in autonomic function and endocrine patterns. Sympathetic arousal changes peristaltic action and can send the intestinal tract into all kinds of dysfunction. Comprehensive stress management programs, including therapeutic massage methods, are often effective in managing these conditions.	12
Rheumatoid arthritis This crippling condition is characterized by swelling of the joints in the hands, feet, and other parts of the body as a result of inflammation and overgrowth of the synovial membranes and other joint tissues.	Because the progression and flare-ups of the disease are often stress related, the generalized gentle stress reduction methods provided by massage therapy may be beneficial in long-term management of the condition, if supervised as part of a total care program. The practitioner should avoid frictioning techniques or any other forms of bodywork that cause inflammation.	8

(Continued)

Disease	Indications/Contraindications of Massage Therapy	*Mosby's Essential Sciences for Therapeutic Massage*
Rickets This disease of bone formation in children most commonly results from vitamin D deficiency and is marked by inadequate mineralization of developing cartilage and newly formed bone, causing abnormalities in the shape, structure, and strength of the skeleton.	Regardless of the cause, a fragile skeletal structure is a contraindication for any type of compressive force or joint movement methods unless the appropriate medical professionals carefully supervise these methods. Light, superficial methods, such as the gentle laying on of hands used in some forms of touch systems, might be indicated with supervision.	7
Rotator cuff tear Tears often are caused by repeated impingement, overuse, or other conditions that weaken the rotator cuff and eventually cause partial or complete tears.	Work on acute myofascial tears is contraindicated. However, massage therapy may be indicated in the rehabilitative process and as part of a supervised treatment protocol. The practitioner can manage and improve compensatory patterns with massage.	9
Scheuermann's disease This disease most commonly is caused by necrosis or inflammation in bone or in a disk of the thoracic vertebrae.	Necrosis usually is a localized condition that requires regional avoidance of the involved bone area. Because massage provides the generalized effect of enhanced circulation, the practitioner might realize indirect benefits with careful use of these methods. However, because these disorders are pathologic conditions, one must give massage with the permission and supervision of the primary health care provider.	7
Schizophrenia Schizophrenia is the most common mental disorder and includes a large group of psychotic disorders characterized by gross distortion of reality; disturbances of language and communication; withdrawal from social interaction; and disorganization and fragmentation of thought, perception, and emotional reaction.	Therapeutic massage is supportive in a multidisciplinary treatment, for such methods influence neurotransmitters. Supervision is necessary.	4
Scoliosis Scoliosis is a lateral S-type curvature of the spine.	Most backaches are preventable. One should not use the back muscles for lifting but should bring the weight close to the body, above the hips if possible, and allow the legs to do the actual lifting. An adequate exercise program is also important.	8
Scurvy Scurvy is the reduction of bone density caused by a vitamin C deficiency.	Regardless of the cause, a fragile skeletal structure is a contraindication for any type of compressive force or joint movement methods unless the appropriate medical professionals carefully supervise these methods. Light, superficial methods, such as the gentle laying on of hands used in some forms of touch systems, might be indicated with supervision.	7
Seizures	The application of massage techniques may decrease the side effects of medications. Massage therapists must remember to refer any clients with any exaggerated or increased symptoms to the prescribing physician.	4

Disease	Indications/Contraindications of Massage Therapy	*Mosby's Essential Sciences for Therapeutic Massage*
Sexually transmitted diseases	As with all acute infections, massage is contraindicated until any disease of the reproductive system runs its course. Most reproductive system conditions present regional contraindications. As with most chronic illness and pain, therapeutic massage offers generalized support for homeostasis and can offer palliative or comfort care for the maintenance of these conditions	12
Shin splints Shin splints are an inflammation of the proximal portion of any of the musculotendinous structures originating from the lower part of the tibia.	Massage approaches may be beneficial as long as they do not increase inflammation and a stress fracture has been ruled out.	9
Skin conditions	Therapeutic massage usually is not contraindicated in localized skin conditions, but local (regional) avoidance of the affected area is necessary. Localized touch can irritate most skin disorders. Massage is contraindicated if the skin is inflamed or if the condition is contagious or transmissible through touch. Malignancy is a contraindication unless the appropriate medical personnel supervise the therapy.	11
Spinal abnormalities: scoliosis, kyphosis, and lordosis Abnormal curvatures of the spine may be congenital, may result from paralysis or weakness or tension in spinal muscles, or may result from rapid growth of the body, especially after puberty.	If skeletal problems create or are part of a permanent condition, supportive care is required. Massage methods are helpful in managing compensatory muscle spasms and connective tissue changes. Any type of compressive force or joint movement methods is contraindicated for fragile skeletal structure, regardless of the causes, unless carefully supervised by the appropriate medical professionals. Light, superficial methods, such as the gentle laying on of hands used in some forms of touch systems, might be indicated, again with supervision.	7
Spinal cord injury	Massage is an effective part of a comprehensive, supervised rehabilitation and long-term care program. Massage and other forms of bodywork can help manage secondary muscle tension resulting from the alteration of posture and the use of equipment such as wheelchairs, braces, and crutches. Specifically focused massage can help manage difficulties with bowel paralysis. The circulation enhancement of massage can assist in managing a decubitus ulcer.	4
Spondylitis Spondylitis is inflammation of more than one vertebra.	Massage therapy modalities are effective in managing backache. The benefits derived are from reduction in protective muscle spasm compensation (guarding) and generalized pain-modulating effects. Be aware that protective spasm provides stabilization. The goal is not to eliminate protective spasm but to support the body in managing dysfunctional patterns. Complex backache involving the joint structures requires the practitioner to incorporate therapeutic massage into a total treatment program supervised by the appropriate health care professional.	8

(Continued)

Disease	Indications/Contraindications of Massage Therapy	*Mosby's Essential Sciences for Therapeutic Massage*
Spondylolisthesis In this condition a part of one vertebra moves forward on another.	Massage therapy modalities are effective in managing backache. The benefits derived are from reduction in protective muscle spasm compensation (guarding) and generalized pain-modulating effects. Be aware that protective spasm provides stabilization. The goal is not to eliminate protective spasm but to support the body in managing dysfunctional patterns. Complex backache involving the joint structures requires the practitioner to incorporate therapeutic massage into a total treatment program supervised by the appropriate health care professional.	8
Spondylosis Spondylosis is the formation of bony spurs at the disk margin of the vertebral bodies and causes degenerative changes in the intervertebral disks.	Massage therapy modalities are effective in managing backache. The benefits derived are from reduction in protective muscle spasm compensation (guarding) and generalized pain-modulating effects. Be aware that protective spasm provides stabilization. The goal is not to eliminate protective spasm but to support the body in managing dysfunctional patterns. Complex backache involving the joint structures requires the practitioner to incorporate therapeutic massage into a total treatment program supervised by the appropriate health care professional.	8
Stomach cancer	Abdominal pain or referred back pain may indicate one of several gastrointestinal disorders. In such cases, referral is necessary for proper diagnosis.	12
Stroke Stroke is sudden loss of neurologic function caused by a vascular injury to the brain.	Stroke is a medical emergency requiring immediate referral. Massage and bodywork is an effective part of a supervised comprehensive care program. Massage and other forms of bodywork can help manage secondary muscle tension resulting from the alteration of posture and the use of equipment such as wheelchairs, braces, and crutches.	4
Tendonitis/tenosynovitis Tendonitis is inflammation of a tendon; tenosynovitis is inflammation of a tendon sheath.	Any methods that could increase the inflammatory response are contraindicated for areas of inflammation. In the acute phase the use of ice and gentle movement are indicated. Chronic conditions may benefit from methods that elongate the connective tissue structures, relieving friction in the area.	9
Thoracic outlet syndrome This syndrome occurs because the brachial plexus and blood supply of the arm become impinged, resulting in shooting pains, weakness, and numbness.	Massage methods help relieve muscle impingement of nerves by relaxing and lengthening the muscles.	9
Thoracic outlet syndrome, sciatica, and carpal tunnel syndrome	Various forms of massage application reduce muscle spasm, lengthen shortened muscles, and soften and stretch connective tissue, restoring a more normal space around the nerve and alleviating impingement. When massage is combined with other appropriate methods, surgery is seldom necessary. If surgery is performed, the practitioner must manage adhesions appropriately to prevent reentrapment of the nerve by maintaining soft tissue suppleness around the	5

Disease	Indications/Contraindications of Massage Therapy	*Mosby's Essential Sciences for Therapeutic Massage*
	healing surgical area and, as healing progresses, extending the soft tissue methods to deal with the forming scar more directly. Before doing any work near the site of a recent incision, one must obtain the physician's approval. In general, work close to the surgical area can begin after the stitches have been removed and all inflammation is gone. Direct work on a new scar usually is safe 8 to 12 weeks into the healing period.	
Thrombosis A thrombus (blood clot) forms within the lumen (open cavity) of the blood vessels or heart.	Thrombosis contraindicates massage. Because obstruction could be a medical emergency, immediate referral is indicated.	11
Thrombus A thrombus is a clot that forms inside a blood vessel. A clot is the conversion of blood from a liquid to a solid through the process of coagulation. A clot that moves inside the vessel is referred to as an embolus (embolism). The presence of atherosclerotic plaque lining blood vessel walls is a significant stimulus for clot formation. Blood clots form from platelets and other elements and may obstruct a blood vessel at its point of formation or travel to other areas of the body. A thrombus that forms in the more surface vessels may create the signs and symptoms of pain, heat, redness and swelling.	Massage therapy is contraindicated regionally and generally because of the potential to move the clot or increased bruising from the medication. Thrombosis can be a medical emergency, and immediate referral is indicated. Treatment may include elevation, the application of heat packs to the affected area, and blood-thinning medications (such as heparin or warfarin).	11
Torticollis Also called wry neck, the condition involves a spasm or shortening of one of the sternocleidomastoid muscles.	Management of torticollis with massage therapy involves relaxing the neck, releasing trigger points, stretching the contracted muscles, and improving range of motion. Avoiding pressure on the vessels under the sternocleidomastoid muscle is important.	9
Tremors Tremors are involuntary muscle twitches.	Because massage has been shown to increase dopamine activity, it is indicated in managing tremor. In addition, the practitioner can manage secondary muscle tension effectively with massage therapy and other forms of soft tissue manipulation.	4
Tuberculosis This systemic disease is caused by the tubercular bacillus.	Massage is contraindicated in infectious disease unless carefully supervised by medical personnel. The therapist always must refer clients with vague pain symptoms for proper diagnosis.	7
Ulcerative colitis This disease primarily affects the sigmoid colon, with symptoms of lower abdominal pain and bloody diarrhea.	Abdominal pain or referred back pain may indicate one of several gastrointestinal disorders. In such cases, referral is necessary for proper diagnosis. The intestinal tract is highly responsive to changes in autonomic function and endocrine patterns. Sympathetic arousal changes peristaltic action and can send the intestinal tract into all kinds of dysfunction. Comprehensive stress management programs, including therapeutic massage methods, are often effective in managing these conditions.	12

(Continued)

Disease	Indications/Contraindications of Massage Therapy	*Mosby's Essential Sciences for Therapeutic Massage*
Urinary incontinence The inability to control urination most often is caused by weak pelvic floor muscles or nerve damage.	Stress is a contributing factor to incontinence. Any form of stress management helps somewhat with stress and urge incontinence. The practitioner needs to consider that incontinent clients require frequent and easy access to the restroom.	12
Vaginitis Vaginitis is inflammation of the vagina. Signs and symptoms are vaginal discharge, itching (pruritus), and irritation.	Most reproductive system conditions present regional contraindications. As with most chronic illness and pain, therapeutic massage offers generalized support for homeostasis and can offer palliative or comfort care for the maintenance of these conditions.	12
Vertebral subluxation; muscle spasms (entrapment) and shortening; disk degeneration; disk herniation	Various forms of massage are important in managing muscle spasm and pain associated with the aforementioned conditions. The student must remember that the muscle spasms serve a stabilizing and protective function called guarding. Without some protective spasm, the nerve could be damaged further, but too much muscle spasm increases the discomfort. Therapeutic intervention seeks to reduce pain and excessive tension and to restore moderate mobility while allowing for the resourceful compensation produced by the muscle tension pattern. Because low back pain is a common disorder, the massage practitioner must be familiar with its causes and treatment protocols.	5
Vertigo Vertigo is the sensation that the body or environment is spinning or swaying.	Movement therapies can help or aggravate vertigo; therefore the practitioner must take care to design an individual therapeutic program based on the client's history. Massage methods can deal effectively with muscle tension and diminish anxiety and nausea, but the benefit is temporary because the symptoms return with a recurrence of vertigo.	5
Whiplash Whiplash is an injury to the soft tissues of the neck caused by sudden hyperextension or flexion (or both) of the neck.	Direct intervention during the acute phase is contraindicated unless closely supervised by a physician or other qualified health professional. Massage methods are valuable as part of rehabilitation in the subacute phase and can help restore function if the condition is chronic. Extension injury is more severe and requires careful intervention.	9

From Fritz S: *Mosby's essential sciences for therapeutic massage*, ed 2, St Louis, 2004, Mosby.

31
Asian Bodywork Methods

The richness of Asian health theory and the unity of its body/mind/spirit connection is based on the energy of life. Life force called Ch'i, or Qi/Ri energy, flows through the body through interconnected pathways as water flows through the streams, rivers, lakes, and oceans of the earth. When Ch'i energy flows through the body like pure water, all of the processes of life are balanced. However, if obstruction or stagnation in the life force develops, it becomes the basis for disease.

The Tao, or "Way," supports the balanced function of all the senses and teaches a lifestyle of moderation that avoids deprivation and excess. Ch'i energy is the vital force of life, and Tao is the path or way to sustain the Ch'i energy.

Some are concerned about taking of pieces from the totality of being expressed in the Tao. Western science has lifted technique from this simultaneously simple but complex all-encompassing system. Often, technique separated from its theoretical basis is less effective. Although technique can stimulate physiologic functions, it cannot support the human experience. The small section presented in this textbook is based on a limited part of the total Asian medicine system commonly found on exams. As you begin to develop an understanding of these methods, be mindful and respectful concerning the larger structure of the body of knowledge from which they have been taken.

Midline Meridians

The body has two midline meridians. The conception or central vessel (yin) meridian starts in the center of the perineum and runs up the midline of the anterior aspect of the body to terminate just below the lower lip and is responsible for all yin meridians (24 points); the governing vessel (yang) meridian starts at the coccyx and runs up the center of the spine, over the midline of the head, and terminates on the front of the upper gum and is responsible for all yang meridians (28 points). See Box 31-1 for the main meridians. If we remove from the acupuncture/meridian phenomenon the concepts of yin and yang and of vital energy or life force (Qi), the explanation provided by neuroanatomy and neurophysiology remains partial. Western research so far has produced no great breakthrough in our understanding of acupuncture.

Sufficient evidence has been acquired regarding acupuncture to explain many of the effects as being neurohumoral chemical mechanisms.

For now, science is beginning to understand the basic concepts of Asian health practices: shu-xue, Qi, and yin/yang. Studying and understanding the Chinese system more fully is helpful for the therapeutic massage student because historic and current Chinese medicine has an important influence on massage practice.

In traditional Chinese medicine, this system of points and meridians is known as jing luo. The term usually is translated into English as "meridians" or "channels and network vessels."

Jing Luo

The channels and network vessels or meridian system form an essential feature of the human body. The jing luo comprises the network of routes for the circulation of Qi and blood. Through this network the entire body is interconnected: the viscera, bowels, the extremities, upper and lower, interior and exterior, and all parts of the body are brought into communication with each other. The jing luo joins the tissues and organs of the body together into an organic whole. The word jing means "warp; channels; longitude; manage; constant, regular; scripture, classic;

347

BOX 31-1   The 12 Main Meridians

---

1. *The lung meridian* (yin; L) begins on the lateral aspect of the chest, in the first intercostal space. It then passes down the anterolateral aspect of the arm to the root of the thumbnail.
   11 points
   Pathologic symptoms: fullness in the chest, cough, asthma, sore throat, colds, chills, and aching of shoulders and back.
2. *The large intestine* (yang; LI) meridian starts at the root of the fingernail of the first finger. It passes up the posterolateral aspect of the arm over the shoulder to the face. It ends at the side of the nostril.
   20 points
   Pathologic symptom: abdominal pain, diarrhea, constipation, nasal discharge, and pain along the crevice of the meridian.
3. *The stomach* (yang; ST) meridian starts below the orbital cavity and runs over the face and up to the forehead from where it passes down the throat, the thorax, and the abdomen and continues down the anterior thigh and leg to end at the root of the second toenail (lateral side).
   45 points
   Pathologic symptom: bloat, edema, vomiting, sore throat, and pain along the crevice of the meridian.
4. *The spleen* (yin; SP) meridian originates at the medial aspect of the great toe. It then travels up the internal aspect of the leg and thigh to the abdomen and thorax, where it finishes on the axillary line in the sixth intercostal space.
   21 points
   Pathologic symptom: gastric discomfort, bloat, vomiting, weakness, heaviness of the body, and pain along the course of the meridian.
5. *The heart* (yin; H) meridian begins in the axilla and runs down the anteromedial aspect of the arm to end at the root of the little fingernail (medial aspect).
   9 points
   Pathologic symptom: dry throat, thirst, cardiac area pain, and pain along course of the meridian.
6. *The small intestine* (yang; SI) meridian starts at the root of the small fingernail (lateral aspect) and then travels up the posteromedial aspect of the arm and over the shoulder to the face, where it terminates in front of the ear.
   19 points
   Pathologic symptom: pain in lower abdomen, deafness, swelling in the face, sore throat, and pain along the course of the meridian.
7. *The bladder* (yang; B) meridian starts at the inner canthus and ascends and passes over the head and down the back and the leg to terminate at the root of the nail of the little toe (lateral aspect).
   67 points
   Pathologic symptom: urinary problem, mania, headaches, eye problems, and pain along the course of the meridian.
8. *The kidney* (yin; K) meridian starts on the sole of the foot. It ascends the medial aspect of the leg and runs up the front of the abdomen to finish on the thorax, just below the clavicle.
   27 points
   Pathologic symptom: dyspnea, dry tongue, sore throat, edema, constipation, diarrhea, motor impairment and atrophy of the lower extremities, and pain along the course of the meridian.
9. *The circulation* (yin; C) meridian (also known as heart constrictor or pericardium) begins on the thorax lateral to the nipple. It runs down the anterior surface of the arm and terminates at the root of the nail of the middle finger.
   9 points
   Pathologic symptom: angina, chest pressure, heart palpation, irritability, restlessness, and pain along the course of the meridian.
10. *The triple heater* (yang; TH) meridian begins at the nail root of the ring finger (ulnar side) and runs up the posterior aspect of the arm over the back of the shoulder and around the ear to finish at the outer aspect of the eyebrow.
    23 points
    Pathologic symptom: abdominal distortion, edema, deafness, tinnitus, sweating, sore throat, and pain along the course of the meridian.
11. *The gall bladder* (yang; GB) meridian starts at the outer canthus and runs backward and forward over the head, passing over the front of the shoulder and down the lateral aspect of the thorax and abdomen. It passes to the hip area and then down the lateral aspect of the leg to terminate on the fourth toe.

(Continued)

BOX 31-1 **The 12 Main Meridians—Cont'd**

44 points
Pathologic symptom: bitter taste in mouth, dizziness, headache, ear problems, and pain along the course of the meridian.

12. *The liver* (yin; LIV) meridian begins on the great toe, runs up the medial aspect of the leg, up the abdomen, and terminates on the costal margin (vertically below the nipple).
14 points
Pathologic symptom: lumbago, digestive problems, retention of urine, pain in lower abdomen, and pain along the course of the meridian.

MIDLINE MERIDIANS

There are two midline meridians. The *conception vessel* (yin; CV) meridian starts in the center of the perineum and runs up the midline of the anterior aspect of the body to terminate just below the lower lip (24 points) and is responsible for all yin meridians; the governor vessel (yang; GV) meridian starts at the coccyx and runs up the center of the spine, over the midline of the head, and terminates on the front of the upper gum and is responsible for all yang meridians (28 points).

From Fritz S: Mosby's fundamentals of therapeutic massage, *ed 3, St Louis, 2004, Mosby.*

---

pass through." The word luo means "something that resembles a net; the subsidiary channels; to hold something in place with a net; to wind or twine."

Disturbances in the meridians are reflected in abnormalities along their course. Acupuncture, acupressure, and cupping largely are based on the theory of the channels and network vessels.

Thus the system of acupuncture points, organized as meridians, is the fundamental infrastructure of Chinese anatomy and physiology. This structure is a comprehensive matrix that passes through the body, connecting all of its parts and serving as an energy/communications grid that generates, propagates, stores, and releases information and forces related to the body and its various components. Every place in the body is permeated by and connected with every other place in the body by means of the jing luo system. Interestingly, new information and understanding of the fascial network and concept of an interconnected fascial web is similar to the Chinese description of jing luo.

The Chinese word-concept that we translate into English as "acupuncture point" is composed of elements conveying the sense of "body transport or communications hole."

Functionally, acupuncture points seem to have two most basic actions: they open and they close. The names of the many points include words that mean gate, pass, or door. In opening, they release information and energy. In closing, they store information and energy.

In clinical use, the meridian point system is the thoroughfare through which the practices of Chinese medicine can influence the condition if the body is restoring the balance of fundamental processes.

Yin/Yang Theory

"Yin-yang theory is one of the oldest doctrines in Chinese culture. The words yin and yang were originally representations of the shady and sunny sides, respectively, of a mountain or a hill. They came to represent two primordial forces that were the fundamental constituents of the universe and everything in it."[*]

When yin and yang were separated from the singularity at the beginning of existence, the resulting potential gave rise to Qi. To the Chinese, Qi is a vital component of everything and everything is sensed or experienced in a manifestation of Qi.

Yin and yang frequently are described as opposites or complementary opposites. In terms of Western science, the notion of opposing forces is a powerful

---

*Excerpt taken from Zhang YH, Rose K: *Who can ride the dragon,* Brookline, Mass, 1999, Paradigm Publications.

---

one, echoing in religious, moral, and ethical concepts of right and wrong, good and evil. However, in Chinese theory, yin and yang are conceived of as being in opposition, but not conflict. Yin and yang nourish and foster the growth of each other; they restrain each other; they support each other; they penetrate each other; they coexist.

Traditional Terminology

The following words describe the additional aspects of Chinese medicine theory.

Cun: A method of measurement that uses a relative standard, usually the length of the second phalange of the second finger. Cun most often is applied in Asian bodywork forms.

Cupping: A method that uses suction to increase blood flow to an area or to remove ingestion.

Disharmony: Distortions in health that result when the functions or systems are neither balanced nor working at their optimum.

Essential substances: The fluids, essences, and energies that maintain balance in the body, mind, and spirit. They include the Qi, or life force; shen, or spirit; jing, or essence; xue, or blood fluids; and jin ye, or fluids.

Han re: Cold and heat. This term refers to two of the eight principal syndromes in differential diagnosis. These are considered to be the primary manifestations of yin and yang, that is, symptoms that evidence a predominance of cold or heat. These two signs of disease are considered of primary importance in herbal ingredients for prescriptions to treat illness. The word han means cold. The word re means heat.

Jin ye: Fluids. This is a general term for all the liquid components of the body other than the blood. Jin ye is one of the basic substances that transforms into blood. It exists extensively within the human body between organs and tissues, serving a nutritive function. Jin ye is composed of two categorically different substances that form a single entity and can transform one into the other.

Jing: The yin essence of life that nurtures growth, reproduction, and development.

Liu fu: The six bowels; the six "hollow" organs; a term given collectively to the gallbladder, stomach, large intestine, small intestine, urinary bladder, and the hard-to-define "triple burner" (san jiao). In contrast to the five zang organs, the six fu organs are considered to be hollow and to be involved in the transportation of substances rather than the storing of essential substances and to decompose food and eliminate waste. The word liu means "six." The word fu means "bowel."

Liu Qi: This term is used to describe the environmental conditions that ancient theorists identified as pathogenic factors of etiology. This concept also is called the Six Pernicious Influences. Liu Qi refers to the wind, cold, summer heat, dampness, dryness, and fire or the six kinds of weather. When changes in weather exceed an individual's tolerance, disease may result. Identifying which of the six Qi are involved in the pathogenesis of a disease is an important step in diagnosing body substances, referring to essence, Qi, liquid, humor, blood, and vessels (or pulse).

Wind diseases are most common in spring, heat diseases in summer, damp diseases in long summer, dryness diseases in autumn, and cold diseases in winter.

Moxibustion: A form of heat therapy in which burning herbs are used to stimulate specific acupuncture points.

Qigong: An ancient Chinese art of exercise and meditation that encourages the flow of Qi and supports homeostasis.

Qi heng zhi fu: Literally, "extraordinary organs." This is a designation given to a group of organs that resemble the fu organs in structure and the zang organs in function, including the bones, blood vessels, gallbladder, and uterus. They are different from the bowels because they do not decompose food or convey waste from the viscera because they do not produce and store excess. The gallbladder is an exception, because it is classed as a bowel and as an extraordinary organ. The gallbladder is considered a bowel because it plays a role in the processing and conveyance of food and stands in interior-exterior relationship with its paired viscus, the liver. However, the bile that the gallbladder produces is regarded as a clear fluid rather than as waste; hence it also is classed among the extraordinary organs.

The brain, marrow, bone, blood vessels, gallbladder, and womb are born of the Qi of the earth. They represent the nature of earth and belong to yin. Thus they can store essence and not release it. The brain and the marrow also are placed in this category.

Qi qing: This word describes seven affects, referring to emotional and mental activities in general and their potential as pathogenic factors in the onset and progress of disease. Ancient theorists recognized that intense or prolonged emotional disturbance can act as a pathogenic factor, and they identified seven such states: anger, melancholy, anxiety, sorrow, terror, fright, and excessive joy. Each of these can act to disturb the normal function of the Qi, blood, and viscera, resulting in disease.

Qi: Also known as Ch'i, Qi refers to the life force.

Shen: The word shen refers to the eternal dimension of life, to the magical or heavenly aspects of being alive. Shen means "God, deity, divinity or divine nature; supernatural; magical expression, look, appearance; smart, clever."

Si shi: The four seasons; a general term for spring, summer, autumn, and winter in which the third month of summer (the sixth month of the Chinese lunar year) is termed "long summer." The four seasons are correlated with the five phases thus: spring-wood; summer-fire; long summer-earth; autumn-metal; winter-water.

Wu xing: The five phases (elements) metal, water, wood, fire, and earth. These phases refer to a theoretical structure that supports much of traditional Chinese thought. Wu xing is an extension or expression of yin/yang theory applied to the nature of material substance and to the various interrelationships that exist between matter in its different phases. These five phases function metaphorically, providing images that ancient theorists used to organize their thinking about the physical world. The five basic processes or phases describe a cycle that represents the inherent capabilities of change, which reflect yin and yang movements as observed in nature. The five element phases, like yin and yang, are representatives of quality and relationship (See Table 31-1). When combined with the principles of Chinese medicine, they are used to determine the diagnosis and treatment of a dysfunction.

Wu zang: The word zang means viscera, internal organ. This is a name given collectively to the solid organs—the heart, liver, spleen, lungs, and kidneys. These organs constitute one category that is distinguished from the six fu organs in structure and function. The zang organs are thought of as solid, essence-containing organs.

Xu shi: This word is translated as deficiency and excess, insubstantial and substantial (particularly in the martial arts), replete and deplete, full and empty; referring to two principles for estimating the condition of the patient's resistance and the pathogenic factors present.

Xue: The word xue is used to mean the blood itself in the same sense as it is understood in modern physiology. The term also is used to mean something specific to Chinese medicine: the substantial fraction of the circulatory system in a unique relationship with the circulation of Qi.

Ying: Construction (Qi), construction nutriment; one of the essential substances for sustaining vital activities. Ying is derived from the digested food and is absorbed by the internal organs. It circulates through the channels as a part of the blood to nourish all parts of the body. Ying is the essential ingredient of the blood and is responsible for the production of blood and the nourishment of body tissues. The blood (xue) and the ying are inseparable. Thus they often are referred to as ying xue.

Zheng xie: Righteous and evil; normal and pathogenic; referring to a distinction between the normal functions of the organism as contrasted to the pathogenic changes accompanying and characterizing disease.

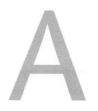

Practice Exams

Practice Test One

1. Which of the following is a quantified outcome goal?

   a. Client will be able to increase range of motion of the lateral flexion of the cervical area by 15 degrees.
   b. Client will be able to resume normal work activities.
   c. Client will be reassessed in 12 sessions.
   d. Client will recover ability to play golf.

2. Condition management involves the use of massage methods to support clients who cannot undergo a therapeutic change but who wish to be as effective as possible within an existing set of circumstances. Which of the following is an example of condition management?

   a. Managing the existing physical compensation patterns
   b. Assisting the client through learning to walk again
   c. Restoring a client's range of motion to preinjury state
   d. Using massage to help a client feel better about self and to change jobs

3. Nerve impingement syndromes occur primarily in plexus areas. A person experiencing an impingement in the cervical plexus would have _____.

   a. Shoulder pain, chest pain, arm pain, wrist pain, and hand pain
   b. Low back discomfort with a belt distribution of pain and pain in lower abdomen, genitals, and thigh
   c. Gluteal pain, leg pain, genital pain, and foot pain
   d. Headaches, neck pain, and breathing difficulties

4. Which of the following is not a general benefit of massage?

   a. Improvement in circulation
   b. Enhanced elimination
   c. Inhibition of homeostasis
   d. Increased levels of endorphins

5. The most effective massage methods to work on impingement syndromes are _____.

   a. Tapotement and shaking
   b. Muscle energy and lengthening
   c. Rapid deep compression
   d. Friction

6. The origin of pain can be somatic or visceral. Somatic pain is defined as _____.

   a. Pain from only stimulation of receptors in the skin
   b. Pain from stimulation of only the receptors in the skeletal muscles, joints, or tendons
   c. Pain resulting from only stimulation of receptors in the internal organs
   d. Pain arising from stimulation of receptors in the skin, skeletal muscles, joints, tendons, and fascia

7. The simplest, most effective deterrent to the spread of disease is _____.

   a. Hand washing
   b. Sterilization technique
   c. Using a towel barrier
   d. Keeping shots up to date

8. The inflammatory response can occur to any tissue injury. This response has four signs: redness, swelling, pain, and _____.

   a. Stickiness
   b. Liquid
   c. Heat
   d. Mucus

9. You are running behind today and your next client has been waiting for 15 minutes. It is most important that you _____.

   a. Maintain your scheduled appointments on time
   b. Have materials and activities available for clients to entertain themselves
   c. Make sure sheets and linens are changed and equipment is disinfected between massages
   d. Apologize to the client for being late

 Answers are on page 405.

10. A client keeps complaining of discomfort at the end of the massage stroke. What is the most logical cause?

    a. The practitioner is not pushing with the legs.
    b. The practitioner is off balance and is using counterpressure.
    c. The skin is being pulled from lack of lubricant.
    d. The compressive force is distributed over a narrow base at the end of the stroke.

11. When stretching the legs of a client by applying a pull against the ankle, the massage practitioner should _____.

    a. Fix the feet and pull with the shoulders
    b. Move to a symmetrical stance and lean back
    c. Maintain an asymmetrical stance and lean back, keeping the back straight
    d. Bend the knees and push back

12. Which of the following is not a safe professional practice?

    a. Assisting the elderly on and off the massage table
    b. Burning candles for atmosphere in the massage room
    c. Maintaining good lighting in massage areas
    d. Regularly checking cables of portable massage tables

13. To prevent allergic reactions, all lubricant should be _____.

    a. Oil based
    b. Water based
    c. Dispensed in sanitary fashion
    d. Scent free

14. A massage professional wants to check to see whether the location for an office being considered for rental is in an appropriate business distinct. Where does one find this information?

    a. Local zoning office
    b. Facility rental agreement
    c. State licensing bureau
    d. County tax office

15. When a practitioner is in a relaxed standing posture supporting the gravitational line with the normal knee-locked position, which muscles are used for balance?

    a. Psoas
    b. Gastrocnemius
    c. Hamstrings
    d. Quadriceps

16. When one is applying compressive force down and forward, weight is most efficient if kept _____.

    a. On the back leg and foot
    b. On the front leg and knee
    c. On the back foot and toes
    d. On the front foot and toes

17. A massage practitioner has been experiencing increasingly severe low back pain. The practice is full time with 20 clients per week. What could the massage practitioner do to reduce back strain?

    a. Bend the knees past 25° while performing massage.
    b. Raise the table height to prevent torso bending.
    c. Keep the head forward and down to change the center of gravity.
    d. Externally rotate the back foot away from the line of force.

18. A massage professional is feeling strain in the knees. Which of the following is the most logical cause?

    a. Doing massage on hard floors
    b. Working with clients in the side-lying position
    c. Keeping the knees flexed and static
    d. Moving whenever the arm reach is beyond 60 degrees

19. The most important stability feature of a portable massage table is the _____.

    a. Frame
    b. Cable support
    c. Adjustable legs
    d. Center hinge

          Answers are on page 405.

20. Regardless of the type of draping material used, which of the following is required?

    a. Disposable
    b. Large
    c. Opaque
    d. Cotton fabric

21. A massage professional has just rented office space and fully decorated the area. The massage room has a window and overhead and indirect lighting. A central thermostat is in another area, but the massage room has a fan and an electric heater to adjust temperature. The small waiting area is bright and comfortable, with many sorts of flowering plants. A private restroom is just off the waiting room. The massage room does not have a closet but does have hooks for the clients' clothing. A closed cabinet holds supplies. The business area is small but has a locked file cabinet and small desk. What suggestion would you make for improving the massage environment?

    a. Add an aromatherapy atomizer.
    b. Put a lock on the massage room door.
    c. Move the file cabinet into the massage room.
    d. Remove the flowering plants.

22. A massage practitioner has been seeing the same client weekly for 3 months. The client often discusses personal issues with the massage practitioner. Last session the massage professional provided some reading information to help the client and talked with the client about how the practitioner had dealt with a similar issue. The client has canceled the last two appointments. What is the most logical cause?

    a. Feedback about the massage broke down.
    b. Conversation with the client overshadowed the massage session.
    c. Gender issues are influencing the session.
    d. The orientation process needs to be repeated.

23. A client complains of a mild general low back pain. Which of the following is most correct?

    a. Use side-lying position with knee support.
    b. Work with client prone, using support under abdomen and ankles.
    c. Work with client supine, using support only under the neck.
    d. Position client in seated position and avoid supports.

24. Massage has been shown to slow formation of scar tissue and helps keep scar tissue pliable. This assists the healing process by _____.

    a. Blocking the action of antihistamines
    b. Counterbalancing the defect in the body
    c. Promoting regeneration and keeping replacement to a minimum
    d. Keeping the functioning energy reserves in place

25. In which situation would you stay in the massage room and assist a client on and off the massage table?

    a. A client in the first trimester of pregnancy
    b. A 65-year-old man with diabetes
    c. An elderly woman with high blood pressure
    d. An adolescent with a wrist cast

26. Massage manipulations are _____.

    a. Skillful use of the hands and forearms to affect the soft tissue directly
    b. Skillful use of the hands to affect the joints directly
    c. Application of methods using heat and equipment to affect soft tissue
    d. Application of compressive forces to affect meridians

 Answers are on page 405.

27. A client has an outcome goal for the massage of increased circulation and range of motion for the knee. Which of the following is the best approach?

    a. Reflexive methods focused on chemical changes
    b. Mechanical methods focused on the area
    c. Mechanical methods to influence neuroactivity reflexively
    d. Reflexive methods to increase compressive force to the viscera

28. Which of the following methods is most beneficial for abdominal massage mechanically to encourage fecal movement in the large intestine?

    a. Effleurage
    b. Resting position
    c. Tapotement
    d. Friction

29. A client reports a sensitivity to lubricant during the history and would like a massage in which no lubricant is used. Which method would be inappropriate?

    a. Shaking
    b. Compression
    c. Kneading
    d. Gliding

30. A client complains of restricted range of motion in the shoulder. The primary outcome for the massage is to increase shoulder mobility. Which massage method would be the best choice?

    a. Tapotement
    b. Muscle energy
    c. Hydrotherapy
    d. Resting stroke

31. Which of the following methods would be best for assessing for the physiologic and pathologic motion barrier?

    a. Passive joint movement
    b. Active resistive movement
    c. Post-isometric relaxation
    d. Concentric isotonic contraction

32. The definition of health is _____.

    a. Prepathologic state
    b. Homeostatic and restorative body mechanisms can no longer adapt
    c. Anatomic and physiologic functioning limits
    d. Optimal functioning with freedom from disease or abnormal processes

33. Which component is essential for effective application of joint movement?

    a. Stabilization to isolate the movement to the targeted joint
    b. Tapotement to stimulate the joint kinesthetic receptors
    c. High-velocity manipulative movement
    d. Cross-directional tissue stretching to cause traction on the joint capsule

34. A client is feeling fatigued and does not wish to participate during the massage. Instead the client wishes to remain passive and quiet. Which of the following muscle energy methods would be appropriate?

    a. Positional release
    b. Pulsed muscle energy
    c. Integrated approach
    d. Approximation

35. A client has been receiving massage weekly for 2 months. The main goal for the massage is increased mobility in the lumbar and hip region. The client has experienced stiffness and reduced ability since a fall off a bike 2 years ago. General massage and muscle energy methods with lengthening have produced mild improvement. Which of the following mechanical methods has the potential to increase results?

    a. Lymphatic drainage
    b. Stretching
    c. Contract/relax
    d. Strain-counterstrain

     Answers are on page 405.

36. A client is requesting extensive massage to the neck and upper shoulders. Which is the most efficient client position to massage these areas easily?

    a. Prone
    b. Supine
    c. Seated
    d. Side-lying

37. A client complains of a stiff and stuck feeling in the lumbar area. Assessment indicates that the fascia in that area is thick and adhered to the underlying tissue. Which method would best restore pliability to this tissue?

    a. Skin rolling
    b. Shaking
    c. Compression
    d. Vibration

38. A major contraindication to massage of the legs is _____.

    a. Acne
    b. Brachial nerve compression
    c. Disk compression
    d. Thrombophlebitis

39. Which of the following methods is best for general broad applications when lubricant is requested?

    a. Petrissage
    b. Compression
    c. Effleurage
    d. Vibration

40. A client is complaining about pain and stiffness in the neck but is particularly sensitive to pressure used in the neck area, flinching and stiffening in a protective stance whenever the neck is massaged. The current approach is primarily to use kneading with the client in the prone position. What is the best alternative?

    a. Change position to supine and use gliding.
    b. Use side-lying position and broad-based compression.
    c. Combine passive range of motion, muscle energy, and friction with client seated.
    d. Have client be seated and then use deep kneading.

41. After tripping down a stair, but not falling, a client describes a sudden onset of pain during twisting and reaching movements. Which type of biomechanical dysfunction is most likely to be occurring?

    a. Neuromuscular
    b. Myofascial
    c. Joint related
    d. Capsular pattern

42. Which of the following body areas is often massaged longer than is effective?

    a. Hands
    b. Abdomen
    c. Legs
    d. Back

43. A client has been receiving massage for a mild peripheral arterial circulation problem. Which of the following would be an appropriate self-help method to teach the client?

    a. Lymphatic drainage
    b. Skin rolling
    c. Alternating applications of hot and cold
    d. Frictioning

44. The secondary effect of a local cold application is _____.

    a. Sedative
    b. Increased localized circulation
    c. Diaphoretic
    d. Decreased systemic circulation

45. A folded towel soaked in water of the desired temperature and placed on a large area of skin is called a _____.

    a. Tonic friction
    b. Vaporizer
    c. Sponge
    d. Pack

 Answers are on page 405.

46. A massage client reports that after the massage she had some itchy areas of skin. Her clothes felt rough against her skin. Which neurotransmitter may be involved?

    a. Histamine
    b. Acetylcholine
    c. Epinephrine
    d. Cholecystokinin

47. A client has mild edema in her lower legs from a long plane fight the previous day. Which of the following is an appropriate treatment plan?

    a. Short, light, gliding strokes focused on the legs. Compression to the soles of the feet. Active and passive joint movement for the ankle, knee, and hip. Placing the legs above the heart.
    b. Compression to the legs focused on the medial side from proximal to distal. Muscle energy and lengthening combined with stretching in the area of the most accumulation of fluid.
    c. Deep gliding strokes from proximal to distal on the legs. Placing the legs above the heart. Limiting movement to encourage drainage.
    d. Superficial and deep compression along the vessels in the lateral leg. Active resistive joint movement combined with shaking.

48. Because of a skin condition, general massage is contraindicated for a client, but he is allowed to have his feet and hands massaged. He complains of neck stiffness. If using foot reflexology theory, where would the massage practitioner focus massage on the foot to affect the neck?

    a. Heel
    b. Tips of the toes
    c. Base of the large toe
    d. Sole of the foot

49. Therapeutic inflammation created by massage is best utilized in situations _____.

    a. In which there is a compromised immune function
    b. Resolving a fibrotic connective tissue dysfunction
    c. In which active inflammation is already present
    d. In which a condition such as fibromyalgia exists

50. A client injured his right shoulder 3 years ago. Assessment indicates decreased mobility of the skin surrounding the shoulder coupled with a painful but normal range of motion. Which is the best treatment option for this client?

    a. Deep transverse friction
    b. Superficial myofascial release
    c. Compression
    d. Lymphatic drainage

51. Deep transverse friction applied correctly will _____.

    a. Inhibit circulation
    b. Create controlled inflammation
    c. Provide broad-based application
    d. Replace broadening contractions

52. An active trigger point that is left untreated for 6 months often will _____.

    a. Become an ashi point
    b. Become hot to the touch
    c. Have fibrotic changes
    d. Only elicit referred pain

53. When treating trigger points, _____.

    a. Direct pressure methods and squeeze methods should be used first
    b. Positional release with lengthening is the first application method
    c. Connective tissue stretching needs to accompany muscle energy application
    d. Lengthening of the tissue housing the trigger point is only effective with a local tissue stretch

 Answers are on page 405.

54. A client is complaining of difficulty hitting a golf ball and describes a sense of timing being off. This could be a result of a disruption in what type of reflex?

    a. Conditioned reflex
    b. Tendon reflex
    c. Stretch reflex
    d. Mono reflex

55. In shiatsu a Qi energy flow that is under energy is called _____.

    a. Tao
    b. Kyo
    c. Jitsu
    d. Ashi

56. Which of the following meridians is yin?

    a. Gallbladder
    b. Stomach
    c. Lung
    d. Large intestine

57. Which of the following meridians is most medial?

    a. Central
    b. Spleen
    c. Liver
    d. Large intestine

58. Which is a correct way to sedate a hyperactive acupuncture point?

    a. Tap the point.
    b. Vibrate the point.
    c. Place sustained pressure on the point.
    d. Stimulate the meridian containing the point.

59. Going clockwise on the five-element wheel, which element is adjacent to the fire element?

    a. Earth
    b. Metal
    c. Water
    d. Wood

60. A client has a cough and nasal mucus, diarrhea, and intestinal cramping. The large intestine meridian is tender to the touch. Which other meridian that is part of the metal element is involved directly?

    a. Pericardium
    b. Lung
    c. Bladder
    d. Heart

61. Which of the following is considered an Ayurvedic dosha?

    a. Pitta
    b. Marma
    c. Governing
    d. Ch'i

62. A dosha is physiologically a(n) _____.

    a. Nerve pathway
    b. Chemical pattern
    c. Electric pattern
    d. Dietary pattern

63. In Ayurveda, the chakras are considered _____.

    a. Seven centers of prana located in the aura
    b. Seven centers of qi located on the central meridian
    c. Seven centers of prana located along the spinal column
    d. Six locations of kyo corresponding to centers of consciousness

64. A system that combines the theory of Asian medicine and Ayurveda is _____.

    a. Polarity
    b. Rolfing
    c. Shiatsu
    d. Reflexology

65. In polarity theory the left side of the body is considered _____.

    a. Ether
    b. Negative
    c. Neutral
    d. Positive

 Answers are on page 405.

66. In polarity theory the color green is associated with which body current?

    a. Ether
    b. Air
    c. Fire
    d. Water

67. In polarity therapy the energy of joints is considered _____.

    a. Chakra areas
    b. Serpentine brain wave currents
    c. Neutral
    d. Negative

68. During the massage, a client often speaks of problems with his children respecting house rules. This is a _____.

    a. Body issue
    b. Mind issue
    c. Spiritual issue
    d. Core issue

69. Wellness programs usually include methods to improve communication. Which of the following best explains why communication is more difficult to improve than diet?

    a. Diet and nutrition are more concrete and objective than subjective communication.
    b. Diet is much more dependent on others, whereas communication is independent of others.
    c. Stress focuses change toward healthful food choices.
    d. Communication skills are highly genetically influenced, but diet is not.

70. When breathing in the normal relaxed pattern, _____.

    a. The inhale is longer than the exhale
    b. Deep inspiration is accentuated
    c. Accessory muscles only work on exhalation
    d. The exhale is longer than the inhale

71. A client feels fatigued all the time. She explains that she does not seem to sleep all night. Which of the following may improve her situation?

    a. An afternoon cup of coffee
    b. Taking a long nap in the afternoon
    c. Going to bed and watching television
    d. Spending at least 30 minutes outdoors

72. A client is in the exhaustion phase of the general adaptation response. When one is considering a treatment plan for massage, which of the following is not appropriate?

    a. Ability of the client to expend energy for active change
    b. The availability of support and resources during the change process
    c. Practitioner must have appropriate knowledge and skills
    d. Completing outcomes in 10 sessions or fewer

73. Science is defined as _____.

    a. Knowing something without going through a conscious process of thinking
    b. The ability to pay attention to a specific area and maintain an unconscious focus and intent
    c. The intellectual process of using all mental and physical resources available to better understand, explain, and predict normal and unusual natural phenomena
    d. Craft, skill, and technique that enable a person to monitor and adjust involuntary or subconscious responses

74. The techniques of therapeutic massage provide manual external sensory stimulation. Which of the following would be a good example?

    a. Entrainment
    b. Rubbing
    c. Centering
    d. Breathing

75. A feeling of connectedness and intimacy in massage is most likely the results of an increased level of _____.

    a. Cortisol
    b. Endorphins
    c. Serotonin
    d. Oxytocin

     Answers are on page 405.

76. A client states a goal of wanting to relax and complains of having headaches, gastrointestinal problems, and high blood pressure. The client is likely to be experiencing _____.

    a. An excessive parasympathetic output
    b. An excessive sympathetic output
    c. An entrainment process normalization
    d. Restorative Sleep

77. A person experiencing fluid retention, muscle weakness, vertigo, hypersensitivity, fatigue, weight gain, and breakdown in connective tissue most likely has _____.

    a. Test anxiety
    b. Long-term high blood levels of cortisol
    c. First-stage/alarm reaction
    d. Conservation withdrawal

78. What type of massage has been demonstrated to be most helpful for a client who has reached the exhaustive reaction phase of stress and has been there for more than 6 months?

    a. Several appointments over 1 month using 15 minutes of tapotement and shaking
    b. A massage using pulling and pressing with light pressure for weekly sessions for 3 months
    c. A massage that primarily focuses on long, slow strokes; broad-based compression; and rocking for weekly appointments for 6 months
    d. A staccato, fast, deep pressure during weekly massage for 6 months

79. Parasympathetic patterns are _____.

    a. Restorative: adrenaline is secreted, mobility is decreased, and the bronchioles are constricted
    b. Physical activity is curtailed, digestion and elimination are increased, and restorative sleep is possible
    c. Physical activity is increased, pupils are dilated, saliva secretion is stopped, and stomach secretion is increased
    d. Restorative: heartbeat speeds up, bladder delays emptying, and saliva secretion increases

80. A massage practitioner identifies an area of restricted tissue and immediately uses skin rolling to increase connective tissue pliability. How did this interfere with assessment processes?

    a. The localized treatment did not prove effective.
    b. The pattern was changed before it was understood.
    c. The therapist did not chart the area before the massage.
    d. The method was not appropriate to the condition.

81. A client becomes very relaxed in response to the music and the rhythm of the strokes used during the massage session. What has occurred?

    a. Mechanical effects
    b. Circulation decrease
    c. Entrainment
    d. Client education

82. There are three main types of proprioceptors: muscle spindles, tendon organs, and _____.

    a. Cervical/lumbar plexus
    b. Spinal nerves
    c. Joint kinesthetic receptors
    d. Sphincter muscles

83. The most common bodywork technique that involves the tendon reflex is _____.

    a. Muscle toning
    b. Post-isometric relaxation
    c. Acupuncture
    d. Counterirritation

84. The gallbladder 30 acupuncture point location correlates with which of the following motor points?

    a. Triceps
    b. Gastrocnemius
    c. Gluteus maximus
    d. Brachioradialis

 Answers are on page 405.

85. The complementary relationship of opposites is described by _____.

   a. Organ and system organization
   b. Responsiveness and metabolism
   c. Yin and yang
   d. Qi and shen

86. The Asian healing theory of the law of five elements relates best to _____.

   a. Muscle tissue structures
   b. Nervous tissue structures
   c. Organs
   d. Prana

87. A massage professional is considering a position at a local day spa. The owner of the business offered an employee position at a salary or a subcontractor position based on commission. Which would be an advantage of the employee position?

   a. Variable income
   b. Stable income
   c. Subject to employer's regulations
   d. Independent ability to set work hours

88. Expenses used to begin new business operations are called _____.

   a. Business plan
   b. Reimbursement
   c. Investments
   d. Start-up costs

89. A massage practitioner has just redesigned his brochure and has included the types of massage provided, what the massage is like, information about the practitioner's qualifications, and client responsibilities. What did he forget?

   a. Tax structures
   b. Type of premise liability insurance
   c. Fees
   d. Client-practitioner agreement

90. The type of insurance needed to protect in case a client falls while in the business location is _____.

   a. Malpractice
   b. Premise liability
   c. Independent contractor liability
   d. Disability

91. A massage professional becomes angry with a client who complains about personal problems during the massage. The massage practitioner is displaying _____.

   a. Transference
   b. Therapeutic relationship
   c. Ethical behavior
   d. Countertransference

92. A massage professional works with three main populations: athletes, those with chronic pain, and clients requiring stress management. The therapist uses a variety of methods. Which of the following best describes the massage application style being used?

   a. Structural and postural approaches
   b. Applied kinesiology
   c. Integrated approaches
   d. Myofascial methods

93. A massage professional with entry-level training has been seeing a client recently diagnosed with diabetes. The massage professional is becoming more uncomfortable providing massage as the client displays more symptoms. What is occurring?

   a. The massage professional is in a dual role now that the client is ill.
   b. The client is more demanding of the professional.
   c. The massage professional has failed to abide by the definition of massage.
   d. The massage professional is functioning outside the personal scope of practice.

 Answers are on page 405.

94. Which of the following would be an appropriate disclosure to a client?

    a. The fact that the massage professional has a cold
    b. Business financial concerns
    c. Discussion about a mutual acquaintance
    d. Marital difficulties

95. A massage professional with 15 years of experience but minimal continuing education is in charge of a massage clinic. A recent massage graduate has obtained a position at the clinic. The new graduate notices that his current skills, particularly in charting and critical thinking, are more sophisticated than those of his supervisor but is hesitant to discuss the issue. What is the best description for this situation?

    a. Power differential
    b. Dual role
    c. Maintenance of professional environment
    d. Reciprocity

96. Which of the following would be the best explanation for a client who is confused over an incident of becoming mildly sexually aware during the last massage?

    a. The massage practitioner was sexualizing the massage.
    b. The client was consciously sexualizing the massage.
    c. The client was experiencing parasympathetic sensations.
    d. The massage practitioner was massaging erotic zones.

97. A client complains of a congested nose and low back stiffness. What is the logical connection between the two?

    a. The respiratory mucus is too thin and allows bacteria to enter the body, causing a kidney infection.
    b. The swell bodies in the nose are not able to function properly, so the normal movement during sleep is disrupted.
    c. The olfactory nerves are increasing parasympathetic arousal, causing an increase in muscle tension.
    d. Nasal congestion is blocking the sinus cavities and inner ear, changing muscle tone in the lower extremities.

98. During assessment a client is observed with mild tachypnea, tension in the muscles of the neck and shoulder, and nervousness. Which of the following is most true?

    a. Nitrogen levels have risen and oxygen levels have decreased, creating a decrease in tidal volume.
    b. Oxyhemoglobin is saturated with carbon dioxide, and the muscles display tetany.
    c. An increase in carbon dioxide in the blood is triggering sympathetic activation.
    d. Oxygen levels have increased and carbon dioxide levels have dropped, predisposing the client to hyperventilation syndrome.

99. Massage methods that modulate breathing pattern disorder also _____.

    a. Predispose a person to pulmonary embolism
    b. Interfere with treatment for sleep apnea
    c. Interact with the autonomic nervous system
    d. Interfere with most meditation methods

100. Which portion of the small intestine contains ducts from the liver, gallbladder, and pancreas?

    a. Ileum
    b. Jejunum
    c. Duodenum
    d. Mesentery

 Answers are on page 405.

101. A major function of the large intestine is to
_____.

   a. Absorb water
   b. Concentrate bile
   c. Remove and store glycogen
   d. Convert amino acids

102. A regular client reports various digestive upsets
including dry mouth and constipation. The
physician who wants a treatment plan and
justification has cleared the client for massage.
Which of the following would be the best plan
to submit to the physician?

   a. Stimulating massage coupled with teaching
   self-help breathing supporting an increase
   in oxygen and a decrease in carbon dioxide
   to support ongoing autonomic nervous
   system sympathetic dominance
   b. General massage combined with deep
   massage to the colon to suppress peristalsis
   and break down concentrated fecal matter
   c. General massage focused to generate
   relaxation with diaphragmatic breathing and
   rhythmic stroking to the colon to stimulate
   peristalsis
   d. General massage to create parasympathetic
   dominance and lymphatic drainage, with
   visceral massage to the liver to increase
   detoxification and support upper chest
   breathing

103. Which of the following pathologic conditions is
considered a medical emergency and requires
immediate referral?

   a. Gastroenteritis
   b. Peptic ulcer disease
   c. Inflammatory bowel disease
   d. Strangulated hernia

104. Cystitis is _____.

   a. Inflammation of the medulla of the kidney
   b. Infection of the glomerulus
   c. Bladder infection
   d. Obstruction of the urethra

105. Thirty minutes into a relaxation massage a
male client has an erection. What is the most
logical physiologic reason for this response?

   a. The client has a sexual intent for the
   massage.
   b. Erection is a parasympathetic response.
   c. Stimulation of the skin shifts blood flow.
   d. Activation of sympathetic reflexes triggers
   the response.

106. During sexual development in the female,
which occurs last?

   a. Hypothalamus matures.
   b. Estradiol is produced.
   c. Adrenal cortex hormone signals pubic hair
   growth.
   d. Ovulation begins.

107. If a female client is in the second trimester of a
pregnancy, which of the following would most
apply?

   a. Massage will be most comfortable if it is
   given with the client prone.
   b. Massage will be most comfortable if the
   client is positioned on the side.
   c. Massage of the feet is contraindicated.
   d. Massage should focus most on lymphatic
   drainage.

108. During massage, a lactating client experiences
the letdown response. What would be the most
likely cause?

   a. Massage stimulates the release of oxytocin.
   b. Massage stimulates the production of
   testosterone.
   c. Massage decreases colostrum.
   d. Massage decreases libido.

109. Which phase of nerve signal conduction is
related to muscle energy methods of massage
that use some sort of muscle contraction to
prepare the muscle to relax and lengthen?

   a. Action potential
   b. Refractory period
   c. Depolarization
   d. Saltatory conduction

    Answers are on page 405.

110. A client reports before the massage that his mind is agitated. He feels like he wants to scream. He is talking loudly and pacing. After the massage he feels calmer and wants a nap. Which neurotransmitter is largely responsible for the mood change?

a. Norepinephrine
b. Dopamine
c. Serotonin
d. Substance P

111. Why do the primary motor and the primary somesthetic sensory areas of the brain interfere with the ability successfully to self-massage areas of the back and limbs?

a. The largest sensory and motor awareness is in these areas.
b. The distribution of sensory and motor function to the hands is too small to stimulate sensation.
c. The distribution of sensory and motor function is larger to the hands than to the back and limbs.
d. The back and limbs have a predominance of sensory distribution over the motor distribution of the hands.

112. A client is experiencing lingering anxiety from a minor auto accident 4 hours ago. What difference between the nervous system and the endocrine system would explain this condition?

a. The nervous system is short acting, and the endocrine system is long acting.
b. The endocrine system is short acting, and the nervous system is long acting.
c. The nervous system transports hormones more consistently through blood and tissues.
d. Neurotransmitters have a long duration of effect, and hormones are short acting.

113. A 38-year-old female client describes symptoms of constipation, increased edema, sensitivity to cold, muscle and joint pain, and hair loss. She indicates that there is an increase in stress in her life; she is tired and seems unable to cope as effectively as before. She had a general physical examination within the last 6 months, but no specific tests were done. Based on these symptoms, which condition might suggest a need for referral?

a. Exophthalmos
b. Hypothyroidism
c. Hyperthyroidism
d. Hypocalcemic tetany

114. A person with type II diabetes wishes to become a client for therapeutic massage. The physician is supportive. Which of the following statements is most accurate as a basic understanding of type II diabetes?

a. There is a disruption of insulin production from the islet cells of the pituitary gland.
b. Insulin is a powerful diuretic, so increased edema is a warning sign of diabetic coma.
c. Insulin is released when levels of blood sugar, amino acids, and fatty acids rise.
d. Glucagon facilitates the ability of insulin to transport glucose across the cell membrane.

115. If an intervertebral disk rupture occurs, what is the possible outcome?

a. Narrowed disk space caused by leakage of the nucleus pulposus
b. Narrowed intervertebral space caused by rupture of the fontanelle
c. Impingement of the nerve from pressure exerted by the sella turcica
d. Increased space in the foramen impinging on the spinal cord

116. A female client, age 67, has a history of smoking. This could indicate caution for compressive force used during massage for which reason?

a. Osteonecrosis
b. Osteomyelitis
c. Osteochondritis dissecans
d. Osteoporosis

 Answers are on page 405.

117. A client complains of fatigue and muscle soreness after attempting to push a car that was stuck. Which of the following best describes this action?

    a. No movement was produced, so static force was generated.
    b. Dynamic force was used because the car did not move.
    c. Static force produced movement and energy expenditure.
    d. Because the car did not move, little energy was expended.

118. A client was a sprinter in high school track and was effective during short and quick runs. Now 10 years later the client is complaining of lacking the endurance to run 5 miles as part of a fitness program. The client is in good physical condition with no apparent reason for the difficulties. Which of the following offers the most plausible explanation for the client's condition?

    a. The person has an abundance of slow-twitch fibers in relationship to fast-twitch fibers.
    b. The person has an increased ability to manage oxygen debt.
    c. The person's legs have a genetic tendency toward a makeup of more white anaerobic fibers.
    d. The person has increased slow-twitch fibers in the postural muscles.

119. Two clients describe accidents in which the muscles of their upper thigh were cut and now healed. Client A has a mobile scar with near normal function. Client B has tissue rigidity and reduced movement. What is the most plausible explanation?

    a. Client A limited exercise and kept the area tightly wrapped during the healing process.
    b. Client B had more satellite cell activity during healing, causing increased scar tissue.
    c. Client A exercised during healing to stimulate satellite cells.
    d. Client B experienced increased circulation and reduced adhesions.

120. A massage practitioner notices that a client's skin has a yellowish gold color. This would be an indication of _____.

    a. Cyanosis
    b. Anemia
    c. Fever
    d. Jaundice

121. A massage professional identifies a few small lumps in the axillary area of a female client. What might be a pathologic concern?

    a. Basal cell carcinoma
    b. Candidiasis
    c. Psoriasis
    d. Fibrocystic disease

122. A client has a history of heart attack and has reduced blood flow to the heart. Which of the following vessels is involved most?

    a. Coronary
    b. Left external carotid
    c. Celiac
    d. Renal

123. What is the first heart chamber to receive blood from the superior and inferior venae cavae?

    a. Right ventricle
    b. Right atrium
    c. Left ventricle
    d. Left atrium

124. A client complains of pooling of blood in the lower extremities. Which of the following circumstances would be a likely cause?

    a. Increased walking
    b. Lying with the feet above the heart
    c. Standing still for extended periods
    d. Regular deep breathing

 Answers are on page 405.

125. During a general massage, the massage practitioner notices that the dorsalis pedis pulse is weaker on the left. Where is the practitioner palpating?

    a. Upper arm
    b. Wrist
    c. Knee
    d. Ankle

126. After a 1-hour massage focused on relaxation, a client becomes dizzy when sitting up. What is the likely cause?

    a. Stimulation of baroreceptors
    b. Increase of sympathetic stimulation
    c. Pulse rate of 65 beats per minute
    d. Decrease in parasympathetic tone

127. The immune function of mucus results because _____.

    a. It is sticky
    b. It creates inflammation
    c. Of phagocytosis
    d. It increases pathogens from the body

128. A client is immune suppressed. The physician has provided approval for massage. What would be the best massage treatment plan?

    a. General massage with specific use of stimulation techniques to encourage sympathetic dominance
    b. General massage with a focus on aggressive lymphatic drainage
    c. General massage with active stretching to encourage parasympathetic dominance
    d. General massage to support nonspecific homeostatic regulation and restorative sleep

129. Joint function is a combined relationship between _____.

    a. Bones and landmarks
    b. Stability and mobility
    c. Articulations and diarthroses
    d. Synovial fluid and pathologic range of motion

130. A client has been participating in a stretching program for more than a year. Initially the program was helpful, but during the last 3 months the program has become more aggressive and the client is complaining of joint pain. Which alteration in connective tissue may explain what has occurred?

    a. The client has experienced a rupture in the connective tissue structures.
    b. The client has exceeded the limits of the elastic range of the tissue, consistently deformed the tissue in the plastic range, and developed lax ligaments.
    c. An avulsion failure of connective tissue has occurred, creating a decrease in mobility.
    d. The tissue has become dehydrated, increasing creep tendency and contributing to stability provided by muscle contraction.

131. A client has been diagnosed with a hypermobile knee joint. Which of the following would be part of an appropriate treatment plan?

    a. Extend the elastic range of connective tissue structures by altering the plastic range.
    b. Elongate the plastic component of connective tissue in the direction of the shortening.
    c. Restore pliability.
    d. Manage muscle contraction around the joint using standard massage methods.

132. A client complains of pain in the region of the low back and buttocks. Which dermatome nerve distribution might indicate where the nerve impingement is located?

    a. C7
    b. T2
    c. C6
    d. L2

133. The sensory receptors most affected by deep compression and slow gliding strokes are _____.

    a. Pacinian corpuscles
    b. Root hair plexuses
    c. Merkel's disks
    d. Ruffini's end organs

 Answers are on page 405.

134. A client reports being prone to headaches from exposure to bright light. Bright light has been a problem only in the last few weeks. The client also reports an increase in workload. What might be the function of the autonomic nervous system that could be responsible for the sensitivity to light?

    a. Parasympathetic dilation of the pupil
    b. Sympathetic dilation of the pupil
    c. Parasympathetic contraction of the pupil
    d. Sympathetic contraction of the pupil

135. A client reports having herpes zoster and is experiencing pain. Which of the following would be the best massage approach?

    a. A full-body 1-hour massage with attention to universal precautions that uses tapotement, active joint movement, and fractioning methods
    b. A full-body massage lasting 1 hour that avoids the area of the rash and that actively engages the client in muscle energy lengthening and stretching
    c. A seated massage that lasts for 15 minutes
    d. A full-body, 1-hour massage that avoids the area of the rash with attention to universal precautions and a focus toward relaxation

136. Which of the following most often would be considered the fulcrum?

    a. Quadriceps muscles
    b. Radius
    c. Deltoid ligament
    d. Glenohumeral joint

137. During normal gait in the adult, the lumbar rotation is countered by a cervical spine rotation in the opposite direction for what reason?

    a. To keep the eyes on a level plane and the head oriented forward with the trunk
    b. To maintain the same-side counterbalance action of the arms and legs
    c. To coordinate the lever action of the elbows with the knees
    d. To activate the second-class lever system of the lift of the heel when moving onto the toes

138. An individual was running up stairs carrying a heavy briefcase in the left hand. Later that day the person felt increased tension in the left biceps muscle. Two days later, during a regular massage session, the client describes weakness and heaviness in one leg when walking up stairs or a hill. If normal gait reflexes are functioning, where would assessment likely find an inhibited muscle pattern?

    a. Right arm extensors
    b. Left hip flexors
    c. Right hip flexors
    d. Left hip extensors

139. Which of the following aspects of the gait cycle would result in most concentric contraction of the plantar flexors?

    a. Heel strike
    b. Midstance
    c. Toe-off preswing
    d. Midswing

140. A massage professional positions the client's body to assess the strength of the hip flexors. Which is the correct position for the hand applying resistance?

    a. Near the hip
    b. At the ankle
    c. At the distal end of the femur
    d. On the tibia

141. The prefix meaning against or opposite is _____.

    a. Circum-
    b. Caud-
    c. Contra-
    d. Brach-

142. The use of abbreviations in charting _____.

    a. Is universally understood
    b. Is more time consuming
    c. Requires a deciphering key
    d. Clearly communicates information

 Answers are on page 405.

143. The cutaneous/visceral reflexes are correlated with which Chinese medicine concept?

    a. Essential substances
    b. Pernicious influences
    c. Organ systems
    d. Five elements

144. The common relationship between yin/yang, the five-element theory, and Ayurvedic dosha is _____.

    a. Entrainment
    b. Somatic
    c. Homeostasis
    d. Etiology

145. Which of the following represent principles of movement?

    a. Pitta
    b. Vata
    c. Kappa
    d. Ether

146. A sensor mechanism, integration/control center, and effector mechanism are part of a _____.

    a. Stress response
    b. Post-isometric relaxation
    c. Stimulus response inhibition
    d. Feedback loop

147. Massage is part of a feedback loop in the _____.

    a. Controlled condition
    b. Control center
    c. Response
    d. Stimulus

148. Biologic rhythms are maintained by _____.

    a. Circadian patterns
    b. Proprioceptive patterns
    c. Negative feedback
    d. Positive feedback

149. Relaxed mood states are experienced by individuals when _____.

    a. Biologic rhythms are entrained to sympathetic patterns
    b. Biologic rhythms are oscillated independently
    c. Biologic rhythms are dysrhythmic to the chakra system
    d. Biologic rhythms are entrained to parasympathetic patterns

150. Relaxation methods that focus on breathing produce entrainment because _____.

    a. Cortisol increases during parasympathetic response
    b. Respiration rate is a major biologic oscillator
    c. Sympathetic mechanisms are generated
    d. Baroreceptors are inhibited

151. A disease with a vague onset that develops slowly and remains active for a long time is considered _____.

    a. Acute
    b. Communicable
    c. Chronic
    d. Idiopathic

152. Systemic inflammatory responses and fibromyalgia are _____.

    a. Indicated for massage that causes inflammation
    b. Indicated for massage that involves extensive stretching and pulling techniques
    c. Contraindicated for massage that causes inflammation
    d. Contraindicated for massage only in the area of the joints

153. Pathogenic disease-causing organisms include _____.

    a. Dirt, sweat, and grime
    b. Paint, tar, and dust
    c. Viruses, bacteria, and funguses
    d. Smoking, drinking, and washing

 Answers are on page 405.

154. A client's low back pain returns within 3 hours of receiving massage. What organ may be the cause of referred back pain?

    a. Heart
    b. Kidney
    c. Stomach
    d. Gallbladder

155. Massage used as a pain management strategy is a form of _____.

    a. Stimulus-induced analgesia
    b. Acupuncture
    c. Dermatomal inhibition
    d. Prostaglandin stimulation

156. Problem-oriented medical records including SOAP method require that _____.

    a. The qualified goals and the outcome of the massage be noted on the record
    b. The facts, possibilities, logical consequences of cause and effect, and impact on clients be noted on the record
    c. The results of palpation assessment but not the client history be recorded
    d. Only the interventions be noted on the record

157. The most important area in terms of determining future intervention procedures based on results is _____.

    a. S: subjective—what the client states
    b. O: objective—what was observed from assessment and examination
    c. A: analysis—what worked/did not work
    d. P: plan—what the client wants to work on and what needs to be done during the next session

158. An individual response to professional therapeutic touch _____.

    a. Is consistent with cultural influences
    b. Cannot be predetermined
    c. Is gender specific
    d. Depends on outcomes

159. The word massage is derived from all the following languages except _____.

    a. English
    b. French
    c. Arabic
    d. Greek

160. The three primary ways pathogens are spread are person-to-person contact, environmental contact, and _____.

    a. Hand washing
    b. Universal precautions
    c. Shoes
    d. Opportunistic invasion

161. What is the massage trend that developed in 1991 that supported acceptance for the benefits of massage?

    a. Increase in valid research
    b. Deregulation of massage education
    c. Decrease in influential women in the profession
    d. Resistance to integrating massage into traditional health care settings

162. A client seems nervous and unwilling to provide information during the history-taking process. The massage therapist is becoming impatient. What is lacking?

    a. Rapport between client and practitioner
    b. Prior information from the physician
    c. State-dependent memory status
    d. Proper clinical reasoning skills

163. When are data collected during the assessment process interpreted as to patterns of dysfunction and methods of massage application?

    a. As the history taking progresses
    b. During the physical assessment
    c. As the information is charted in the subjective section
    d. After the data have been collected and analyzed

                    Answers are on page 405.

164. During the initial greeting, a client seems generally healthy and in good spirits; however, when the client is speaking, the breathing pattern seems strained. What assessment process is being used?

    a. Palpation
    b. Physical assessment
    c. Interviewing
    d. Observation

165. A massage practitioner asks a client the following question, "Please explain to me how you would like to feel after the massage." What is correct about this communication?

    a. The massage practitioner used an open-ended question.
    b. The massage practitioner directed the response to reduce rapport.
    c. The practitioner was formulating a response during listening to the answer.
    d. A closed-ended interview was used to use time effectively.

166. A massage practitioner carefully listens to a client during the interview portion of the assessment process and then proceeds to the physical assessment. What communication step was forgotten?

    a. Open-ended questions and analysis
    b. Charting and treatment plan development
    c. Summarizing and restating information
    d. Using understandable language

167. A vacationing client will have only one massage from the massage practitioner. Which is the appropriate assessment process?

    a. Subjective history taking for possible referral combined with a physical assessment for symmetry and gait assessment for optimal movement patterns
    b. Palpation assessment of soft tissues to identify treatment areas
    c. Subjective and objective assessment for contraindications
    d. Interviewing for client's quantitative goals based on physician referral

168. During postural assessment, the massage professional observes that the client's shoulder girdle is rotated to the left. Which of the following histories is most likely to be the cause?

    a. The client regularly reaches to the left when answering the phone.
    b. The client often wears boots when riding horses.
    c. The client does weight-bearing exercise with machines 3 times a week.
    d. The client wears tight clothing.

169. A regular client has a grade 2 left ankle sprain and is using a crutch to maintain balance when walking. During assessment of posture, the massage therapist notices an elevated right shoulder. What is happening to cause this?

    a. The client is closing an open kinetic chain pattern.
    b. The muscles of the right lower leg are inhibited.
    c. The symmetrical stance is enhanced.
    d. The body is displaying compensation patterns.

170. When one is observing for symmetry, which of the following is correct?

    a. The shoulders should roll forward evenly, leveling the clavicles.
    b. The circumference of the muscle mass in the legs should be similar.
    c. The ribs should be fixed more on the left and springy on the right.
    d. The patella should be pointed more medially.

171. Which of the following is part of a normal gait pattern?

    a. The arms swing freely opposite the leg swing.
    b. The knee is maintained in the "screw-home" mechanism.
    c. The toes contact the floor first and then roll to the heel.
    d. During push-off, the foot is dorsiflexed.

 Answers are on page 405.

172. In which area would additional study be required when working with any population with special needs?

    a. Massage methods
    b. Environmental situations
    c. Psychology
    d. Relaxation methods

173. An adult male client has many surgical scars on his chest and abdomen. History indicates that the client had surgical intervention as a child to repair congenital malformations. The client enjoys massage on the limbs and back in the prone position but appears distant and unsettled when turned to the supine position. What is the most logical explanation for this response?

    a. An abusive family history
    b. Reenactment
    c. Dissociation
    d. Integration

174. A college football player is seeking massage as part of a healing program for an injured knee that required surgical intervention. The athletic trainer is supervising the massage. The massage consists of general full-body massage that addresses any developing compensation caused by the gait change while the knee is healing. Specific applications of kneading and myofascial release are being used to maintain pliability in the soft tissue of the upper and lower leg. What type of massage is being performed?

    a. Post-event massage
    b. Recovery massage
    c. Pre-event massage
    d. Rehabilitation massage

175. In which of the following circumstances would massage of breast tissue be most appropriate?

    a. General massage
    b. Adjunct to breast cancer treatment
    c. Scar tissue management
    d. Examination for lumps

176. In which of the following circumstances would massage without supervision by a health care professional best benefit children?

    a. Growing pains
    b. Anxiety disorder
    c. Touch sensitivity
    d. Attention deficit disorder

177. A massage professional has been working with a client who has chronic pain syndrome. The massage helps when combined with physical therapy, judicious use of pain medications, and support group attendance. Improvement in the condition begins after 6 or 7 massage sessions. After 10 to 12 sessions the client misses 3 or 4 sessions and then returns for massage and indicates that she is right back where she started. She states that she does not feel like the situation will ever improve. What is the most logical explanation for this behavior?

    a. Dual role
    b. Decrease in hardiness
    c. Secondary gain
    d. Acute pain

178. A client has been working on a project that required gripping a hammer for an extended period. Now the client is complaining of weakness when attempting to extend the wrist. Which of the following is the most likely explanation?

    a. The flexor muscle group of the hand and wrist increased tone levels, resulting in inhibition of the extensor group of muscles in the forearm.
    b. The flexor digitorum superficialis and profundus are weak from fatigue, so the wrist extensors have been facilitated.
    c. The deep layer of the posterior wrist extensor group is antagonistic to the superficial layer of this same muscle group, resulting in weakness in the wrist extensors.
    d. The flexor carpi ulnaris and the extensor carpi ulnaris are in spasm, resulting in inhibition of the abductor pollicis longus.

 Answers are on page 405.

179. While observing a client walk, the massage professional notices that the pelvis does not move evenly. The client complains of focused pain in the right sacral area. Which of the following is most correct?

    a. Create a massage treatment plan describing specific treatment for sacroiliac dysfunction.
    b. This information combined with other data may indicate the need for referral, with current massage focused on general nonspecific approaches.
    c. Design a massage to lengthen the left leg to balance the pelvic rotation.
    d. Immediately refer the client to a chiropractor for sacroiliac dysfunction.

180. A client is taking an anticoagulant. Which of the following would be contraindicated?

    a. Resting stroke
    b. Friction
    c. Muscle energy
    d. Rocking

181. During the massage, the massage professional notices a temperature difference in the tissue of the lumbar area. One area the size of a quarter is warmer than the surrounding area. Which type of assessment is being used?

    a. Postural assessment
    b. Gait assessment
    c. Palpation
    d. Muscle testing

182. Which of the following is the most effective way to assess for potential areas of muscle hyperactivity when the focus of the palpation is on the surface of the skin?

    a. Compressing until the striations of the underlying muscles are felt
    b. Light fingertip stroking to assess for areas of dampness or drag
    c. Skin rolling to assess for any adherence of superficial fascia to the skin
    d. Moving the skin on top of the superficial fascia to locate areas of bind

183. Sensory stimulation of massage causes a chemical change in a neuron called _____.

    a. Action potential
    b. Refractory period
    c. Depolarization
    d. Saltatory conduction

184. Which of the following statements is most correct?

    a. The body has no actual anatomic or physiologic functioning limits.
    b. The body has only anatomic functioning limits.
    c. The body has only physiologic functioning limits.
    d. The body has anatomic and physiologic functioning limits.

185. A person is clumsy and has a dull or foggy mind in terms of understanding information and making decisions. Which of the following neurotransmitters may be involved?

    a. Norepinephrine
    b. Histamine
    c. Glutamate
    d. Dopamine

186. In relation to anatomy and physiology, the phrase "structure and function" involves _____.

    a. Gross anatomy translates to regional anatomy
    b. Anatomy guides physiology and is modified by function
    c. Systemic physiology involves organizational anatomy
    d. Duality of wholeness represented in catabolism and anabolism

187. A client experienced an accident in which the trunk was thrust into extension. Which of the following structures might have been injured?

    a. Deltoid ligament
    b. Anterior longitudinal ligament
    c. Anterior superior iliac spine
    d. Linea aspera

 Answers are on page 405.

188. The process of homeostasis is a logical, well-coordinated pattern of balance. When balance is disrupted, patterns of dysfunction occur. What level of body organization is most basic?

    a. Chemical
    b. Cellular
    c. Tissue
    d. Organ

189. The concept of yang as compared with atomic structure is the _____.

    a. Nucleus
    b. Protons
    c. Electrons
    d. Neutrons

190. Which of the following is a description of burning pain?

    a. Short-lived but intense and easily localized
    b. Constant but not well localized
    c. Slow to develop, lasts longer, and less accurately localized
    d. Blood supply to the muscle is occluded, and contraction causes pain.

191. Which type of atomic bond holds together DNA?

    a. Ionic bond
    b. Anabolic bond
    c. Polar covalent bond
    d. Catabolic bond

192. Feedback is an essential aspect of homeostasis because of _____.

    a. Afferent discharge
    b. Effector response
    c. Information exchange
    d. Efferent signaling

193. If a client complains of pain in the buttocks and into the lateral side of the leg, which plexus is a potential site of nerve impingement?

    a. Cervical
    b. Brachial
    c. Lumbar
    d. Dorsal

194. Pain, tingling, and numbness in the arm and hand may be the result of nerve damage in which plexus?

    a. Cervical
    b. Brachial
    c. Lumbar
    d. Sacral

195. A compressive massage method is applied to the belly of a muscle with the intent of reducing a muscle spasm brought on by a cramp. The receptors most affected are _____.

    a. Joint kinesthetic
    b. Golgi tendon organ
    c. Muscle spindles
    d. Meissner's corpuscles

196. Sacral plexus nerve impingement is indicated by _____.

    a. Gluteal pain, leg pain, genital pain, and foot pain
    b. Headaches, neck pain, and breathing difficulties
    c. Shoulder pain, chest pain, arm pain, wrist pain, and hand pain
    d. Low back discomfort with a belt distribution of pain and with pain in lower abdomen, genitals, thigh, and medial lower leg

197. As slow, deep effleurage is applied to the left upper thigh, the practitioner notices and the client describes a twitching of the muscles in the back of the opposite leg. What type of reflex has been stimulated?

    a. Stretch reflex
    b. Tendon reflex
    c. Ipsilateral reflex
    d. Contralateral reflex

 Answers are on page 405.

198. A client complains of a sensation of thickness and stiffness in the myofascial structures of the body. Slow, sustained stretching provides the most benefit. What is the most plausible reason for this effect?

    a. The neuromuscular unit is deprived of calcium, allowing the actin and myosin to disengage.
    b. The viscous nature of connective tissue responds to this method by becoming more pliable.
    c. The colloid connective tissue ground substance decreases water binding with these methods.
    d. The compression against the capillaries increases blood flow.

199. A client is complaining of pain when straightening the elbow. Palpation of the triceps at the musculotendinous junction indicates more tenderness at the insertion/distal attachment when the muscle is activated. What is the most likely reason for this?

    a. The insertion is the fixed attachment and would be more tender during movement.
    b. The insertion is the proximal attachment and is straining at the intermuscular septa.
    c. The belly of the muscle located at the insertion is highly innervated.
    d. The insertion is the more movable attachment, so it would produce more tenderness upon motion.

200. A client unexpectedly lifted a box that was much too heavy. Now the client is experiencing residual weakness in the biceps and brachialis muscles and tension in the triceps muscle group. Which of the following reflexes best explains this situation?

    a. Stretch reflex
    b. Tendon reflex
    c. Withdrawal reflex
    d. Crossed extensor reflex

                    Answers are on page 405.

Practice Test Two

1. Which of the following is a violation of confidentiality?

   a. Maintaining client records in a secure location

   b. Asking the client questions about the work environment

   c. Approaching and speaking to a client in a restaurant

   d. Speaking to a client's chiropractor with appropriate releases

2. A client complains of pain in the tibia. The client completed a marathon 24 hours before the massage session. What contraindication to massage may account for the pain?

   a. Stress fracture

   b. Compound fracture

   c. Dislocation

   d. Whiplash

3. A massage professional has been working with a particular client for 12 months. Recently, the client has been experiencing increasing difficulties with the family communications. The biggest problem is stress and tension between son and father. Discussions during massage are centered around solving this problem. Which of the following best describes this situation?

   a. Massage professional is having difficulty maintaining informed consent.

   b. Scope of practice violations, particularly with psychology, are occurring.

   c. The client should be referred for acupuncture or chiropractic.

   d. The client is engaged in countertransference.

4. Research indicates that massage increases the availability of the following neurotransmitters: norepinephrine, serotonin, and dopamine. Which central nervous system disorder would be most benefited by massage?

   a. Stroke

   b. Cerebral palsy

   c. Depression

   d. Schizophrenia

5. During massage, pain that is not related to specific symptoms radiates around the ear. This indicates excessive pressure on which nerve?

   a. Greater auricular

   b. Thoracodorsal

   c. Medial cutaneous

   d. Pudendal

6. Which of the following receptors is most likely to adapt and cease responding to the sustained compression during massage on one specific area of the body?

   a. Meissner's corpuscles

   b. Thermal receptors

   c. Type II cutaneous mechanoreceptors

   d. Nociceptors

7. A client is complaining of a recent inability to sleep and a feeling of agitation and reports concern over a change in management systems at work. The physician diagnosis was exogenous anxiety. Which of the following treatment plans is most appropriate?

   a. Mild exercise program, therapeutic massage, and a stimulant medication to control symptoms

   b. A hypoventilation syndrome management program including massage and chiropractic manipulation

   c. A mild exercise program, cognitive behavioral therapy, short-term use of diazepam, and relaxation massage

   d. Therapeutic massage, meditation, increase in caffeine consumption, and bed rest

 Answers are on page 406.

8. A client who is a marathon runner developed an inflammatory condition of the knee. As part of the treatment process, the client received an injection of corticosteroid into the area of the knee. The client wishes to have a deep massage of the area to reduce the pain. Why is this not appropriate?

   a. The massage could decrease the inflammatory response and concentrate the medication at the injection site.
   b. Deep massage increases the potential for localized inflammation and would disturb the action of the corticosteroid injection.
   c. Deep massage would increase the tension of the muscles, causing instability, and inflammation would decrease.
   d. Corticosteroids reduce inflammation and increase tissue repair; because massage increases the tendency for tissue repair, excessive scarring could result.

9. A client is experiencing pain on palpation of many points along the kidney meridian. Which element of the five elements contains the kidney meridian?

   a. Fire
   b. Water
   c. Wood
   d. Earth

10. A client has just experienced a job shift change from days to nights and is having difficulty adjusting to the sleep pattern. The client indicates feeling disconnected and out of sorts. Which endocrine gland initially might be affected, and which massage approach would be most beneficial?

   a. Pineal gland; a massage that focuses on sympathetic stimulations with active participation by the client
   b. Adrenal glands; a massage that generates localized inflammatory areas, such as is found with direct pressure and friction on trigger points
   c. Thymus gland; a massage that uses sufficient pressure but pain-free compression and rhythmic gliding methods to support parasympathetic dominance
   d. Pineal gland; a massage that uses sufficient pressure but pain-free compression and rhythmic gliding methods to support parasympathetic dominance

11. A young male client is experiencing a growth spurt. He complains that the bones in his legs ache. What is responsible for this phenomenon?

   a. Increased testosterone promotes long bone growth.
   b. Increased estrogen promotes long bone growth.
   c. Decreased estrogen supports long bone growth.
   d. Decreased testosterone promotes long bone growth.

12. A client complains of pain in the lower back. Observation indicates an excessive lumbar curve. This is called _____.

   a. Scoliosis
   b. Kyphosis
   c. Lordosis
   d. Talipes

 Answers are on page 406.

13. A client is complaining of a feeling of shortening and pulling in the area of the low back and sacroiliac joints. Assessment indicates decreased pliability in the connective tissue structures in this area. Which of the following massage applications is most appropriate to achieve an increase in short-term mobility without compromising stability or creating a remodeling process of the tissue?

    a. Application of massage methods that slowly introduce creep, increasing pliability at the plastic range of the tissue
    b. Application of therapeutic inflammation coupled with stretching to exceed the plastic range of the tissue
    c. Application of elongation stretching to breach the plastic range of the tissue, creating inflammation to restore an appropriate creep pattern
    d. Application of abrupt bending of the connective tissue to support the increase in ligament laxity, thereby increasing mobility

14. We now know that biochemicals are responsible for most problems in behavior, mood, and perception of stress and pain. Which of the following is an example of this type of problem?

    a. Anxiety
    b. Obstructive sleep apnea
    c. Eczema
    d. Farsightedness

15. A client is experiencing spasms in the left thigh flexor muscles. An attempt to muscle test the area could result in a cramp. The massage professional remembers that activation of the gait reflexes can facilitate or inhibit muscle contraction. Which group of muscles would the massage professional have the client contract in order to inhibit the left thigh flexors?

    a. Left arm flexors
    b. Right arm flexors
    c. Left arm extensors
    d. Right thigh extensors

16. A client is experiencing muscle spasms and reduced mobility around a shoulder joint that has a history of dislocation. Which of the following applications of massage would be best in assisting this client?

    a. Increase the plastic range of the ligament structures and stretch tense muscles.
    b. Use friction on tendons and ligaments, and then incorporate a stretching program to increase flexibility.
    c. Reduce muscle spasms to the point that mobility is supported but stability is not compromised.
    d. Use massage methods and stretching to eliminate muscle spasms.

17. A massage practitioner has obtained required licenses and permits for her business location. The type of business set up was a sole proprietorship with a DBA. She has her business checking account and tax plan developed with an attorney. She also contacted a local insurance agent for appropriate insurance. She is a member of a professional organization that supplies professional liability insurance. She has a marketing plan and client practitioner agreements. What did she forget?

    a. Retirement investment plan
    b. Zoning approval
    c. Salary structure
    d. Business plan

18. A client has a history of a broken wrist. The wrist was in a cast for an extended period of time because bone repair was slower than normal. The client now is experiencing a decrease in range of motion of the wrist. What might be the cause?

    a. Hypomobility caused by contracture
    b. Hypomobility caused by reduced muscle tension
    c. Hypermobility caused by increased muscle tension
    d. Hypomobility caused by increased anatomic range of motion

	Answers are on page 406.

19. During assessment, the massage professional realizes that a client has extremely mobile joints. Which muscle functions would seem to be impaired?

    a. Produce movement
    b. Generate heat
    c. Maintain posture
    d. Stabilize joints

20. A client is complaining of tender areas in the postural muscles along the spine. Assessment indicates a series of trigger points in these muscles. The massage professional must determine how much compressive force to apply to the trigger points and how long to hold the contraction. Which of the following will affect this decision?

    a. These muscles contain more slow-twitch red fibers that are fatigue resistant.
    b. These muscles are prone to oxygen debt.
    c. These muscles have an abundance of fast-twitch and intermediate fibers.
    d. These muscles require a maximal stimulus to respond to treatment.

21. A client with fibromyalgia has been referred from the physician for massage. A treatment plan has been requested for approval before treatment begins. Which of the following would be the best approach?

    a. General massage with active assisted joint movement and stretching
    b. General massage with friction methods to active tender points
    c. Localized massage to the feet and ischemic compression to active trigger points
    d. General massage to support restorative sleep and symptomatic pain management

22. A client experienced an auto accident 4 years ago that resulted in a bulging disk at L4. The injury since has healed with minimal difficulties. During assessment, palpation indicates a moderate decrease in pliability of the lumbar dorsal fascia and mild shortening in the lumbar muscles. Forward flexion and rotation of the lumbar area are mildly impaired. Massage was focused to reduce the muscle shortening in the lumbar area and increase connective tissue pliability. Immediately after the massage the client reported increased mobility but within 15 minutes began to complain of lower back pain. What is the most likely explanation for this occurrence?

    a. A shift of the condition from second-degree functional stress to first-degree functional tension
    b. Increase in stability around the past injury
    c. Decrease in mobility in the area around the past injury
    d. Destabilization of resourceful compensation in lumbar area around the past injury

23. A client complains of joint pain in the knee, and assessment indicates hypermobility with pain on passive movement. Which of the following would be the most appropriate treatment plan?

    a. General massage to the body with specific muscle energy work and lengthening of the extensors and flexors of the knee
    b. General massage with regional contraindications to the knee area and referral for more appropriate diagnosis of possible capsular dysfunction
    c. Referral for diagnosis before any massage
    d. General massage with attention to friction methods at the joint capsule

24. A client is experiencing an upper chest breathing pattern. Which of the following muscle(s) may test as short and too strong from this type of breathing?

    a. Diaphragm
    b. Suprahyoid muscles
    c. Scalene muscles
    d. Infraspinalis

 Answers are on page 406.

25. A client complains of pain and tension in the lower back more to the left side. Physical assessment indicates that the pelvis is elevated on the left compared with the right. The client also indicates difficulty raising the left arm over the head. Which of the following muscles may be involved?

    a. Psoas
    b. Rectus abdominis
    c. Latissimus dorsi
    d. Semispinalis

26. If the scapula remains fixed and immobile, what would result at the glenohumeral joint?

    a. Range of motion would be limited.
    b. Internal and external rotation would be enhanced.
    c. Flexion would be unaffected.
    d. Horizontal abduction would be the only limitation.

27. Which of the following functions of the integumentary system is supported by maintaining sanitary procedures?

    a. Protecting against water loss
    b. Detecting sensory stimuli
    c. Preventing entry of bacteria and viruses
    d. Excreting sweat and salts

28. Which of the following heart valves controls the flow of blood from the ventricles into the aorta?

    a. Atrioventricular
    b. Mitral
    c. Tricuspid
    d. Semilunar

29. When one feels confident with commitment, control, and challenge in life, one is _____.

    a. Coping well
    b. Using behavior modification
    c. Functioning from an external locus of control
    d. Reliant on defense mechanisms

30. A client is shy and modest. Which of the following draping methods would be the best choice?

    a. Contoured draping with towels
    b. Partial body towel draping
    c. Full body sheet and towel draping
    d. Sheet draping with no towels

31. Which of the following would be an indication for referral?

    a. A radial pulse of 85 beats per minute
    b. A femoral pulse of 55 beats per minute
    c. A carotid pulse of 70 beats per minute
    d. A dorsalis pedis pulse of 52 beats per minute

32. A massage professional has been working 12-hour days, 6 days a week, for 2 years. She is seeing 40 clients per week. Lately she finds herself tired and out of sorts. She does not attempt to rebook clients who cancel. What is the most logical explanation for her behavior?

    a. Motivation
    b. Coping mechanisms
    c. Burnout
    d. Infection

33. In polarity theory, how many major body currents exist?

    a. Two
    b. Three
    c. Five
    d. Seven

34. What is the water temperature for a neutral bath?

    a. 65° to 92° F
    b. 98° to 104° F
    c. 92° to 98° F
    d. 56° to 65° F

35. A client has had surgery for varicose veins in the legs. Which vein was targeted?

    a. Azygous
    b. Brachiocephalic
    c. Hepatic
    d. Saphenous

 Answers are on page 406.

36. Characteristics of life involve _____.

    a. Physiology
    b. Coping skills
    c. Anatomy
    d. Tissue

37. Which of the following is a temporary deficiency or diminished supply of blood to a tissue?

    a. Aneurysm
    b. Embolus
    c. Blockage of a vessel
    d. Ischemia

38. Both lymphatic ducts empty lymph fluid into the _____.

    a. Mediastinal nodes
    b. Subclavian veins
    c. Mesenteric artery
    d. Cisterna chyli

39. Massage that provides a pumping compression to the foot encourages lymphatic flow because _____.

    a. The palmar plexus is stimulated
    b. The parotid nodes are drained
    c. The plantar plexus is stimulated
    d. The mammary plexus is stimulated

40. A person had the measles as a child and is no longer susceptible. This is called _____.

    a. Nonspecific immunity
    b. Immune deficiency
    c. Specific immunity
    d. Phagocytosis

41. Which of the following is most correct in application of trigger point therapy?

    a. 15-minute application in combination with lengthening and stretching
    b. 45-minute application with hydrotherapy cold applications
    c. Limiting application to active trigger points only
    d. Using pressure methods first and limiting lengthening

42. A client has been experiencing ongoing work and family stress and cannot seem to recover from an upper respiratory infection. What is the most logical cause?

    a. Ongoing stress increases natural killer cells.
    b. Ongoing stress supports the development of autoimmune disease.
    c. Ongoing stress suppresses T cell activity.
    d. Decrease in cortisol suppresses the immune system.

43. A client is having difficulty being comfortable with the touch of draping material during the massage. He says that he cannot get used to the scratchy feeling. The client may be displaying a reduced ability of sensory receptors to _____.

    a. Send impulses
    b. Adapt to sensation
    c. Remain monosynaptic
    d. Initiate reciprocal inhibition

44. Myofascial methods are focused most specifically on change in the _____.

    a. Motor point
    b. Lymph nodes
    c. Gait control mechanism
    d. Ground substance

45. A client with a diagnosis of asthma is referred for massage. What would be the most likely benefits of massage?

    a. Activation of the sympathetic nervous system, which would support bronchoconstriction
    b. Reduction in anxiety and increased mobility of the ribs
    c. Stimulation of the client's ability to inhale but inhibition of excessive exhalation
    d. Increase in tone of respiratory muscles, supporting effective exhalation

46. A client has severely limited all dietary fat. Which of the following might occur?

    a. Inability to digest protein
    b. Difficulty with hormone production
    c. Interference with the absorption of water-soluble vitamins
    d. Decreased conversion of galactose

    Answers are on page 406.

47. Massage in Ayurvedic theory concentrates on
_____.

    a. Manipulation of the doshas
    b. Tapping, rubbing, and squeezing points
    called Kappa
    c. Movement of fluid along the Vata centers
    d. Tapping, rubbing, and squeezing points on
    the body called marmas

48. Of the following, which is contagious?

    a. Appendicitis
    b. Hepatitis
    c. Reflux esophagitis
    d. Irritable bowel syndrome

49. Appropriate massage for the colon _____.

    a. Begins at the ascending colon, ends at the
    rectum, and moves toward the cecum
    b. Begins at the sigmoid colon and ends at the
    cecum, with directional flow toward the
    rectum
    c. Begins at the rectum and ends at the cecum,
    with a directional flow toward the cecum
    d. Begins at the splenic flexure and ends at the
    hepatic flexure, with directional flow toward
    the sigmoid colon

50. Erectile tissue is able to become firmer because
_____.

    a. This tissue engorges with blood
    b. Muscles contract, stiffening the tissue
    c. The tissue absorbs water from the lymph
    d. Smooth muscles encircle the tissue, acting as
    a diffuser

51. The alkaline nature of semen is to _____.

    a. Stimulate orgasm
    b. Counteract the acid nature of vaginal fluid
    c. Thin the protective coating of the ovum
    d. Lubricate the ejaculatory duct

52. During muscle strength testing, the flexors and
the extensors of the elbow seem equally strong.
Why is this a dysfunctional pattern?

    a. Gait patterns should inhibit the flexors.
    b. Flexors should be about 25% stronger than
    extensors.
    c. Extensors should be 30% stronger than
    adductors.
    d. Postural muscles are inhibited by gait reflexes.

53. A massage client does not provide effective
feedback about the amount of pressure
requested for massage. The client asks for very
deep pressure. As the massage professional, you
keep asking if the pressure is causing pain, and
the client says no. It seems that any deeper
pressure may cause bruising and other tissue
damage. This client may be exhibiting _____.

    a. Counterirritation facilitator
    b. Reduced influence of beta-endorphins
    c. High pain tolerance
    d. Hyperstimulation analgesia

54. A 56-year-old male client complains of difficulty
voiding urine. What would be the most likely
diagnosis from his physician?

    a. Endometriosis
    b. Trichomonas vaginitis
    c. Bartholin cyst
    d. Benign prostatic hypertrophy

     Answers are on page 406.

55. A client is getting ready to play a tournament tennis game in 60 minutes. She wants to increase circulation and prepare her muscles for the game. Which of the following treatment plans is the best option?

    a. Long gliding strokes from distal to proximal focused toward the heart combined with rocking. Duration of the massage: 45 minutes.
    b. Broad-based compression to the soft tissue of the limbs generally focused from proximal to distal combined with shaking and tapotement. Duration of the massage: 20 minutes.
    c. Full-body massage with muscle energy methods and lengthening. Duration of the massage: 45 minutes.
    d. Compression, superficial myofascial release, and trigger point work focused on the limbs combined with passive joint movement and shaking. Duration of the massage: 15 minutes.

56. A client is experiencing weakness and exhaustion; impaired concentration, memory, and performance; disturbed sleep; and emotional sweating. A complete physical has ruled out any existing pathologic condition. Stress is indicated as a probable cause. Which of the following treatment plans would best reverse the stress response?

    a. Massage to promote lymphatic drainage and stimulate arterial circulation
    b. Massage to support proper breathing function and reverse breathing pattern disorder
    c. Massage to reduce scar tissue and prevent adhesions
    d. Massage to stimulate increase in heart rate and blood pressure

57. A massage professional needs an understanding of disease processes. This study of disease processes is called _____.

    a. Pathogenesis
    b. Pathology
    c. Epidemiology
    d. Pharmacology

58. Which of the following meridians is located on the lateral side of the body beginning at the ear and ending at the toes?

    a. Pericardium
    b. Bladder
    c. Liver
    d. Gallbladder

59. A massage therapist feels restless on days off and finds it more difficult to sleep. What is the most logical reason for this phenomenon?

    a. Providing massage usually promotes a parasympathetic response in the client and the practitioner; on days when no massage is performed, the practitioner does not stimulate relaxation responses as effectively.
    b. Providing massage is fatiguing; on days off the massage practitioner has more energy.
    c. Providing massage interferes with natural entrainment responses, and on days off the practitioner is more in tune with biorhythms.
    d. Providing massage increases adrenaline and other stimulating hormones and neurotransmitters; when this occurs, hyperventilation is common, resulting in restlessness and sleep disturbances.

60. A middle-aged client is reluctant to work with a 22-year-old massage therapist. This is an example of _____.

    a. Gender issues
    b. Genetic predisposition
    c. Age issues
    d. Body sensitivity

61. Which of the following is a form of touch technique?

    a. Socially stereotyped touch
    b. Mechanical touch
    c. Inadvertent touch
    d. Ritualized touch

 Answers are on page 406.

62. The practice of acupuncture involves _____.

    a. The stimulation of specific points along the body, usually by the insertion of tiny, solid needles
    b. The stimulation of specific points along the body, usually by the pressing of the thumb into the point
    c. The stimulation of broad points along the body, usually by accomplishing a series of ever-deepening compressive strokes
    d. Using counterirritation, such as scraping, cutting, or burning of skin, to relieve pain

63. In shiatsu the points are called _____.

    a. Hara
    b. Meridians
    c. Jitsu
    d. Tsubo

64. A massage professional does not regularly drape all clients in a modest and professional manner. Which of the following best describes this conduct?

    a. The massage professional practices a dual role.
    b. The massage professional has breached a standard of practice.
    c. The massage professional is involved in misuse of the scope of practice.
    d. The massage professional needs additional training in draping.

65. Ayurvedic theory classifies physiologic functions by _____.

    a. Elements
    b. Visceral function
    c. Feedback
    d. Doshas

66. A massage professional has been asked to work with a support group for persons with cerebral palsy. The therapist is well trained and has 7 years of experience but is uncomfortable with persons with disabilities, especially if communication is problematic. Which of the following is grounds for refusal on the part of the massage professional?

    a. Lack of skills
    b. Lack of peer support
    c. Inability to serve without bias
    d. Only wishes to work with females

67. PRICE applications for first aid are appropriate for _____.

    a. Infection care of abrasion
    b. Grade 2 and 3 sprains and strains
    c. Neural injury
    d. Shock

68. Which of the following is the best example of transference?

    a. A massage professional is biased toward a client because of political beliefs.
    b. A massage professional is receiving small gifts from a client expressing affection.
    c. A massage professional asks a client to attend a meeting about a nutritional product with him.
    d. A client is frustrated with the massage professional for being late for the last three appointments.

69. Massage sensations travel on which spinal cord tracts?

    a. Sensory ascending tracts
    b. Motor descending tracts
    c. Corticospinal tracts
    d. Lateral reticulospinal tracts

70. In Ayurvedic theory, bones, flesh, skin, and nerves belong to which element?

    a. Ether
    b. Air
    c. Earth
    d. Water

 Answers are on page 406.

71. Record keeping for clients involves what documents?

   a. Charting each session of the ongoing process
   b. Having the client fill out a general information packet for marketing
   c. Written record of intake procedures, informed consent, needs assessments, recording of each session, and release of information
   d. Filing each piece of information received from physicians, insurance companies, or payments received from clients

72. Allergy is a condition of _____.

   a. Immune system suppression
   b. Lack of T cell activity
   c. Overactive immune response
   d. Immune deficiency

73. Which of the following would be recorded in the objective data section of a SOAP note?

   a. Client states she has interrupted sleep.
   b. Client is currently taking melatonin.
   c. Observation and palpation indicate upper chest breathing.
   d. Client wishes to have weekly appointments.

74. The purpose of valid research in massage is to _____.

   a. Generate more questions about massage
   b. Objectively research the physiologic process
   c. Subjectively research the massage process
   d. Justify massage as an art

75. A massage practitioner notices that he becomes a bit aloof if he gets behind and is late for scheduled massage sessions. This is a(n) _____.

   a. Denial measure
   b. Defensive measure
   c. Exhaustion phase response
   d. Lack of purpose

76. Wellness usually involves simplification of lifestyle to reduce demands. A stressful psychologic outcome of this process is often _____.

   a. Breathing pattern disorder
   b. Financial stability
   c. Dealing with loss and letting go
   d. Increased social support

77. In relationship to ancient chakra theory, if someone is concerned with not having enough money to pay bills, surviving a job change, and staying focused learning a new computer skill, which endocrine gland is likely to be affected?

   a. Pituitary
   b. Thyroid
   c. Adrenal
   d. Pineal

78. Which methods directly affect (stimulate) the nervous system?

   a. Mechanical methods
   b. Circulatory methods
   c. Reflexive methods
   d. Connective tissue methods

79. Massage can increase a person's fine motor movements such as handwriting. Which neurotransmitter is influenced?

   a. Serotonin
   b. Oxytocin
   c. Dopamine
   d. Growth hormone

80. Massage has been demonstrated to reduce some individual's craving for food and/or to reduce hunger. Which neurotransmitter is responsible?

   a. Epinephrine
   b. Serotonin
   c. Dopamine
   d. Norepinephrine

 Answers are on page 406.

81. If I wanted my employees to be more attentive, I would do massage for _____.

    a. 5 minutes
    b. 45 minutes
    c. 15 minutes
    d. 60 minutes

82. An objective measurement of connective tissue shortening in the lumbar area would be _____.

    a. Measuring a skinfold by lifting the tissue
    b. Placing the client in the prone position and having her lift her chest off the table into extension
    c. Measurements of hot and cold skin temperature
    d. Palpation of adjacent pulse points for evenness

83. In the human body, what initiates entrainment?

    a. Digestive glands
    b. Autonomic nerves
    c. Sweating
    d. Biologic oscillators

84. The Arndt-Shultz law states that weak stimuli activate physiologic processes; very strong stimuli inhibit them. What are the implications for massage?

    a. Massage is a strong sensory stimulant.
    b. Techniques have to be intense to produce responses.
    c. It is difficult to figure out whether a pain originates from a joint or surrounding tissue.
    d. To encourage a specific response, use gentler methods; to shut off the response, use deeper methods.

85. The best way to increase arterial flow circulation enhancement during massage is _____.

    a. A 50-minute massage using gliding but not heavy pressure
    b. A 45-minute compressive massage against the arteries proximal to the heart and moving in a distal direction
    c. A 50-minute massage using short, pumping kneading and gliding toward the heart
    d. A 30-minute massage emphasizing gliding strokes to passive/active joint movement distal to proximal

86. During the interview process, a client continues to grab the tissue at the back of the neck and pull it. What is the most logical explanation for this gesture?

    a. Nerve entrapment
    b. Joint compression
    c. Trigger point
    d. Connective tissue shortening

87. The triple heater meridian location corresponds with which nerve?

    a. Ulnar nerve
    b. Tibial nerve
    c. Sciatic nerve
    d. Lateral plantar nerve

88. A client enters the massage room complaining of a bad back from working at the computer. There are no stated contraindications. This is a stage one dysfunction. The client wants to reverse the condition. Which approach is the best process?

    a. Refer client to low back specialist
    b. Therapeutic change
    c. Condition management
    d. Palliative care

89. Which of the following persons may require only palliative care from a massage therapist?

    a. An athlete with a sprained ankle
    b. A 48-year-old woman with a broken arm
    c. A man with cancer
    d. A pregnant woman in the first trimester

          Answers are on page 406.

90. Pathology can be defined best as _____.

    a. The in-between state of not healthy but not sick
    b. Anatomic and physiologic functioning limits
    c. The study of disease
    d. Processes of inflammatory tissue repair

91. The root word pneum(o)- means _____.

    a. Vein
    b. Lung or gas
    c. Chest
    d. Breathing

92. Homeostasis can be defined as _____.

    a. The process of counterbalancing a defect in body structure or function
    b. A group of signs and symptoms
    c. The relative constancy of the internal environment of the body
    d. The subjective abnormalities felt by the patient

93. What is it called when new cells are similar to those that they replace?

    a. Egestion
    b. Fibrosis
    c. Inflammation
    d. Regeneration

94. Inflammation that persists beyond beneficial healing is considered an inflammatory disease. This chronic form of inflammation may be helped with what form of massage?

    a. Extensive application of deep transverse friction
    b. Light surface stroking
    c. Controlled use of friction, stretching, and pulling
    d. Brisk beating and pounding

95. The generally accepted definition of chronic pain is _____.

    a. A symptom of a disease condition or a temporary aspect of medical treatment
    b. Pain frequently experienced by clients who have had a limb removed
    c. Pain that persists or recurs for indefinite periods, usually longer than 6 months
    d. Pain that often subsides with or without therapy

96. If a client is experiencing pain in a surface area away from the stimulated organ, this is called _____.

    a. Muscle pain
    b. Referred pain
    c. Deep pain
    d. Acute pain

97. Cold applications of hydrotherapy to reduce swelling are called _____.

    a. Analgesic
    b. Antipyretic
    c. Antispasmodic
    d. Antiedemic

98. Neck pain on the right side can be indicative of referred pain from what organs?

    a. Appendix and kidney
    b. Colon and bladder
    c. Heart and lungs
    d. Liver and gallbladder

99. Relaxed, ordered entrainment is produced by massage in response to _____.

    a. The practitioner's direct application of methods
    b. The practitioner's calm presence and rhythmic application
    c. The practitioner's educational status
    d. The practitioner's specific choice of methods that address the chakra system

 Answers are on page 406.

100. Intervention is different for managing acute versus chronic pain. Acute pain is managed _____.

    a. With inhibitory methods
    b. Using aggressive rehabilitation approach
    c. Less invasively and is focused to support current healing process
    d. By compression on a nerve in a bony structure

101. What is the major reason that massage practitioners need to be aware of endangerment sites?

    a. These are soft areas that are unable to tolerate any pressure or movement.
    b. These sites may be a sign of a life-threatening disorder.
    c. The remaining proximal portions of sensory nerves are exposed here.
    d. These areas are not well protected by muscle or connective tissue, so deep sustained pressure could damage vessels, nerves, or other structures.

102. Predisposing conditions that may make the development of disease more likely by the client than by another person are called _____.

    a. Metastasis
    b. Pathology
    c. Signs
    d. Risk factors

103. A massage professional is troubled over a client's responses during the last four massage sessions. There is nothing specific about the client's behavior, but something has changed in the client's response to the massage. What could be helpful to the massage professional?

    a. Credentialing review with certification
    b. Managing intimacy issues
    c. Changing body language
    d. Problem solving with peer support

104. A doctor referral is indicated if the _____.

    a. Client has mild edema in the lower legs after a plane flight
    b. Client complains about care at the local outpatient client
    c. Client bruises easily and cannot explain why
    d. Client is beginning a new medication

105. A group of simple parasitic organisms that are similar to plants but have no chlorophyll and live on skin or mucous membranes are _____.

    a. Viruses
    b. Fungi
    c. Bacteria
    d. Protozoa

106. *Pathogens are spread by three main routes. Which of the following is one of these?*

    a. Opportunistic invasion
    b. Clean uniform
    c. Intact skin
    d. Aseptic technique

107. Pressurized steam bath would be an example of what common aseptic technique?

    a. Isolation
    b. Sterilization
    c. Disinfections
    d. Standard precautions

108. Acquired immunodeficiency syndrome is defined as _____.

    a. An inflammatory process caused by a virus
    b. Human immunodeficiency virus
    c. A group of clinical symptoms caused by a dysfunction in the immune system
    d. A disease contracted by casual contact such as shaking hands or sharing bathroom facilities

 Answers are on page 406.

109. Standard precautions are defined as _____.

    a. Emergency care given to all ill or injured persons before medical help arrives
    b. Procedures developed by the Centers for Disease Control and Prevention to prevent the spread of contagious disease
    c. The process by which all microorganisms are destroyed
    d. The process by which pathogens are destroyed

110. What is the most efficient standing position?

    a. Symmetrical and static
    b. Wide stance (feet 3 feet apart)
    c. Asymmetrical with weight transfer
    d. Lead foot with the pressure on it

111. Most massage applications use a force generated _____.

    a. Downward only
    b. Forward only
    c. Downward and forward
    d. Forward and across

112. A massage professional is feeling strain in the shoulders and arms after doing four massage sessions. Which of the following is the most logical reason?

    a. The massage professional is using muscle strength in the arms to exert force.
    b. The massage professional is standing in an asymmetrical stance.
    c. The client is positioned for best mechanical advantage.
    d. The massage professional effectively is leaning uphill.

113. A massage professional is complaining of pain in the wrist and near the elbow. Which of the following is an appropriate corrective action?

    a. Maintain the hands in a clenched fist to promote stability.
    b. Increase the movement of the stroke at the shoulder joint.
    c. Relax the hand and fingers during massage.
    d. Shift the compressive force to the fingers and thumb.

114. Observation of a fellow massage practitioner indicates that the shoulder girdle is aligned with the pelvic girdle, the pressure-bearing arm opposite the weight-bearing leg, the fingers relaxed, the head up, the back straight, the elbows bent, and the stance asymmetrical. Which of these areas needs correction?

    a. Elbows
    b. Stance
    c. Back position
    d. Shoulder position

115. In the earth element, if the stomach is yang, then what is yin?

    a. Spleen
    b. Bladder
    c. Liver
    d. Triple heater

116. Increasing levels of pressure are achieved by _____.

    a. Moving closer to the massage table
    b. Moving away from the massage table
    c. Standing on the toes
    d. Shifting the weight-bearing foot to the front

117. A client is particularly concerned with safety and is afraid of falling. Of the following massage equipment, which would make the client most comfortable?

    a. Mat
    b. Stationary table
    c. Portable table
    d. Chair

118. To maintain sanitary practice, draping material must be _____.

    a. Laundered in hot soapy water with a disinfectant such as bleach
    b. Sterilized and heat pressed
    c. Professionally laundered
    d. Warm, large enough to cover the client, and different colors

 Answers are on page 406.

119. The purpose of lubricant is _____.

    a. To moisturize the skin
    b. To reduce drag on the skin
    c. To transport nutrients
    d. Counterirritation

120. A client comes to you complaining of an aching pain just under the ribs right of the midline, under the right scapula, and in the right neck and shoulder area. The pain has been occurring more frequently and is now almost constant. The referred pain pattern might indicate problems with what organ?

    a. Bladder
    b. Kidney
    c. Stomach
    d. Gallbladder

121. A massage professional is preparing an orientation process for a new client. The professional has developed the following checklist: Show client massage area, where to change and hang clothes, demonstrate massage table draping and positioning, how to get on and off the massage table, music choices, and restrooms. Explain charts and equipment, lubricant types, sanitary procedures, and privacy methods. What did the massage professional forget?

    a. To explain the general pattern of massage flow
    b. To provide a centering meditation with the client
    c. To provide education on self-help
    d. To introduce the client to products for sale

122. The history-taking interview provides data for which part of the SOAP note charting process?

    a. Subjective data
    b. Objective data
    c. Analysis/assessment
    d. Plan

123. Which of the following is contraindicated for application of deep sustained compression?

    a. Lymph nodes
    b. Trigger points
    c. Dermatomes
    d. Ground substance

124. A massage practitioner uses massage manipulations in a brisk and specific way. Which of the following client goals is best served by this approach?

    a. Decreased alertness
    b. Increased parasympathetic response
    c. Decreased sensory awareness
    d. Increased alertness

125. Many ancient healing practices were developed based on _____.

    a. Measurement of concrete functions
    b. Experiential observation
    c. Scientific methods
    d. Meridian system

126. A massage client is unhappy with the massage. The main complaint is a feeling of choppiness and lack of continuity. Which of the following qualities of touch is most responsible?

    a. Depth of pressure
    b. Drag
    c. Rhythm
    d. Direction

127. Which of the following methods has as its primary effect a lifting of the tissue away from underlying structures?

    a. Compression
    b. Kneading
    c. Gliding
    d. Vibration

128. In which pathologic process would massage be most beneficial in assisting in the movement of body fluids?

    a. Spinal cord injury
    b. Anxiety
    c. Aneurysm
    d. Chorea

          Answers are on page 406.

129. A couple has experienced difficulties conceiving a third child. The doctors can find no reason for the difficulties. The man is a regular client. He asks whether massage could be of help. The answer is yes. Which of the following justification statements is most logical?

   a. Massage can assist in the success of sexual intercourse by encouraging adrenaline secretion.

   b. Massage can increase the rate of ovulation by stimulating the hypothalamus to secrete follicle-stimulating hormone.

   c. Massage can encourage more efficient homeostatic mechanism in the body, promoting general health, including fertility.

   d. Massage can increase the levels of testosterone, prolactin, and progesterone, promoting ovulation.

130. When the outcome for the massage is to produce parasympathetic dominance, which combination of methods would be the best choice?

   a. Gliding, rocking, and passive joint movement

   b. Compression, shaking, and friction

   c. Active joint movement, reciprocal inhibition, and rocking

   d. Tapotement, compression, and vibration

131. The main therapeutic focus of polarity therapy is to _____.

   a. Balance the tridosha system

   b. Restore balance in the yin/yang system

   c. Remove structural imbalance

   d. Locate blocked energy and release it

132. Many benefits of massage are a result of _____.

   a. Nonspecific stimulus that encourages feedback response to more optimum function

   b. Precise application of selected stimulus creating positive feedback

   c. Positive feedback response to return function to homeostasis

   d. Afferent transmission to the sensory mechanism with the disrupted homeostasis reduced by the control center

133. A client requests that tapotement be used at the end of the massage to stimulate the nervous system. Which is the best choice for the face?

   a. Hacking

   b. Cupping

   c. Tapping

   d. Slapping

134. Which of the following is produced voluntarily?

   a. Joint play

   b. Arthrokinematic movement

   c. Osteokinematic movement

   d. Joint end-feel

135. A client's muscles cramp when the massage professional attempts to use post-isometric relaxation to lengthen a shortened group of muscles. Which of the following methods would be a better choice to lengthen the muscle group?

   a. Skin rolling

   b. Active resistive joint movement

   c. Reciprocal inhibition

   d. Stretching

136. Which method is being described? Isolate the target muscle in passive contraction. Have the client contract the antagonist group. Have the client relax and then lengthen the target muscles.

   a. Post-isometric relaxation

   b. Reciprocal inhibition

   c. Contract-relax antagonist contract

   d. Pulsed muscle energy

137. A client is ticklish, particularly on the chest. Which method would be the best choice to use in this area?

   a. Compression over the client's own hand

   b. Friction

   c. Gentle effleurage

   d. Fingertip compression

    Answers are on page 406.

138. Which method is beneficial to use on the hands and feet to stimulate lymphatic movement?

    a. Superficial gliding
    b. Skin rolling
    c. Vibration
    d. Pumping compression

139. A client has a lot of body hair on his back. During the first massage, lubricant was used. At the return visit the client requests that lubricant not be used on his body where there are large amounts of hair. Which method could be used?

    a. Gliding
    b. Kneading
    c. Compression
    d. Petrissage

140. A client likes to have the back massaged and asks that most of the massage time be focused on the back. The client continues to complain that the massage is not effective in reducing back pain. What explanation can be given to the client?

    a. The soft tissue of the back often is long and taut because of extensive pulling and shortening of the tissues in the chest; massage of the chest may help.
    b. Massage to the back limits blood flow, so the soft tissues remain in contracture.
    c. Massage on the extremities would be better to reduce the pain in this area because the mechanical effect is more concentrated.
    d. The connective tissues of the back respond best to reflexive measures, and using a more generalized approach would provide relief.

141. If a pathologic condition occurs because of a state of "too much" or "not enough," then health would occur because of _____.

    a. Increased immune activity
    b. Decreased sympathetic arousal response
    c. Effective feedback and adaptive capacity
    d. General adaptation syndrome

142. A client notices that the massage office is clean, neat, and efficient and that licenses and certifications are posted on the wall. The client is impressed with the massage practitioner's abilities in _____.

    a. Applications of massage
    b. Communication skills
    c. Marketing
    d. Management

143. During the history interview, a client reports that she almost fell down stairs but caught herself and was able to regain her balance. What type of reflex action was required to accomplish this?

    a. Monosynaptic
    b. Polysynaptic
    c. Patellar
    d. Pacinian

144. Which of the following is of most concern when massaging the face?

    a. Proximity to mucous membranes and transmission of pathogens.
    b. The skin of the face is thin.
    c. Facial muscles are weak.
    d. Compression damages underlying cranial sutures.

145. Which of the following body areas requires special attention to draping?

    a. Hand
    b. Leg
    c. Chest
    d. Shoulder

146. A client arrives late for a massage appointment. The remaining time is 30 minutes. The goal for the session is general relaxation. Which combination is the best choice to achieve desired outcomes in the allotted time?

    a. Back, gluteals, and hips
    b. Face, hands, and feet
    c. Hands, arms, and back
    d. Face, neck, and shoulders

          Answers are on page 406.

147. When one is using passive joint movement as an assessment method, which of the following is being identified?

    a. End-feel
    b. Viscosity
    c. Vessels
    d. Pilomotor reflex

148. A client is experiencing pain on palpation of many points along the kidney meridian. Which element of the five elements contains the kidney meridian?

    a. Fire
    b. Water
    c. Wood
    d. Earth

149. Bilateral assessment of the dorsalis pedis pulse would provide information about _____.

    a. Respiration
    b. Abdominal viscera
    c. Lymph nodes
    d. Arterial circulation

150. During palpation assessment, the massage practitioner wishes to assess for the status of the acupuncture meridians. Where would the practitioner focus the assessment?

    a. Tendons at the proximal attachment
    b. Ligament of synovial joints
    c. Grooves in fascial sheaths
    d. Myotomes

151. Which of the following is incorrect when using muscle strength testing?

    a. Isolate muscles and position attachments as close together as is comfortable.
    b. Use a force sufficient to recruit a full response of the tested muscles and the surrounding muscles.
    c. Use a slow and even counterpressure to pull or push the muscle out of the isolated position.
    d. Compare muscle tests bilaterally for symmetry.

152. A client is complaining of weakness and heaviness in the muscles that flex the left thigh. During muscle testing, the muscle group is found to be inhibited. Based on gait patterns, which of the following muscle groups also should be inhibited?

    a. Right arm flexors
    b. Left arm flexors
    c. Right thigh flexors
    d. Left thigh extensors

153. If the area between C7 and T12 is pulled forward, making the chest concave, with a right rotation pattern making the right shoulder more forward than the left, where are the shortened soft tissues?

    a. Anterior thorax on the right
    b. Right lumbar posterior
    c. Left thorax posterior
    d. Lower abdominal on the right

154. Which of the following is contraindicated for application of deep sustained compression?

    a. Popliteal space
    b. Trigger points
    c. Dermatomes
    d. Ground substance

   Answers are on page 406.

155. A physician refers a client for massage for circulation enhancement to the limbs. The client complains of cold hands and feet. Assessment indicates decreased pliability of the tissues around the elbows and knees. Work-related activities require repetitive movement in these areas. The massage professional presents three main approaches for the physician to consider:

    1. *General massage and rest*
    2. *General massage with connective tissue stretching in the restricted areas*
    3. *Compression focused specifically to the arteries to encourage circulation*

    After considering all three options, the physician eliminates number 1 as too time consuming. Option 2 seems viable, but the client does not respond well to methods that may be painful. Option 3 seems too limited an approach to the massage professional. The decision is to begin with option 3 and expand to connective tissue methods when the client is able to tolerate them. Which part of this process best reflects brainstorming possibilities?

    a. Data collection
    b. Elimination of options based on pros and cons
    c. Generating the options
    d. Assessment for more facts

156. A client experienced an episode of severe low back pain 3 years ago. The diagnosis was a compressed disk at L4. The condition has stabilized, and the client experiences pain only occasionally. Assessment indicates shortened lumbar fascia, increased lateral flexion to the right, and a high shoulder on the right. The massage professional specifically addressed these areas and noted improvement following the massage. The next day the client called complaining that the low back was in spasm. What is the most logical reason for what happened?

    a. The phasic muscles were too weak to maintain posture.
    b. The gait shifted so that there was a more normal heel strike.
    c. Facilitated segments in the skeletal muscles went into spasm.
    d. Resourceful compensation patterns were disturbed.

157. When one is evaluating a treatment plan for successful client compliance, which of the following would provide the best information?

    a. Any referral information from the heath care provider
    b. Completing a comprehensive physical assessment
    c. Generating multiple treatment options
    d. Indications of enthusiasm for the plan by the client and any support system

158. Bodywork methods that focus on meridians and points fall into which category?

    a. Eastern and Asian
    b. Cognitive
    c. State dependent
    d. Structural

159. Which environment is the most difficult for maintaining professional boundaries?

    a. Public events
    b. Private office commercial building
    c. On-site residence
    d. Home office

160. Reflexology can be beneficial because _____.

    a. The complex structure of the foot is highly innervated and sensitive to changes in pressure and position, making it highly responsive to massage manipulation
    b. The flexor withdrawal mechanism of the foot is inhibited with pressure to the foot, and this inhibits neural activity in the dorsal horn of the spinal cord
    c. The specific mapped areas of reflex activity in the foot to organs have a direct relationship to visceral/cutaneous responses
    d. Stimulation of the zone therapy points on the bottom of the foot activates meridian energy movement in the chakra system

            Answers are on page 406.

161. A client is experiencing pain with any activity involving external or lateral rotation of the right shoulder. Range of motion is limited to 40 degrees. This condition has been coming on gradually. Muscle testing indicates weakness when resistance is applied to move the shoulder from external rotation to internal rotation. There is shortening in the muscles of internal rotation. Which of the following would be the most logical treatment plan?

    a. Muscle energy methods to support lengthening of the infraspinatus and methods to increase tone in the subscapularis
    b. Deep massage to the rhomboids and stretching of the lumbar fascia
    c. Traction of the scapulothoracic junction
    d. Massage to reduce tension in the pectoralis major and latissimus dorsi with tapotement to increase tone in the infraspinatus and teres major

162. Why might massage be contraindicated for those with renal insufficiency?

    a. Massage causes an increase in blood pressure.
    b. Massage increases blood volume through the kidneys.
    c. Massage spreads bacteria through the urinary system.
    d. Massage increases the difficulty with incontinence.

163. A client is experiencing pain on palpation of many points along the kidney meridian. Which element of the five elements contains the kidney meridian?

    a. Fire
    b. Water
    c. Wood
    d. Earth

164. In the five-element theory, what is the relationship of water to fire?

    a. Yin
    b. Yang
    c. Inhibiting
    d. Facilitating

165. Heat, redness, swelling, and pain are signs of _____.

    a. Cancer
    b. Degeneration
    c. Counterirritation
    d. Inflammation

166. A system of health and medicine developed in India is called _____.

    a. Prana
    b. Elements
    c. Polarity
    d. Ayurveda

167. Lung and diaphragm pain may be referred to which cutaneous area?

    a. Left side of the neck
    b. Right side of the chest
    c. Right side of the neck
    d. In the hip girdle area

168. A client complains of increased hunger and thirst, feels hot, and has a bad temper lately. Which of the Ayurvedic elements is out of balance?

    a. Earth
    b. Fire
    c. Water
    d. Ether

169. If an area of blocked energy is located, a simple polarity method is to _____.

    a. Place the left hand on the painful area and the right hand opposite the painful area
    b. Rub the area with specialized oil preparations
    c. Press into the area with the first finger and hold
    d. Stimulate the corresponding marma

 Answers are on page 406.

170. In polarity therapy, the heel of the foot is in a reflex relationship with the _____.

    a. Shoulders and chest
    b. Pelvis
    c. Head and brain
    d. Abdomen

171. An interesting similarity between the traditional chakra system and biologic oscillators is _____.

    a. Rhythm patterns
    b. Vibratory rate
    c. Shared location
    d. Size comparison

172. When one is considering the wellness components of balanced body, mind, and spirit, in which of the following intervention areas is massage most effective?

    a. Promoting exercise
    b. Inhibition of an appropriate eating and sleep cycle
    c. Normalization of breathing mechanisms
    d. Promoting belief system changes

173. The law of facilitation states that when an impulse has passed through a certain set of neurons to the exclusion of others one time, it will tend to take the same course on a future occasion, and each time it travels this path, the resistance will be smaller. What are the implications for massage?

    a. If a sensory receptor is activated, it will respond in a certain way.
    b. Methods must override a sensation to produce a response.
    c. The body likes sameness; after a pattern has been established, less stimulation is required to activate the response.
    d. For a massage method to change a sensory perception, the intensity of the method must match and then exceed the existing sensation.

174. A massage therapist is involved with developing a promotional campaign to increase his massage business since taking on a part-time massage employee. What is this called?

    a. Marketing
    b. Business plan
    c. Resume
    d. Management

175. Gross income minus expenses equals _____.

    a. Deductions
    b. Deposits
    c. Net income
    d. A draw

176. In which situation would you stay in the massage room and assist a client on and off the massage table?

    a. A client in the first trimester of pregnancy
    b. A 65-year-old man with diabetes
    c. An elderly woman with high blood pressure
    d. An adolescent with a wrist cast

177. Trigger points commonly are located in the belly of_____.

    a. Ligaments
    b. Tendons
    c. The joint capsule
    d. Muscles

178. A client has increased internal rotation of the right shoulder. Which of the following is the best massage approach to reverse the condition?

    a. Frictioning and traction to the external rotators
    b. Muscle energy methods with lengthening and then stretching of the internal rotators
    c. Compression and tapotement to the internal rotators
    d. Stretching of the flexors and extensors with lengthening to the external rotators

          Answers are on page 406.

179. The attachment of myosin to cross-bridges on actin requires _____.

    a. Calcium
    b. Maximal stimulus
    c. Endomysium
    d. Potassium

180. An adult male client has many surgical scars on his chest and abdomen. History indicates that the client had surgical intervention as a child to repair congenital malformations. The client enjoys massage on the limbs and back in the prone position but appears distant and unsettled when turned to the supine position. What is the most logical explanation for this response?

    a. An abusive family history
    b. Reenactment
    c. Dissociation
    d. Integration

181. A massage practitioner has been asked by a group of mental health professionals to begin working at a residential facility. She would need to be most concerned over which of the following?

    a. Reversal of mental health issues
    b. Obtaining informed consent
    c. Learning specific massage protocols for each condition
    d. Frequency and duration of the massage

182. The nervous system and the endocrine system reflect quantum properties because _____.

    a. Predictable physiologic outcomes are constant
    b. Feedback loops reliably affect outcomes
    c. Linear pathways of affect are constant
    d. Tendency for response is most accurate

183. Which aspect of bone structure supports the shape of bone?

    a. Fluid mineral
    b. Organic material
    c. Trabeculas
    d. Endoskeleton

184. Which of the following ancient healing systems most correlates with the endocrine system?

    a. Meridian system
    b. Five elements
    c. Doshas
    d. Chakra system

185. Massage therapy benefits conditions by encouraging the body through the phases involved in rehabilitation, restoration, and _____ of anatomic and physiologic function.

    a. Secretion
    b. Normalization
    c. Dysregulation
    d. Circulation

186. A client is experiencing a limitation in range of motion of the hip into abduction. Assessment indicates shortening and tension in the adductor group of muscles. Which of the following is the most likely source of the limited range of motion?

    a. Agonists
    b. Synergists
    c. Antagonists
    d. Fixators

187. Which of the following conditions is most likely to benefit directly from a nonspecific general massage session?

    a. Contusion
    b. Anterior compartment syndrome
    c. Muscle tension headache
    d. Spasticity

188. The external intercostal muscles create a vacuum in the thorax in which way?

    a. The upper ribs expand
    b. The ribs are pulled together
    c. The lower ribs are lifted up and out
    d. The diaphragm muscle arches upward

 Answers are on page 406.

189. Joints in which stability is reduced because of increased laxity of supportive ligaments also will have an increase in _____.

    a. Joint play
    b. Hypomobility
    c. Muscle relaxation
    d. Plasma membrane

190. A client requests an outcome from the massage session that includes a good night's sleep and less fidgeting. The massage session then would need to be designed to accomplish what?

    a. Cranial sacral plexus inhibition
    b. Parasympathetic inhibition
    c. Sympathetic inhibition
    d. Sympathetic dominance

191. Should there be an injury to the sternoclavicular joint that limits its range of motion, what other structure will be affected?

    a. Radius
    b. Olecranon
    c. Scapula
    d. Deltoid ligament

192. A client seeks massage after a diagnosis of neuralgia in the left leg. Which of the following would be a realistic therapeutic massage outcome?

    a. Reduction of pain and regeneration
    b. Long-term symptom increase
    c. Short-term pain management
    d. Short-term regeneration

193. An elderly client with a history of slow tissue healing and gradual weight loss begins to stabilize her weight and increase her ability to heal skin abrasions after receiving a weekly massage for 3 months. Which of the following offers the most concrete explanation for this outcome?

    a. Massage influences positive feedback mechanism to decrease adrenal output.
    b. Massage supports hypothalamic release of growth hormone–releasing hormone.
    c. Massage changes sleep patterns to increase dopamine influence.
    d. Massage beneficially influences tissue transport systems of neurotransmitters from endocrine tissues.

194. A client sprained the joint in one of the fingers. What is going to be the most comfortable position for the joint and why?

    a. The closed packed position because this is the most stable position of the joint
    b. The loose packed position so that movement can occur most easily
    c. The least packed position to accommodate swelling
    d. The closed packed position to accommodate increased synovial fluid

195. The sympathetic chain ganglia are located in an area similar to the back-shu points on which meridian?

    a. Spleen
    b. Kidney
    c. Liver
    d. Bladder

196. Neurotransmitters work in excitatory and inhibitory pairs. Which of the following would provide a balancing action for enkephalin?

    a. Somatostatin
    b. Substance P
    c. Serotonin
    d. Gamma-aminobutyric acid

     Answers are on page 406.

197. During assessment, you want the client to rotate the hip externally. What instructions would you give the client?

    a. Please move your leg so that you cross it over the other leg at the ankles.
    b. Please straighten your legs and turn the entire leg so that you point your toes toward each other.
    c. Please straighten your legs and turn the entire leg so that you point your toes away from each other.
    d. Please bring your knee toward your chest.

198. The massage method that most affects the inner ear balance mechanisms is _____.

    a. Tapotement
    b. Compression
    c. Friction
    d. Rocking

199. The purpose of therapeutic (feel good) pain during massage to manage undesirable pain is to stimulate which neurotransmitters?

    a. Serotonin and endorphin
    b. Epinephrine and histamine
    c. Acetylcholine and dopamine
    d. Histamine and substance P

200. Muscle uses which of the following to produce mechanical energy to exert force?

    a. Myoglobin
    b. Adenosine triphosphate
    c. Perimysium
    d. Cholecystokinin

 Answers are on page 406.

B

Answer Keys to Practice Exams

Answer key to Practice Exam One

1. A	51. B	101. A	151. C
2. A	52. C	102. C	152. C
3. D	53. B	103. D	153. C
4. C	54. A	104. C	154. B
5. C	55. B	105. B	155. A
6. D	56. C	106. D	156. B
7. A	57. A	107. B	157. C
8. C	58. C	108. A	158. B
9. C	59. A	109. B	159. A
10. D	60. B	110. C	160. D
11. C	61. A	111. C	161. A
12. B	62. B	112. A	162. A
13. D	63. C	113. B	163. D
14. A	64. A	114. C	164. D
15. B	65. B	115. A	165. A
16. A	66. B	116. D	166. C
17. B	67. C	117. A	167. C
18. C	68. B	118. C	168. A
19. B	69. A	119. C	169. D
20. C	70. D	120. D	170. B
21. D	71. D	121. D	171. A
22. B	72. D	122. A	172. C
23. B	73. C	123. B	173. C
24. C	74. B	124. C	174. D
25. C	75. D	125. D	175. C
26. A	76. B	126. A	176. A
27. B	77. B	127. A	177. C
28. A	78. C	128. D	178. A
29. D	79. B	129. B	179. B
30. B	80. B	130. B	180. B
31. A	81. C	131. D	181. C
32. D	82. C	132. D	182. B
33. A	83. B	133. D	183. C
34. D	84. C	134. B	184. D
35. B	85. C	135. D	185. D
36. D	86. C	136. D	186. B
37. A	87. B	137. A	187. B
38. D	88. D	138. B	188. A
39. C	89. C	139. C	189. B
40. B	90. B	140. C	190. C
41. A	91. D	141. C	191. C
42. D	92. C	142. C	192. C
43. C	93. D	143. C	193. C
44. B	94. A	144. C	194. B
45. D	95. A	145. B	195. C
46. A	96. C	146. D	196. A
47. A	97. B	147. D	197. D
48. C	98. D	148. A	198. B
49. B	99. C	149. D	199. D
50. B	100. C	150. B	200. B

Answer Key to Practice Exam Two

1. C	51. B	101. D	151. B
2. A	52. B	102. D	152. A
3. B	53. C	103. D	153. A
4. C	54. D	104. C	154. A
5. A	55. B	105. B	155. C
6. A	56. B	106. A	156. D
7. C	57. B	107. B	157. D
8. B	58. D	108. C	158. A
9. B	59. A	109. B	159. C
10. D	60. C	110. C	160. A
11. A	61. B	111. C	161. D
12. C	62. A	112. A	162. B
13. A	63. D	113. C	163. B
14. A	64. B	114. A	164. C
15. A	65. D	115. A	165. D
16. C	66. C	116. B	166. D
17. A	67. B	117. A	167. A
18. A	68. B	118. A	168. B
19. D	69. A	119. B	169. A
20. A	70. C	120. D	170. B
21. D	71. C	121. A	171. C
22. D	72. C	122. A	172. C
23. B	73. C	123. A	173. C
24. C	74. B	124. D	174. A
25. C	75. B	125. B	175. C
26. A	76. C	126. C	176. C
27. C	77. C	127. B	177. D
28. D	78. C	128. A	178. B
29. A	79. C	129. C	179. A
30. C	80. B	130. A	180. C
31. A	81. C	131. D	181. B
32. C	82. A	132. A	182. D
33. C	83. D	133. C	183. C
34. C	84. D	134. C	184. D
35. D	85. B	135. C	185. B
36. A	86. D	136. B	186. C
37. D	87. A	137. A	187. C
38. B	88. B	138. D	188. C
39. C	89. D	139. C	189. A
40. C	90. C	140. A	190. C
41. A	91. B	141. C	191. C
42. C	92. C	142. D	192. C
43. B	93. D	143. B	193. B
44. D	94. C	144. A	194. C
45. B	95. C	145. C	195. D
46. B	96. B	146. B	196. B
47. D	97. D	147. A	197. C
48. B	98. D	148. B	198. D
49. B	99. B	149. D	199. A
50. A	100. C	150. C	200. B

Glossary

Abbreviation Shortened forms of words or phrases.

Abduction Lateral movement away from the midline of the trunk.

Absorption The movement of food molecules from the digestive tract to the circulatory or lymphatic systems.

Abuse Exploitation, misuse, mistreatment, molestation, neglect.

Acetylcholine A neurotransmitter that stimulates the parasympathetic nervous system and the skeletal muscles and is involved in memory.

Acne A chronic inflammation of the sebaceous glands and hair follicles caused by interactions between bacteria, sebum, and sex hormones.

Acquired immunodeficiency syndrome A dysfunction in the immune system, which defends the body against disease. Abbreviated AIDS.

Active assisted movement Movement of a joint in which the client and the therapist produce the motion.

Active joint movement Movement of a joint through its range of motion by the client.

Active range of motion Movement of a joint by the client without any type of assistance from the massage practitioner.

Active resistive movement Movement of a joint by the client against resistance provided by the therapist.

Active transport The transport of substances into or out of a cell using energy.

Acupressure Methods used to tone or sedate acupuncture points without the use of needles.

Acupuncture The practice of inserting needles at specific points on meridians, or channels, to stimulate or sedate energy flow to regulate or alter body function. A branch of Chinese medicine, acupuncture is the art and science of manipulating the flow of Qi, the basic life force, and xue, the blood, body fluids, and nourishing essences. Western medicine uses acupuncture primarily to reduce pain. Acupressure, which uses digital pressure, follows the same Asian principles.

Acupuncture point Asian term for a specific point that correlates with a neurologic motor point.

Acute A term that describes a condition in which the signs and symptoms develop quickly, last a short time, and then disappear.

Acute disease Disease that has a specific beginning, signs, and symptoms that develop quickly, last a short time, and then disappear.

Acute illness A short-term illness that resolves by means of the normal healing process and, if necessary, supportive medical care.

Acute pain A symptom of a disease condition or a temporary aspect of medical treatment. Acute pain acts as a warning signal because it can activate the sympathetic nervous system. It usually is temporary, of sudden onset, and easily localized. The client frequently can describe the pain, which often subsides without treatment.

Adaptation A response to a sensory stimulation in which nerve signaling is reduced or ceases.

Adduction A medial movement toward the midline of the body.

Adenosine triphosphate A compound that stores energy in the muscles. When adenosine triphosphate is broken down during catabolic reactions, it releases energy. Abbreviated ATP.

Adrenergic Stimulation of the sympathetic nervous system causing a release of epinephrine and similar neurotransmitters and hormones.

Aerobic exercise training An exercise program focused to increase fitness and endurance.

Afferent Toward a center or point of reference.

407

Afferent nerves Sensory nerves that link sensory receptors with the central nervous system and transmit sensory information.

Agonist A muscle that causes or controls joint motion through a specified plane of motion; also known as the primary or prime mover.

Alimentary canal The tube-shaped portion of the digestive system known as the gastrointestinal tract; the alimentary canal is about 30 feet long and contains several special structures throughout its length.

Allied health A division of medicine in which the professional receives training in a specific area of medicine to serve as support for the physician.

All-or-none response The property of a muscle fiber (cell) contraction by which, when contraction is initiated, the fiber contracts to its full ability or does not contract at all.

Alopecia Hair loss or baldness on parts or all of the body

Amphiarthrosis A slightly movable joint that connects bone to bone with fibrocartilage or hyaline growth cartilage. The two types in the human body are symphyses and synchondroses.

Amyotrophic lateral sclerosis A progressive disease that begins in the central nervous system and involves the degeneration of motor neurons and the subsequent atrophy of voluntary muscle. Also called Lou Gehrig disease.

Anabolism Chemical processes in the body that join simple compounds to form more complex compounds of carbohydrates, lipids, proteins, and nucleic acids. The processes require energy supplied from adenosine triphosphate.

Anaplasia Meaning without shape, the term describes abnormal or undifferentiated cells that fail to mature into specialized cell types. Anaplasia is a characteristic of malignant cells.

Anatomic barriers Anatomic structures determined by the shape and fit of the bones at the joint.

Anatomic position A standard position in which the person stands upright with the feet slightly apart, arms hanging at the sides, and palms facing forward with thumbs outward.

Anatomic range of motion The amount of motion available to a joint based on the structure of the joint and determined by the shape of the joint surfaces, joint capsule, ligaments, muscle bulk, and surrounding musculotendinous and bony structures.

Anatomy The study of the structures of the body and the relationship of its parts.

Androgens Male sex hormones.

Anemia A decrease in the normal number of red blood cells or in the amount of hemoglobin or iron in the blood.

Aneurysm A permanent dilation of part of a blood vessel caused by weakness or damage to its structure. The most common sites of aneurysms are the aorta and the arteries of the brain.

Antagonism Opposition, as when massage produces the opposite effect, such as with medications.

Antagonist A muscle usually located on the opposite side of a joint from the agonist and having the opposite action. The muscle that opposes the movement of the prime movers.

Anterior pelvic rotation Anterior movement of the upper pelvis; the iliac crest tilts forward in a sagittal plane.

Antibody A specific protein produced to destroy or suppress antigens.

Antigen Any substance that causes the body to produce antibodies.

Anxiety A feeling of uneasiness, usually connected with an increase in sympathetic arousal responses.

Aorta The large artery that carries oxygen- and nutrient-enriched blood out of the heart.

Apical surface The surface of epithelial cells that is exposed to the external surface such as the atmosphere or a passage in the body.

Apocrine A type of sweat gland that discharges a thicker and more odoriferous form of sweat.

Aponeurosis A broad, flat sheet of fibrous connective tissue.

Appendicular skeleton The part of the skeleton composed of the limbs and their attachments.

Applied kinesiology Methods of evaluation and bodywork that use a specialized type of muscle testing and various forms of massage and bodywork for corrective procedures.

Approximation The technique of pushing muscle fibers together in the belly of the muscle.

Art Craft, skill, technique, and talent.

Arterial circulation Movement of oxygenated blood under pressure from the heart to the body through the arteries.

Arterioles The smallest arteries.

Arteriosclerosis A term meaning hardening of the arteries and referring to arteries that have become brittle and have lost their elasticity.

Artery A blood vessel that transports oxygenated blood from the heart to the body or deoxygenated blood from the heart to the lungs.

Arthritis The most common type of joint disorder, arthritis literally means inflammation of the joint.

Arthrokinematic movement Accessory movements that occur as a result of inherent laxity or joint play that exists in each joint. The joint play allows the ends of the bones to slide, roll, or spin smoothly on one another. These essential movements occur passively with movement of the joint and are not under voluntary control.

Articulation Another word for a joint, the structure created when bones connect to each other.

Ascending tracts Tracts that carry sensory information to the brain.

Aseptic technique Procedures that kill or disable pathogens on surfaces to prevent transmission.

Asian approaches Methods of bodywork that have developed from ancient Chinese methods.

Assessment The collection and interpretation of information provided by the client, the client's family and friends, the massage practitioner, and referring medical professionals.

Asymmetrical stance The position in which the body weight is shifted from one foot to the other while standing.

Atherosclerosis A condition in which fatty plaque is deposited in medium and large arteries.

Athlete A person who participates in sports as an amateur or a professional. Athletes require precise use of their bodies.

Atom The smallest particle of an element that retains and exhibits the properties of that element. Atoms are made up of protons, neutrons, and electrons.

Atrium One of the two small, thin-walled upper chambers of the heart; the right and left atria are separated by a thin interatrial septum.

Atrophy A decrease in the size of a body part or organ caused by a decrease in the size of the cells.

Attachments Connections of skeletal muscles to bones; often referred to as the origin and insertion.

Autonomic nervous system A division of the peripheral nervous system composed of nerves that connect the central nervous system to the glands, heart, and smooth muscles to maintain the internal body environment. The body system that regulates involuntary body functions using the sympathetic "fight-flight-fear response" and the restorative parasympathetic "relaxation response." The sympathetic and parasympathetic systems work together to maintain homeostasis through a feedback loop system.

Autoregulation Control of homeostasis through alteration of tissue or function.

Avulsion Injury to a ligament or tendon involving tearing off of its attachment.

Axial skeleton The axis of the body; the axial skeleton consists of the head, vertebral column (the spine), and the ribs and sternum and provides the body with form and protection.

Axon A single elongated projection from the nerve cell body that transmits impulses away from the cell body.

Ayurveda A system of health and medicine that grew from East Indian roots.

Bacteria Primitive cells that have no nuclei. Bacteria cause disease by secreting toxic substances that damage human tissues, by becoming parasites inside human cells, or by forming colonies in the body that disrupt normal function.

Balance The ability to control equilibrium. Two types of balance are static or still balance and dynamic or moving balance.

Balance point The point of contact between the practitioner and client.

Ball-and-socket joint Joint that allows movement in many directions around a central point. Ball-and-socket joints are ball-shaped convex surfaces fitted into concave sockets. This type of joint gives the greatest freedom of movement but also is the most easily dislocated.

Basal metabolic rate The rate of energy expenditure of the body under normal, relaxed activities.

Basal surface The tissue surface that faces the inside of the body.

Basement membrane A permeable membrane that attaches epithelial tissues to the underlying connective tissues.

Beating A form of heavy tapotement involving use of the fist.

Benign A term that describes the type of tumor that remains localized within the tissue from which it arose and does not undergo malignant changes. Benign tumors usually grow slowly.

Biologic rhythms The internal, periodic timing component of an organism, also known as a biorhythm. Circadian rhythms work on a 24-hour period to coordinate internal functions such as sleep. Ultradian rhythms repeat themselves from every 90 minutes to every few hours, whereas seasonal rhythms are annual functions.

Biomechanics The study of mechanical principles, movements, and actions applied to living bodies.

Blood A thick, red fluid that provides oxygen, nourishment, and protection to the cells and carries away waste products. Whole blood consists of two components: the formed cellular elements and the liquid plasma. Blood is a form of connective tissue.

Blood pressure The measurement of pressure exerted by the heart on the walls of the blood vessels. The highest pressure exerted is called systolic pressure, which results when the ventricles are contracted. Diastolic pressure, the lowest pressure, results when the ventricles are at rest. Blood forced into the aorta during systole sets up a pressure wave that travels down the arteries. The wave expands the arterial wall, and the expansion can be palpated by pressing the artery against tissue; the waves constitute the pulse rate.

Body mechanics Use of the body in an efficient and biomechanically correct way.

Body segment The area of the body between joints that provides movement during walking and balance.

Body supports Pillows, folded blankets, foam forms, or commercial products that help contour the flat surface of a massage table or mat.

Body/mind The interaction between thought and physiology that is connected to the limbic system, hypothalamic influence on the autonomic nervous system, and the endocrine system.

Bodywork A term that encompasses all the various forms of massage, movement, and other touch therapies.

Boundary Personal space that exists within an arm's length perimeter. Personal emotional space is designated by morals, values, and experience.

Brain The largest and most complex unit of the nervous system, the brain is responsible for perception, sensation, emotion, intellect, and action.

Brainstem The primitive portion of the brain that contains centers for vital functions and reflex actions, such as vomiting, coughing, sneezing, posture, and basic movement patterns.

Breathing pattern disorders A complex set of behaviors that lead to overbreathing in the absence of a pathologic condition. These disorders are considered a functional syndrome because all the parts are working effectively; therefore a specific pathologic condition does not exist.

Buffers Compounds that prevent the hydrogen ion concentration from fluctuating too much and too rapidly to alter the pH.

Burnout A condition that occurs when a person uses up energy faster than it can be restored.

Bursa A flat sac of synovial membrane in which the inner sides of the sac are separated by fluid film. Bursas are located where moving structures are apt to rub.

Bursitis Inflammation of a bursa.

Callus An area of thickened, hardened skin that develops in an area of friction or region of recurrent pressure.

Cancer Malignant, nonencapsulated cells that invade surrounding tissue. They often break away, or metastasize, from the primary tumor and form secondary cancer masses.

Capillary One of the small blood vessels found between arteries and veins that allows the exchange of gases, nutrients, and waste products. The walls of capillaries are thin, allowing molecules to diffuse easily.

Carbohydrates Sugars, starches, and cellulose composed of carbon, hydrogen, and oxygen.

Cardiac cycle A synchronized sequence of events that takes place during one full heartbeat.

Cardiac muscle fibers Smaller, striated, involuntary muscle fibers (cells) in the heart that contract to pump blood.

Cardiac output The amount of blood pumped by the left ventricle in 1 minute.

Care or treatment plan The plan used to achieve therapeutic goals. It outlines the agreed objectives; the frequency, duration, and number of visits; progress measurements; the date of reassessment; and massage methods to be used.

Career A chosen pursuit; a life's work.

Carotene A yellow pigment found in the dermis that provides a natural yellow tint to the skin of some individuals.

Cartilage A form of flexible connective tissue. Types of cartilage include hyaline, fibrocartilage, and elastic cartilage.

Catabolism Chemical processes in the body that release energy as complex compounds are broken down into simpler ones.

Catecholamines A group of neurotransmitters involved in sleep, mood, pleasure, and motor function.

Cell The basic structural unit of a living organism. A cell contains a nucleus and cytoplasm and is surrounded by a membrane.

Center of gravity An imaginary midpoint or center of the weight of a body or object, where the body or object could balance on a point.

Centering The ability to focus the mind by screening out sensation.

Central nervous system The brain and spinal cord and their coverings.

Cerebellum The second largest part of the brain, the cerebellum is involved with balance, posture, coordination, and movement.

Cerebrospinal fluid A clear, colorless fluid that flows throughout the brain and around the spinal cord, cushioning and protecting these structures and maintaining proper pH balance.

Cerebrum The largest of the brain divisions, the cerebrum consists of two hemispheres that occupy the uppermost region of the cranium. The cerebrum receives, interprets, and associates incoming information with past memories and then transmits the appropriate motor response.

Certification A voluntary credentialing process that usually requires education and testing; tests are administered privately or by government regulatory bodies.

Cerumen A sticky substance released by glands in the ear. Also known as earwax, cerumen protects the ear from the entry of foreign material and repels insects.

Ceruminous glands Modified apocrine glands found in the external ear canal that secrete cerumen.

Chakra Energy fields or centers of consciousness within the body.

Challenge Living each day knowing that it is filled with things to learn, skills to practice, tasks to accomplish, and obstacles to overcome.

Charting The process of keeping a written record of a client or patient. The most effective charting methods follow clinical reasoning, which emphasizes a problem-solving approach. Many systems of charting are used, but all these models have similar components: POMR (problem-oriented medical record) and SOAP (subjective, objective, analysis, and plan—the four parts of the written record).

Chemical effects The effects of massage produced by the release of chemical substances in the body. These substances may be released locally from the massaged tissue, or they may be substances released into the general circulation.

Chemical properties Properties that demonstrate how a substance reacts with other substances or responds to a change in the environment.

Chronic A term that describes the type of disease that develops slowly and lasts for a long time, sometimes for life.

Chronic disease Disease with a vague onset that develops slowly and lasts for a long time, sometimes for life.

Chronic illness A disease, injury, or syndrome that shows little change or slow progression.

Chronic pain Pain that continues or recurs over a prolonged time, usually for more than 6 months. The onset may be obscure, and the character and quality of the pain may change over time. Chronic pain usually is poorly localized and not as intense as acute pain, although for some the pain is exhausting and depressing. Chronic pain usually does not activate the sympathetic nervous system.

Circulatory Systems that depend on the pumping action of the skeletal muscle (i.e., the arterial, venous, lymphatic, respiratory, cerebrospinal fluid circulatory systems).

Circumduction Circular movement of a limb, combining the movements of flexion, extension, abduction, and adduction, to create a cone shape.

Client information form A document used to obtain information from the client about health, preexisting conditions, and expectations for the massage.

Client outcome The results desired from the massage and the massage therapist.

Client/practitioner agreement and policy statement A detailed written explanation of all rules, expectations, and procedures for the massage.

Closed kinematic chain The positioning of joints in such a way that motion at one of the joints is accompanied by motion at an adjacent joint.

Close-packed position The position of a synovial joint in which the surfaces fit precisely together and maximal contact between the opposing surfaces occurs. The compression of joint surfaces permits no movement, and the joint possesses its greatest stability.

Coalition A group formed for a particular purpose.

Cognition Conscious awareness and perception, reasoning, judgment, intuition, and memory.

Collagen A protein substance composed of small fibrils that combine to create the connective tissue of fascias, tendons, and ligaments. When combined with water, collagen forms gelatin. Collagen constitutes approximately one fourth of the protein in the body.

Collagenous fibers Strong fibers with little capacity for stretch. They have a high degree of tensile strength, which allows them to withstand longitudinal stress.

Collaterals Branches from an axon that allow communication among neurons.

Combining vowel A vowel added between two roots or a root and a suffix to make pronunciation of the word easier.

Comfort barrier The first point of resistance short of the client's perceiving any discomfort at the physiologic or pathologic barrier.

Commitment The ability and willingness to be involved in what is happening around us so as to have a purpose for being.

Communicable disease A disease caused by pathogens that are spread easily; a contagious disease.

Compact (dense) bone The hard portion of bone that protects spongy bone and provides the firm framework of the bone and the body. The osteocytes in this type of bone are located in concentric rings around a central haversian canal, through which nerves and blood vessels pass.

Compensation The process of counterbalancing a defect in body structure or function.

Compression Pressure into the body to spread tissue against underlying structures. (This massage manipulation sometimes is classified with petrissage.) Also, the exertion of inappropriate pressure on nerves by hard tissue (e.g., bone).

Compressive force The amount of pressure exerted against the surface of the body in order to apply pressure to the deeper body structures; pressure directed in a particular direction.

Concentric contraction The action of a prime mover or agonist by which a muscle develops tension as it shortens to provide enough force to overcome resistance, described as positive contraction.

Concentric isotonic contraction Application of a counterforce by the massage therapist while allowing the client to move, which brings the origin and insertion of the target muscle together against the pressure.

Condition management The use of massage methods to support clients who are unable to undergo a therapeutic change but who wish to function as effectively as possible under a set of circumstances.

Condyle A rounded projection at the end of a bone.

Condyloid (condylar) joint Joint that allows movement in two directions, but one motion predominates. The joint resembles a condyle, which is a rounded protuberance at the end of a bone forming an articulation.

Confidentiality Respect for the privacy of information.

Conflict An expressed struggle between at least two interdependent parties who perceive incompatible goals, scarce resources, and/or interference from the other party in achieving their goals.

Connective tissue The most abundant type of tissue in the body, connective tissue supports and holds together the body and its parts, protects the body from foreign matter, and is organized to transport substances throughout the body.

Conservation withdrawal A parasympathetic survival pattern that is similar to playing "possum" or hibernation.

Contamination The process by which an object or area becomes unclean.

Contractility The ability of a muscle to shorten forcibly with adequate stimulation. This property sets muscle apart from all other types of tissue.

Contracture The chronic shortening of a muscle, especially the connective tissue component.

Contraindication Any condition that renders a particular treatment improper or undesirable.

Control The belief that we can influence events by the way we feel, think, and act.

Contusion A bruise.

Corn A painful, conical thickening of skin over bony prominences of the feet caused by continued pressure and friction on normally thin skin. Soft corns are those located in moist areas, such as between the toes.

Coronary arteries The arteries that supply oxygenated blood to the heart muscle itself; they are located in grooves between the atria and ventricles and between the two ventricles.

Coronary veins Veins that return the deoxygenated blood from the heart to the right atrium.

Cortisol A glucocorticoid, also known as hydrocortisone. Levels of stress often are measured by cortisol levels. A stress hormone produced by the adrenal glands that is released during long-term stress. An elevated level indicates increased sympathetic arousal.

Counterirritation Superficial stimulation that relieves a deeper sensation by stimulating different sensory signals.

Counterpressure Force applied to an area that is designed to match exactly (isometric contraction) or partly (isotonic contraction) the effort or force produced by the muscles of that area.

Countertransference The personalization of the professional relationship by the therapist in which the practitioner is unable to separate the therapeutic relationship from personal feelings and expectations for the client.

Cramps Painful muscle spasms or involuntary twitches that involve the whole muscle.

Cranial nerves Twelve pairs of nerves that originate from the olfactory bulbs, thalamus, visual cortex, and brainstem. They transmit information to and from the sensory organs of the face and the muscles of the face, neck, and upper shoulders.

Craniosacral and myofascial approaches Methods of bodywork that work reflexively and mechanically with the fascial network of the body.

Cream A type of lubricant that is in a semisolid or solid state.

Credential A designation earned by completing a process that verifies a certain level of expertise in a given skill.

Creep The slow movement of viscoelastic materials back to their original state and tissue structure after release of a deforming force.

Cross-directional stretching Tissue stretching that pulls and twists connective tissue against its fiber direction.

Cryotherapy Therapeutic use of ice.

Culture The arts, beliefs, customs, institutions, and all other products of human work and thought created by a specific group of people at a particular time.

Cupping The type of tapotement that involves the use of a cupped hand; it often is used over the thorax.

Cutaneous sensory receptors Sensory nerves in the skin.

Cytoplasm Material enclosed by the cell membrane.

Cytoskeleton A framework of proteins inside the cell providing flexibility and strength.

Cytosol The fluid that surrounds the nucleus or organelles inside the cell membrane.

Database All the information available that contributes to therapeutic interaction.

Deep fascia A coarse sheet of fibrous connective tissue that binds muscles into functional groups and forms partitions, called intermuscular septa, between muscle groups.

Deep inspiration Movement of air into the body by hard breathing to meet an increased demand for oxygen. Any muscles that can pull the ribs up are called into action.

Deep transverse friction A specific rehabilitation technique that creates therapeutic inflammation by creating a specific, controlled reinjury of tissues by applying concentrated therapeutic movement that moves the tissue against its grain over only a small area.

Defensive measures The means by which our bodies defend against stressors (e.g., production of antibodies and white blood cells or through behavioral or emotional means).

Degenerative joint disease Progressive change to joint surfaces commonly called osteoarthritis.

Dendrites Branching projections from the nerve cell body that carry signals to the cell body.

Denial The ability to retreat and to ignore stressors.

Deoxyribonucleic acid Genetic material of the cell that carries the chemical "blueprint" of the body. Abbreviated DNA.

Depression 1. A condition characterized by a decrease in vital functional activity and by mood disturbances of exaggerated emptiness, hopelessness, and melancholy or of unbridled high energy with no purpose or outcome. 2. Downward or inferior movement.

Depth of pressure Compressive stress that can be light, moderate, deep, or varied.

Dermatitis A general term for acute or chronic skin inflammation characterized by redness, eruptions, edema, scaling, and itching. The three main types are atopic dermatitis, seborrheic dermatitis, and contact dermatitis. Eczema is a form of dermatitis.

Dermatome Cutaneous (skin) distribution of spinal nerve sensation.

Dermis The inner layer of skin that contains collagen and elastin fibers, which provide much of the structure and strength of the skin, and is much thicker than the epidermis.

Descending tracts Tracts that carry sensory information from the brain to the spinal cord.

Diagnosis A labeling of signs and symptoms by a licensed medical professional.

Diagonal abduction Movement of a limb through a diagonal plane directly across and away from the midline of the body.

Diagonal adduction Movement of a limb through a diagonal plane toward and across the midline of the body.

Diaphragm A dome-shaped sheet of muscle attached to the thoracic wall that separates the lungs and thoracic cavity from the abdominal cavity. As the chest cavity enlarges, the diaphragm moves downward and flattens to create a vacuum that allows air to flow into the lungs. As the chest contracts and the diaphragm relaxes, the diaphragm arches upward, helping air to flow out of the lungs.

Diarthrosis A freely movable synovial joint.

Diffusion Movement of ions and molecules from an area of higher concentration to that of a lower concentration.

Digestion The mechanical and chemical breakdown of food from its complex form into simple molecules.

Direction Flow of massage strokes from the center of the body outward (centrifugal) or from the extremities inward toward the center of the body (centripetal). Direction can be circular motions; it can flow from origin to insertion of the muscle, following the muscle fibers, or can flow transverse to the tissue fibers.

Direction of ease The position the body assumes with postural changes and muscle shortening or weakening, depending on how it has balanced against gravity.

Disclosure Acknowledging and informing the client of any situation that interferes with or affects the professional relationship.

Disease An abnormality in functions of the body, especially when the abnormality threatens well-being.

Disharmony Distortions in health that result when the functions or systems are neither balanced nor working at their optimum. In Chinese medicine, disharmony can be created by the imbalance of the Six Pernicious Influences or the Seven Emotions.

Disinfection The process by which pathogens are destroyed.

Disk herniation A pathologic condition that occurs when the fibrocartilage that surrounds the intervertebral disk ruptures, releasing the nucleus pulposus that cushions the vertebrae above and below. The resultant pressure on spinal nerve roots may cause pain and damage the surrounding nerves.

Dissociation Detachment, discontentedness, separation, isolation.

Dopamine A neurochemical that influences motor activity involving movement (especially learned fine movement, such as handwriting), conscious selectivity (what to pay attention to), mood (in terms of inspiration), possibility, intuition, joy, and enthusiasm. If the dopamine level is low, the opposite effects are seen, such as lack of motor control, clumsiness, inability to decide what to attend to, and boredom.

Dorsal root One of two roots that attaches a spinal nerve to the spinal cord.

Dorsiflexion (dorsal flexion) Movement of the ankle that results in the top of the foot moving toward the anterior tibia.

Dosha An Ayurvedic concept that describes chemical processes in the body. The three types are Vata, Pitta, and Kappa.

Drag The amount of pull (stretch) on the tissue (tensile stress).

Drape Fabric used to cover the client and keep the individual warm while the massage is given.

Draping The procedures of covering and uncovering areas of the body and turning the client during the massage.

Draping material Coverings that provide the client with privacy and warmth. The most commonly used coverings are standard bed linens because they are large enough to cover the entire body and are easy to use for most draping procedures.

Dual role Overlap in the scope of practice, with one professional providing support in more than one area of expertise.

Duration The length of time a method lasts or stays in the same location.

Dynamic force Force applied to an object that produces movement in or of the object.

Dysfunction An in-between state in which one is "not healthy" but also "not sick" (i.e., experiencing disease).

Eccentric The action of an antagonist by which a muscle lengthens while under tension and changes in tension to control the descent of the resistance. Eccentric movement may be thought of as controlling movement against gravity or resistance and are described as negative contractions.

Eccentric isotonic contraction Application of a counterforce while the client moves the jointed area, which allows the origin and insertion to separate. The muscle lengthens against the pressure.

Eccrine A type of sweat gland that releases a watery fluid known as sweat, which cools the body and provides minor elimination of metabolic waste.

Edema The accumulation of abnormal amounts of fluid in tissue spaces.

Efferent Away from a center or point of reference.

Efferent nerves Motor nerves that link the central nervous system to the effectors outside it and transmit motor impulses.

Effleurage Gliding strokes; horizontal strokes applied with the fingers, hand, or forearm that usually follow the fiber direction of the underlying muscle, fascial planes, or dermatome pattern.

Effort The force applied to overcome resistance.

Elastic fibers Connective tissue fibers that are extensible and elastic. They are made of a protein called elastin, which returns to its original length after being stretched.

Elasticity The ability of a muscle to recoil and resume its original resting length after being stretched.

Elastin A connective tissue fiber type that has elastic properties and allows flexibility of connective tissue structures.

Electrical-chemical functions Physiologic functions of the body that rely on or produce body energy; often called Ch'i, prana, and meridian energy.

Element Substance containing only a single kind of atom.

Elevation Upward or superior movement.

Elimination (egestion) Removal and release of solid waste products from food that cannot be digested or absorbed.

Employee A person who works for another for a wage.

Endangerment site Any area of the body where nerves and blood vessels surface close to the skin and are not well protected by muscle or connective tissue; therefore deep, sustained pressure into these areas could damage these vessels and nerves. The kidney area is included because the kidneys are loosely suspended in fat and connective tissue, and heavy pounding is contraindicated in that area.

End-feel The perception of the joint at the limit of its range of motion. The end-feel is soft or hard. (See *joint end-feel*.)

Endocrine gland A ductless gland that secretes hormones directly into the bloodstream.

Endocytosis The cellular process of engulfing particles located outside the cell membrane into a cell by forming vesicles.

Endogenous Made in the body.

Endoplasmic reticulum A network of intracellular membranes in the form of tubes that is connected to the nuclear membrane.

Endorphins Peptide hormones that mainly work like morphine to suppress pain. They influence mood, producing a mild euphoric feeling such as is seen in runner's high.

Endoskeleton The bony support structure found inside the human body that accommodates growth.

Endosteum A thin membrane of connective tissue that lines the marrow cavity of a bone.

Endurance A measure of fitness. The ability to work for prolonged periods and the ability to resist fatigue.

Energetic approaches Methods of bodywork that work with subtle body responses.

Energy The capacity to work, and work is the movement of or a change in the physical structure of matter.

Enkephalins and endorphins Neurochemicals that elevate mood, support satiety (reduce hunger and cravings), and modulate pain.

Entrainment A coordination or synchronization to an internal or external rhythm, especially when a person responds to certain patterns by moving in a coordinated manner to those patterns.

Entrapment Pathologic pressure placed on a nerve or vessel by soft tissue.

Environmental contact Contact with pathogens found in the environment in food, water, and soil and on various surfaces.

Epicondyle A bony projection above a condyle.

Epidermis The outer or top layer of skin composed of sublayers called strata. The epidermis contains no nerves or blood vessels.

Epilepticus A continuous seizure.

Epinephrine A catecholamine released by the nervous system and involved in fight-or-flight responses such as dilation of blood vessels to the skeletal muscles. Epinephrine is classified as a hormone when secreted by the adrenal gland.

Epinephrine/adrenaline A neurochemical that activates arousal mechanisms in the body; the activation, arousal, alertness, and alarm chemical of the fight-or-flight response and all sympathetic arousal functions and behaviors.

Epithelial tissues A specialized group of tissues that cover and protect the surface of the body and its parts, line body cavities, and form glands. Epithelial tissue usually is found in areas that move substances into and out of the body during secretion, absorption, and excretion.

Erythrocytes Red blood cells that contain hemoglobin and function to transport oxygen to the cells and carbon dioxide away from the cells.

Essential touch Vital, fundamental, and primary touch that is crucial to well-being.

Essential tremor A chronic tremor that does not proceed from any other pathologic condition.

Ethical behavior Right and good conduct that is based on moral and cultural standards as defined by the society in which we live.

Ethical decision making The application of ethical principles and professional skills to determine appropriate behavior and resolve ethical dilemmas.

Ethics The science or study of morals, values, or principles, including ideals of autonomy, beneficence, and justice; principles of right and good conduct.

Etiology The study of the factors involved in the development of disease, including the nature of the disease and the susceptibility of the person.

Eversion Movement of the sole of the foot outward away from the midline.

Excitability The ability of a muscle to receive and respond to a stimulus.

Exemption A situation in which a professional is not required to comply with an existing law because of educational or professional standing.

Exocrine gland A gland that secretes hormones through ducts directly into specific areas. Exocrine glands are part of the endocrine system.

Exocytosis The movement of substances out of a cell.

Experiment A method of testing a hypothesis.

Expressive touch Touch applied to support and convey awareness and empathy for the client as a whole.

Extensibility The ability of a muscle to be stretched or extended.

Extension A movement that increases the angle between two bones, usually moving the body part back toward the anatomic position.

External respiration The exchange of oxygen and carbon dioxide between the lungs and the bloodstream.

External rotation Rotary movement around the longitudinal axis of a bone away from the midline of the body. Also known as rotation laterally, outward rotation, and lateral rotation.

External sensory information Stimulation from an origin exterior to the surface of the skin that is detected by the body.

Facet A smooth, flat surface on a bone.

Facilitated diffusion The transport of substances by carriers to which the substance binds to move the substance into a cell along the concentration gradient without energy.

Facilitation The state of a nerve in which it is stimulated but not to the point of threshold, the point at which it transmits a nerve signal.

Fascia A fibrous membrane covering, supporting, and separating muscles; the subcutaneous tissue that connects the skin to the muscles.

Fascial sheath A flat sheet of connective tissue used for separation, stability, and muscular attachment points.

Feedback A method of autoregulation to maintain internal homeostasis that interlinks body functions; a noninvasive, continual exchange of information between the client and the professional.

Feedback loop A self-regulating control system in the body that receives information, integrates that information, and provides a response to maintain homeostasis. Negative feedback reverses the original stimulus, whereas positive feedback enhances and maintains the stimulus.

Fibrocartilage A connective tissue that permits little motion in joints and structures, is found in places such as the intervertebral disks, and forms our ears.

Fibromyalgia A syndrome with symptoms of widespread pain or aching, persistent fatigue, generalized morning stiffness, nonrestorative sleep, and multiple tender points. A disrupted sleep pattern, coupled with the dysfunction of myofascial repair mechanisms, seems to be a factor.

Fibrous joint An articulation in which fibrous tissue connects bone directly to bone.

Fistula A tract that is open at both ends through which abnormal connection occurs between two surfaces.

Fitness A general term used to describe the ability to perform physical work.

Fixator One of the stabilizing muscles surrounding a joint or body part that contracts to fixate, or stabilize, the area, enabling another limb or body segment to exert force and move.

Flaccid A term used to describe a muscle with decreased or absent tone.

Flexion A movement that decreases the angle between two bones as the body part moves out of the anatomic position.

Fontanels Areas of the skull of an infant in which the bone formation is incomplete. The fontanels allow for compression of the skull as the infant travels through the birth canal and expansion as the brain grows.

Foramen An opening in a bone, such as the foramen magnum of the skull.

Force Any push or pull on an object in an attempt to affect motion or shape.

Forced expiration Movement of air out of the body, produced by activating muscles that can pull down the ribs and muscles that can compress the abdomen, forcing the diaphragm upward.

Forced inspiration Movement of air into the body that occurs when an individual is working hard and needs a great deal of oxygen. This involves not only the muscles of quiet and deep inspiration but also the muscles that stabilize and/or elevate the shoulder girdle in order to elevate the ribs directly or indirectly.

Fossa A depression in the surface or at the end of a bone.

Free nerve endings Sensory receptors that detect itch and tickle sensations.

Frequency The number of times a method repeats itself in a time period.

Friction Specific circular or transverse movements that do not glide on the skin and that are focused on the underlying tissue.

Frontal (coronal) plane A vertical plane that divides the body into anterior and posterior (front and back) parts.

Funguses A group of simple parasitic organisms that are similar to plants but that have no chlorophyll (green pigment). Most pathogenic funguses live on tissue on or near the skin or mucous membranes.

Gait The rhythmic and alternating motions of the legs, trunk, and arms resulting in the propulsion of the body.

Gait The walking pattern.

Gait cycle Subdivided into the stance phase and swing phase, this cycle begins when the heel of one foot strikes the floor and continues until the same heel strikes the floor again.

Gallbladder A small 3- to 4-inch sac that stores and concentrates bile.

Ganglion Cystic, round, usually nontender swellings located along tendon sheaths or joint capsules.

Gate-control theory A hypothetical gating mechanism that functions at the level of the spinal cord; a "gate" through which pain impulses reach the lateral spinothalamic system. Painful impulses are transmitted by large-diameter and small-diameter nerve fibers. Stimulation of large-diameter fibers prevents the small-diameter fibers from transmitting signals. Stimulating (rubbing, massaging) large-diameter fibers helps to suppress the sensation of pain, especially sharp pain.

General adaptation syndrome The method the body uses to mobilize different defense mechanisms when threatened by actual or perceived harmful stimuli. The process that calls into play the three stages of response to stress (i.e., the alarm reaction, the resistance reaction, and the exhaustion reaction).

General contraindications Factors that require a physician's evaluation to rule out serious underlying conditions before any massage is indicated. If the physician recommends massage, the physician must help develop a comprehensive treatment plan.

Gestation The period of fetal growth from conception until birth.

Gestures The way a client touches the body while explaining a problem. These movements may indicate whether the problem is a muscle problem, a joint problem, or a visceral problem.

Gibbus An angular deformity of a collapsed vertebra, the causes of which include metastatic cancer and tuberculosis of the spine.

Gliding joints Known also as synovial planes, gliding joints allow only a gliding motion in various planes.

Goals Desired outcomes.

Golgi tendon receptors Receptors in the tendons that sense tension.

Gray matter Unmyelinated nervous tissue, particularly that found in the central nervous system.

Gross anatomy The study of body structures visible to the naked eye.

Ground substance The medium in which the cells and protein fibers are suspended. Ground substance is usually clear and colorless and has the consistency of thick syrup.

Growth hormone A hormone that promotes cell division; in adults it is implicated in the repair and regeneration of tissue.

Guarding Contraction of muscles in a splinting action, surrounding an injured area.

Hacking A type of tapotement that alternately strikes the surface of the body with quick, snapping movements.

Half-life The amount of time required for half of a hormone to be eliminated from the bloodstream.

Hardening A method of teaching the body to deal more effectively with stress; sometimes called *toughening*.

Hardiness The physical and mental ability to withstand external stressors.

Healing The restoration of well-being.

Health A condition of homeostasis resulting in a state of physical, emotional, social, and spiritual well-being. Optimal functioning with freedom from disease or abnormal processes.

Heart The pump of the cardiovascular system; the heart is hollow, cone-shaped, and about the size of a fist and is located in the mediastinum of the thoracic cavity. The myocardium is the heart muscle itself, the endocardium is the thin inner lining, and the epicardium is the outer membrane.

Heart rate The number of cardiac cycles in 1 minute. In the average, healthy person the rate works out to be 60 to 70 cycles or beats per minute.

Heart sounds The two main sounds resulting from the closure of the valves. Murmurs are extra sounds, such as those resulting from faulty valves.

Heart valves Four sets of valves that keep the blood flowing in the correct direction through the heart.

Heavy pressure Compressive force that extends to the bone under the tissue.

Hemoglobin The oxygen-carrying, red-colored molecule in the blood.

Hemorrhage The passage of blood outside of the cardiovascular system.

Hepatitis A viral inflammatory process and infection of the liver.

Hernia Weakness in a muscle or structure that allows for protrusion of a muscle, organ, or structure through the resulting opening.

Herpes simplex A DNA virus that causes painful blisters and small ulcers in and around the mouth and on the genital area.

High-energy bonds Covalent bonds created in specific organic substrates in the presence of enzymes.

Hinge joint Joint that allows flexion and extension in one direction, changing the angle of the bones at the joint, like a door hinge.

Histamine A chemical produced by the body that dilates the blood vessels. A neurotransmitter that is considered a stimulant. Histamine is released by the mast cells as part of the inflammatory process and can cause itching.

History Information from the client about past and present medical conditions and patterns of symptoms.

Homeostasis Dynamic equilibrium of the internal environment of the body through processes of feedback and regulation. The relatively constant state of the internal environment of the body that is maintained by adaptive responses. Specific control and feedback mechanisms are responsible for adjusting body systems to maintain this state.

Horizontal abduction Movement of the humerus in the horizontal plane away from the midline of the body. Also known as the horizontal extension or transverse abduction.

Horizontal adduction Movement of the humerus in the horizontal plane toward the midline of the body. Also known as horizontal flexion or transverse adduction.

Hormone A messenger chemical in the bloodstream.

Human immunodeficiency virus The virus that appears to be responsible for acquired immunodeficiency syndrome. Abbreviated HIV.

Hyaline cartilage The thin covering of articular connective tissue on the ends of the bones in freely movable joints in the adult skeleton. Hyaline cartilage forms a smooth, resilient, low-friction surface for the articulation of one bone with another, distributes forces, and helps absorb some of the pressure imposed on the joint surfaces.

Hydrotherapy The use of various types of water applications and temperatures for therapy.

Hygiene Practices and conditions that promote health and prevent disease.

Hyperalgesia An increased sensitivity to pain.

Hyperextension A movement that takes the body part farther in the direction of the extension and farther out of anatomic position.

Hypermobility A range of motion of a joint greater than would be permitted normally by the structure. Hypermobility results in instability.

Hyperplasia An uncontrolled increase in the number of cells of a body part.

Hypersecretion The excessive release of a hormone.

Hyperstimulation analgesia Diminishing the perception of a sensation by stimulating large-diameter nerve fibers. Some methods used are application of ice or heat, counterirritation, acupressure, acupuncture, rocking, music, and repetitive massage strokes.

Hypertension An increase in systolic and diastolic pressures.

Hypertrophy An increase in the size of a cell, which results in an increase in the size of a body part or organ.

Hyperventilation Abnormally deep or rapid breathing in excess of physical demands.

Hypomobility A range of motion of a joint less than what would be permitted normally by the structure.

Hyposecretion The insufficient release of a hormone.

Hypotension A decrease in systolic and diastolic pressures. Hypotension is an important manifestation of shock, which causes inadequate blood supply to vital organs.

Hypothesis The starting point of research; it is based on the statement, "If this happens, then that will happen."

Immunity Resistance to disease provided by the body through specific or nonspecific immunity. The immune system is a functional system rather than an organ system in the anatomic sense. The most important immune cells are lymphocytes and macrophages. The key to immunity is the ability of the body to distinguish self from nonself.

Impermeable The quality of not permitting entry of a substance.

Impingement syndromes Conditions that involve pathologic pressure on nerves and vessels; the two types of impingement are compression and entrapment.

Incontinence The inability to control urination or defecation, most often because of weak pelvic floor muscles or nerve damage.

Indication A therapeutic application that promotes health or assists in a healing process.

Inertia The reluctance of matter to change its state of motion.

Inflammation A protective response of the tissues to irritation or injury that may be chronic or acute. The four primary signs are redness, heat, swelling, and pain.

Inflammatory response A sequence of events that involves chemical and cellular activation that destroys pathogens and aids in repairing tissues.

Informed consent Client authorization for any service from a professional based on adequate information provided by the professional. Obtaining informed consent is a consumer protection process that requires that clients have knowledge of what will occur, that their participation is voluntary, and that they are competent to give consent. Informed consent is an educational procedure that allows clients to make knowledgeable decisions about whether they want to receive a massage.

Ingestion Taking food into the mouth.

Inhibition A decrease in or the cessation of a response or function.

Initial treatment plan A plan that states therapeutic goals, the duration of the sessions, the number of appointments necessary to meet the agreed goals, costs, the general classification of intervention to be used, and the objective progress measurement to be used to identify attainment of goals.

Inorganic compounds Chemical structures that do not have carbon and hydrogen atoms as the primary structure.

Insertion The distal attachment of a muscle; the part of a muscle that attaches farthest from the midline, or center, of the body. The muscle attachment point that is closest to the moving joint.

Integrated approaches Combined methods of various forms of massage and bodywork styles.

Integration The process of remembering an event while being able to remain in the present moment, with an awareness of the difference between then and now, to bring some sort of resolution to the event.

Integument The skin and its appendages: hair, sebaceous and sweat glands, nails, and breasts.

Intercompetition massage Massage provided during an athletic event.

Internal respiration The exchange of gases between the tissues and blood.

Internal rotation Medial rotary movement of a bone. Also known as rotation medially, inward rotation, and medial rotation.

Interphase The period during which a cell grows and carries on its activities.

Intimacy A tender, familiar, and understanding experience between beings.

Intractable pain The continuation of chronic pain without active disease present or when chronic pain persists even with treatment.

Intuition Knowing something by using subconscious information.

Inversion Movement of the sole of the foot inward toward the midline.

Ion pumps Carriers that transport substances into or out of a cell using energy.

Ischemia A temporary deficiency or decreased supply of blood to a tissue.

Isometric contraction The action of the prime mover that occurs when tension develops within the muscle but no appreciable change occurs in the joint angle or the length of the muscle. Movement does not occur.

Isotonic contraction A contraction in which the effort of the target muscle or group of muscles is matched partly by counterpressure, allowing a degree of resisted movement. The action of the prime mover that occurs when tension develops in the muscle while it shortens or lengthens.

Job A regular activity performed for payment.

Joint capsule A connective tissue structure that indirectly connects the bony components of a joint.

Joint end-feel The sensation felt when a normal joint is taken to its physiologic limit. (See *end-feel.*)

Joint kinesthetic receptors Receptors in the capsules of joints that respond to pressure and to acceleration and deceleration of joint movement. The two main types of joint kinesthetic receptors are type II cutaneous mechanoreceptors and pacinian (lamellated) corpuscles.

Joint movement The movement of the joint through its normal range of motion.

Joint play The inherent laxity present in a joint. The involuntary movement that occurs between articular surfaces that is separate from the range of motion of a joint produced by muscles. Joint play is an essential component of joint motion and must occur for normal functioning of the joint.

Keratin The fibrous protein produced in the epidermis that protects our skin and makes it waterproof.

Kinematics A branch of mechanics that involves the time, space, and mass aspects of a moving system.

Kinesiology The study of movement that combines the fields of anatomy, physiology, physics, and geometry and relates them to human movement.

Kinetic chain An integrated functional unit. The kinetic chain is made up of the myofascial system (muscle, ligament, tendon, and fascia), articular (joint) system, and nervous system. Each of these systems works interdependently to allow structural and functional efficiency in all three planes of motion: sagittal, frontal, and transverse. The process by which each individual joint movement pattern is part of an interconnected aspect of the neurologic coordination pattern of muscle movement.

Kinetics Those forces causing movement in a system.

Kyphosis A condition of exaggeration of the thoracic curve.

Lateral flexion (side bending) Movement of the head or trunk laterally away from the midline. Abduction of the spine.

Lateral recumbency (side-lying) Lying horizontally on the right or left side.

Law A scientific statement that is true uniformly for a whole class of natural occurrences.

Lengthening The process in which the muscle assumes a normal resting length by means of the neuromuscular mechanism.

Leukocytes White blood cells that protect the body from pathogens and remove dead cells and substances.

Lever A solid mass, such as a crowbar or a person's arm, that rotates around a fixed point called the fulcrum. The rotation is produced by a force applied to a lever at some distance from the fulcrum.

Leverage Leaning with the body weight to provide pressure.

License A type of credential required by law; licenses are used to regulate the practice of a profession to protect the public health, safety, and welfare.

Ligaments Dense bundles of parallel connective tissue fibers, primarily collagen, that connect bones and strengthen and stabilize the joint.

Lipids Fats and oils; organic compounds that have carbon, hydrogen, and oxygen atoms but in a different proportion than that of carbohydrates.

List A lateral tilt of the spine.

Locomotion Moving from one place to another; walking.

Longitudinal stretching A stretch applied along the fiber direction of the connective tissues and muscles.

Loose-packed position The position of a synovial joint in which the joint capsule is most lax. Joints tend to assume this position when inflammation occurs to accommodate the increased volume of synovial fluid.

Lordosis A condition of exaggeration of the normal lumbar curve.

Lower respiratory tract The larynx, trachea, bronchi, and alveoli.

Lubricant A substance that reduces friction on the skin during massage movements.

Lungs The primary organs of respiration, the lungs are soft, spongy, highly vascular structures separated into the left and right lungs by the mediastinum. Each lung is separated into lobes. The right lung has three lobes: an upper, middle, and lower; the left, two lobes: an upper and lower.

Lymph A clear interstitial tissue fluid that bathes the cells. Lymph contains lymphocytes, which provide immune response; returns plasma proteins that have leaked out through capillary walls; and transports fats from the gastrointestinal system to the bloodstream.

Lymph nodes Small, round structures distributed along the network of lymph vessels that provide a filtering system for removing waste products and transferring them to the bloodstream for removal to the spleen, intestines, and kidneys for detoxification. Lymph nodes are centers for lymphocyte production. Their main function is to prevent bacteria and viruses from gaining access to the bloodstream. Generally clustered at the joints for assistance in pumping when the joint moves, they are especially numerous in the axillas, groin, and neck and along certain blood vessels of the pelvic, abdominal, and thoracic cavities.

Lymph system A specialized component of the circulatory system responsible for waste disposal and immune response.

Lymphatic drainage A specific type of massage that enhances lymphatic flow.

Lysosome Cell organelle that is part of the intracellular digestive system.

Malignant The type of tumor (cancer) that tends to spread to other regions of the body.

Manipulation Skillful use of the hands in a therapeutic manner. Massage manipulations focus on the soft tissues of the body and are not to be confused with joint manipulation using a high-velocity thrust.

Manual lymph drainage Methods of bodywork that influence lymphatic movement.

Marketing The advertising and other promotional activities required to sell a product or service.

Massage The scientific art and system of assessment of and manual application of certain techniques to the superficial soft tissue of skin, muscles, tendons, ligaments, and fascia and the structures that lie within the superficial tissue. The hand, foot, knee, arm, elbow, and forearm are used for the systematic external application of touch, stroking (effleurage), friction, vibration, percussion, kneading (petrissage), stretching, compression, or passive and active joint movements within the normal physiologic range of motion. Massage includes adjunctive external applications of water, heat, and cold for the purposes of establishing and maintaining good physical condition and health by normalizing and improving muscle tone, promoting relaxation, stimulating circulation, and producing therapeutic effects on the respiratory and nervous systems and the subtle interactions among all body systems. These intended effects are accomplished through the physiologic energetic and mind/body connections in a safe, nonsexual environment that respects the client's self-determined outcome for the session.

Massage chair A specially designed chair that allows the client to sit comfortably during the massage.

Massage environment An area or location where a massage is given.

Massage equipment Tables, mats, chairs, and other incidental supplies and implements used during the massage.

Massage mat A cushioned surface that is placed on the floor.

Massage routine The step-by-step protocol and sequence used to give a massage.

Massage table A specially designed table that allows massage to be done with the client lying down.

Matrix The basic substance between the cells of a tissue. Matrix is composed of amorphous ground substance consisting of molecules that expand when water molecules and electrolytes bind to them. Up to 90% of connective tissue is ground substance. Fibers make up the other component of matrix.

Maximal stimulus The point at which all motor units of a muscle have been recruited and the muscle is unable to increase in strength.

Mechanical methods Techniques that directly affect the soft tissue by normalizing the connective tissue or moving body fluids and intestinal contents.

Mechanical receptors Sensory receptors that detect changes in pressure, movement, temperature, or other mechanical forces.

Mechanical response A response that is based on a structural change in the tissue. The tissue change is caused directly by application of the technique.

Mechanical touch Touch applied with the intent of achieving a specific anatomic or physiologic outcome.

Mechanics The branch of physics dealing with the study of forces and the motion produced by their actions.

Medications Substances prescribed to stimulate or inhibit a body process or replace a chemical in the body.

Meiosis A type of cell division in which each daughter cell divides again. In the second division, each daughter cell receives half the normal number of chromosomes, forming two reproductive cells (a total of four reproductive cells from one meiotic cycle).

Melanin The pigment that colors our skin and works as a natural sunscreen to protect us from ultraviolet rays by darkening our skin.

Membrane A thin, sheetlike layer of tissue that covers a cell, an organ, or some other structure; that lines a tube or a cavity; or that divides or separates one part from another.

Mental impairment Any mental or psychologic disorder, such as mental retardation, developmental disabilities, organic brain syndrome, emotional or mental illness, and specific learning disabilities.

Mentoring Career support by someone more experienced.

Metabolism Chemical processes in the body that convert food and oxygen into energy to support growth, distribution of nutrients, and elimination of waste.

Metabolites Molecules synthesized or broken down inside the body by chemical reactions.

Metastasis Migration of cancer cells.

Microorganisms Small life forms that may be damaging to the body or interfere with its function.

Microvilli Small projections of the cell membrane that increase the surface area of the cell.

Micturition The clinical term for urination or voiding.

Mitochondria Cell organelles of rod or oval shape.

Mitosis Cell division in which the cell duplicates its DNA and divides into two identical daughter cells.

Mixed nerves Nerves that contain sensory and motor axons.

Moderate pressure Compressive pressure that extends to the muscle layer but does not press the tissue against the underlying bone.

Mole Also known as a nevus, a mole is a benign pigmented skin growth formed of melanocytes.

Molecule A combination of two or more atoms. A molecule is the smallest portion of a substance that can exist separately without losing the physical and chemical properties of that substance.

Monoplegia Paralysis of a single limb or a single group of muscles.

Motivation The internal drive that provides the energy to do what is necessary to accomplish a goal.

Motor point The location where the motor neuron enters the muscle and where a visible contraction can be elicited with a minimal amount of stimulation. Motor points most often are located in the belly of the muscle.

Motor unit A motor neuron and all of the muscle fibers it controls.

Movement cure Term used in the nineteenth and early twentieth centuries for a system of exercise and massage manipulations focused on treating a variety of ailments.

Multiple isotonic contractions Movement of the joint and associated muscles by the client through a full range of motion against partial resistance applied by the massage therapist.

Muscle energy techniques Neuromuscular facilitation; specific use of active contraction in individual muscles or groups of muscles to initiate a relaxation response; activation of the proprioceptors to facilitate muscle tone, relaxation, and stretching.

Muscle spindles Structures located primarily in the belly of the muscle that respond to sudden and prolonged stretches.

Muscle testing procedures An assessment process that uses muscle contraction. Strength testing is done to determine whether a muscle responds with sufficient strength to perform the required body functions. Neurologic muscle testing is designed to determine whether the neurologic interaction of the muscles is working smoothly.

Muscle tissue A specialized form of tissue that contracts and shortens to provide movement, maintain posture, and produce heat.

Musculotendinous junction The point where muscle fibers end and the connective tissue continues to form the tendon; a major site of injury.

Myasthenia gravis A disorder that usually affects muscles in the face, lips, tongue, neck, and throat, which are innervated by the cranial nerves, but that can affect any muscle group.

Myelin A white, fatty, insulating substance formed by the Schwann cells that surrounds some axons. Also produced in the central nervous system by oligodendrocytes.

Myofascial approaches Styles of bodywork that affect the connective tissues; often called deep tissue massage, soft tissue manipulation, or *myofascial release.*

Myofascial release A system of bodywork that affects the connective tissue of the body through various methods that elongate and alter the plastic component and ground matrix of the connective tissue.

Myotome A skeletal muscle or group of skeletal muscles that receives motor axons from a particular spinal nerve.

Needs assessment History taking using a client information form and physical assessment using an assessment form. The information is evaluated to develop a care plan.

Negative feedback system A control mechanism that provides a stimulus to decrease a function, such as a fire alarm, which causes a series of reactions that work to reduce the fire.

Neoplasm The abnormal growth of new tissue. Also called a *tumor,* a neoplasm may be benign or malignant.

Nerve A bundle of axons or dendrites or both.

Nerve impingement Pressure against a nerve by skin, fascia, muscles, ligaments, or joints.

Nervous tissue A specialized tissue that coordinates and regulates body activity and can develop more excitability and conductivity than other types of tissue.

Neurilemma The outer cell membrane of a Schwann cell that is essential in the regeneration of injured axons. The thin membrane spirally wraps the myelin layers of certain fibers, especially of peripheral nerves, or the axons of certain unmyelinated nerve fibers. Also called Schwann's membrane, sheath of Schwann, and endoneural membrane.

Neuroglia Specialized connective tissue cells that support, protect, and hold neurons together.

Neurologic muscle testing Testing designed to determine whether the neurologic interaction of the muscles is proceeding smoothly.

Neuromuscular A term describing the interaction between nervous system control of the muscles and the response of the muscles to the nerve signals.

Neuromuscular approaches Methods of bodywork that influence the reflexive responses of the nervous system and its connection to muscular function.

Neuromuscular mechanism The interplay and reflex connection between sensory and motor neurons and muscle function.

Neurons Nerve cells that conduct impulses.

Neurotransmitters Chemical compounds that generate action potentials when released in the synapses from presynaptic cells.

Nociceptors Sensory receptors that detect painful or intense stimuli.

Norepinephrine A catecholamine primarily involved in emotional responses. Norepinephrine is found in the central nervous system and the sympathetic division of the autonomic nervous system and causes constriction of blood vessels in the skeletal muscles.

Norepinephrine/noradrenaline A neurochemical that functions in a manner similar to epinephrine but that is more concentrated in the brain.

Nucleic acids The two types of nucleic acid are deoxyribonucleic acid (DNA) and ribonucleic acid (RNA).

Nutrients Essential elements and molecules obtained from the diet that are required by the body for normal body function.

Nutrition The use of food for growth and maintenance of the body.

Occupation A productive or creative activity that serves as a regular source of livelihood.

Oil A type of liquid lubricant.

Open kinematic chain A position in which the ends of the limbs or parts of the body are free to move without causing motion at another joint.

Open-ended question A question that cannot be answered with a simple, one-word response.

Opportunistic invasion Potentially pathogenic organisms that are found on the skin and mucous membranes of nearly everyone but do not cause disease until they have the opportunity, such as in depressed immunity.

Opportunistic pathogens Organisms that cause disease only when the immunity is low in a host.

Opposition Movement of the thumb across the palmar aspect to make contact with the fingers.

Organelles The basic components of a cell that perform specific functions within the cell.

Organic compounds Substances that have carbon and hydrogen as part of their basic structure.

Origin The attachment point of a muscle at the fixed point during movement. The proximal attachment of a muscle; the part that attaches closest to the midline (center) of the body; the least movable part of a muscle.

Osmosis Diffusion of water from a region of lower concentration of solution to a region of higher concentration of solution across the semipermeable membrane of a cell.

Osteokinematic movements The movements of flexion, extension, abduction, adduction, and rotation; also known as physiologic movements.

Osteokinematics The movement of bones as opposed to the movement of articular surfaces; also known as range of motion.

Osteoporosis A disorder of the bones in which a lack of calcium and other minerals and a decrease in bone protein leaves the bones soft, fragile, and more likely to break.

Overload principle A stress on an organism that is greater than the one regularly encountered during everyday life.

Oxygen debt The extra amount of oxygen that must be taken in to convert lactic acid to glucose or glycogen.

Oxytocin A hormone that is implicated in pair or couple bonding, parental bonding, feelings of attachment, and caretaking, along with its more commonly known functions in pregnancy, delivery, and lactation.

Pain An unpleasant sensation. Pain is a complex, private experience with physiologic, psychologic, and social aspects. Because pain is subjective, it is often difficult to explain or describe.

Pain and fatigue syndromes Multicausal and often chronic nonproductive patterns that interfere with well-being, activities of living, and productivity.

Pain-spasm-pain cycle Steady contraction of muscles, which causes ischemia and stimulates pain receptors in muscles. The pain, in turn, initiates more spasms.

Palliative care Care intended to relieve or reduce the intensity of uncomfortable symptoms but that cannot effect a cure.

Palpation Assessment through touch.

Panic An intense, sudden, and overwhelming fear or feeling of anxiety that produces terror and immediate physiologic change resulting in immobility or senseless, hysteric behavior.

Paraplegia Paralysis of the lower portion of the body and of both legs.

Parasympathetic autonomic nervous system The restorative part of the autonomic nervous system. The parasympathetic response often is called the relaxation response.

Parasympathetic nervous system The energy conservation and restorative system associated with what commonly is called the relaxation response.

Passive joint movement Movement of a joint by the massage practitioner without the assistance of the client.

Passive range of motion Movement of a joint in which the therapist, not the client, effects the motion.

Passive transport Transportation of a substance across the cell membrane without the use of energy

Pathogenesis The development of a disease.

Pathogenic animals Large, multicellular organisms sometimes called metazoa. Most metazoa are worms that feed off human tissue or cause other disease processes.

Pathogenicity The ability of the infectious agent to cause disease.

Pathogens Microorganisms capable of producing disease.

Pathologic barrier An adaptation of the physiologic barrier that allows the protective function to limit rather than support optimal functioning.

Pathologic range of motion The amount of motion at a joint that fails to reach the normal physiologic range or exceeds normal anatomic limits of motion of that joint.

Pathology The study of disease as observed in the structure and function of the body.

Peer support Interaction among those involved in the same pursuit. Regular interaction with other massage practitioners creates an environment in which technical information and dilemmas and interpersonal dilemmas can be sorted out.

Pericardium A double membranous, serous sac surrounding the heart. The pericardium secretes a lubricating fluid to prevent friction from the movement of the heart.

Periosteum The thin membrane of connective tissue that covers bones except at articulations.

Peripheral nervous system The system of somatic and autonomic neurons outside the central nervous system. The peripheral nervous system comprises the afferent (sensory) division and the efferent (motor) division.

Peristalsis Rhythmic contraction of smooth muscles that propel products of digestion along the tract from the esophagus to the anus.

Peritoneum The mucous membrane that lines the abdominal cavity to prevent friction from the organs.

Person-to-person contact Pathogens often can be carried in the air from one person to another.

Petrissage Kneading; rhythmic rolling, lifting, squeezing, and wringing of soft tissue.

Phagocytosis The process of endocytosis followed by digestion of the vesicle contents by enzymes present in the cytoplasm.

Phantom pain A form of pain or other sensation experienced in the missing extremity after a limb amputation.

Pharynx The throat.

Phasic muscles The muscles that move the body.

Phospholipid bilayer Cell membrane made up of lipids, carbohydrates, and proteins.

Physical assessment Evaluation of body balance, efficient function, basic symmetry, range of motion, and ability to function.

Physical disability Any physiologic disorder, condition, cosmetic disfigurement, or anatomic loss that affects one or more of the following body systems: neurologic, musculoskeletal, special sense organ, respiratory (including speech organs), cardiovascular, reproductive, digestive, genitourinary, hemic and lymphatic, skin, and endocrine.

Extremes in size and extensive burns also may be considered physical impairments.

Physiologic barriers The result of the limits in range of motion imposed by protective nerve and sensory functions to support optimal performance.

Physiologic range of motion The amount of motion available to a joint determined by the nervous system from information provided by joint sensory receptors. This information usually prevents a joint from being positioned so that injury could occur.

Physiology The study of the processes and functions of the body involved in supporting life.

Piezoelectric The quality of bones that allows them to deform slightly and vibrate when electric currents pass through them. Bone formation patterns follow lines of stress load directed by the piezoelectric currents.

Piezoelectricity The production of an electric current by application of pressure to certain crystals such as mica, quartz, Rochelle salt, and connective tissue.

Pivot joint A bony projection from one bone fits into a "ring" formed by another bone and ligament structure to allow rotation around its own axis.

Placebo A treatment for an illness that influences the course of the disease even if the treatment is not specifically validated.

Plantar flexion An extension movement of the ankle that results in the foot and toes moving away from the body.

Plasma A thick, straw-colored fluid that makes up about 55% of the blood.

Plastic range The range of movement of connective tissue that is taken beyond the elastic limits. In this range the tissue permanently deforms and cannot return to its original state.

Plexus A network of intertwining nerves that innervates a particular region of the body.

Polarity A holistic health practice that encompasses some of the theory base of Asian medicine and Ayurveda. Polarity is an eclectic, multifaceted system.

Polio (or poliomyelitis) A viral infection that affects the nerves that control skeletal muscle movement.

Positional release A method of moving the body into the direction of ease (the way the body wants to move out of the position that causes the pain); the proprioception is taken into a state of safety and may stop signaling for protective spasm.

Posterior pelvic rotation Posterior movement of the upper pelvis; the iliac crest tilts backward in a sagittal plane.

Post-event massage Massage provided after an athletic event.

Post-isometric relaxation The state that occurs after isometric contraction of a muscle; it results from the activity of minute neural reporting stations called the Golgi tendon bodies.

Post-traumatic stress disorder A disorder characterized by episodes of flashback memory, state-dependent memory, somatization, anxiety, irritability, sleep disturbance, concentration difficulties, times of melancholy or depression, grief, fear, worry, anger, and avoidance behavior.

Postural muscles Muscles that support the body against gravity.

Powder A type of lubricant that consists of a finely ground substance.

Prefix A word element added to the beginning of a root to change the meaning of the word.

Premassage activities Any activity that is involved in preparation for a massage, including setting up the massage room, obtaining supplies, and determining the temperature of the room.

Pressure Compressive force. The amount of force on a specific area.

PRICE first aid Protection, rest, ice, compression, elevation.

Prime movers The muscles responsible for movement.

Principle A basic truth or rule of conduct

Process Any prominent bony growth that projects out from the bone.

Profession An occupation that requires training and specialized study.

Professional A person who practices a profession.

Professional touch Skilled touch delivered to achieve a specific outcome; the recipient in some way reimburses the professional for services rendered.

Professionalism The adherence to professional status, methods, standards, and character.

Pronation Internal rotary movement of the radius on the ulna that results in the hand moving from the palm-up to the palm-down position.

Prone Lying horizontal with the face down.

Proprioceptive neuromuscular facilitation Specific application of muscle energy techniques that uses strong contraction combined with stretching and muscular pattern retraining.

Proprioceptors Sensory receptors that provide the body with information about position, movement, muscle tension, joint activity, and equilibrium.

Proteins Substances formed from amino acids.

Protozoa One-celled organisms that are larger than bacteria and can infest human fluids and cause disease by parasitizing (living off) or directly destroying cells.

Protraction Forward movement remaining in a horizontal plane.

Psoriasis A common, chronic skin disease characterized by reddened skin covered by dry, silvery scales. Psoriasis most often is found on the scalp, elbows, knees, back, or buttocks.

Pulmonary trunk The large artery that carries blood to the lungs to release carbon dioxide and take in oxygen.

Pulmonary veins The four veins from the lungs that bring oxygen-rich blood to the left atrium.

Pulsed muscle energy Procedures that involve engaging the barrier and using minute, resisted contractions (usually 20 in 10 seconds), which introduces mechanical pumping as well as post-isometric relaxation or reciprocal inhibition.

Qi Also known as Ch'i, Qi refers to the life force.

Quadriplegia Paralysis or loss of movement of all four limbs.

Qualified Criteria that indicate when the goal is achieved.

Quantified Goals measured in terms of objective criteria, such as time, frequency, 1 to 10 scale, measurable increase or decrease in the ability to perform an activity, or measurable increase or decrease in a sensation, such as relaxation or pain.

Quiet expiration Movement of air out of the body through passive action. This occurs through relaxation of the external intercostals and the elastic recoil of the thoracic wall and tissue of the lungs and bronchi, with gravity pulling the rib cage down from its elevated position.

Quiet inspiration Movement of air into the body while resting or sitting quietly. The diaphragm and external intercostals are the prime movers.

Range of motion Movement of joints.

Rapport The development of a relationship based on mutual trust and harmony.

Reciprocal inhibition The effect that occurs when a muscle contracts, obliging its antagonist to relax in order to allow normal movement to take place.

Reciprocal innervation The circuitry of neurons that allows reciprocal inhibition to take place. One can use reciprocal innervation therapeutically to assist in muscle relaxation.

Reciprocity The exchange of privileges between governing bodies.

Recovery massage Massage structured primarily for the uninjured athlete who wants to recover from a strenuous workout or competition.

Reduction Return of the spinal column to the anatomic position from lateral flexion. Adduction of the spine.

Reenactment Reliving an event as though it were happening at the moment.

Referral Sending a client to a health care professional for specific diagnosis and treatment of a disease.

Referred pain Pain felt in a surface area far from the stimulated organ.

Reflex An involuntary response to a stimulus. Reflexes are specific, predictable, adaptive, and purposeful. Reflexive methods work by stimulating the nervous system (sensory neurons), and tissue changes occur in response to the adaptation of the body to the neural stimulation.

Reflex arc The pathway that a nerve impulse follows in a reflex action.

Reflexive methods Massage techniques that stimulate the nervous system, the endocrine system, and the chemicals of the body.

Reflexology A massage system directed primarily toward the feet and hands.

Refractory period The period after a muscle contraction during which the muscle is unable to contract again.

Regional anatomy The study of the structures of a particular area of the body.

Regional contraindications Contraindications that relate to a specific area of the body.

Rehabilitation massage Massage used for severe injury or as part of intervention after surgery.

Remedial massage Massage used for minor to moderate injuries.

Remission A reversal of signs and symptoms in chronic disease that can be temporary or permanent.

Resourceful compensation Adjustments made by the body to manage a permanent or chronic dysfunction.

Respiration The movement of air in and out of the lungs, the exchange of oxygen and carbon dioxide between the lungs and blood, and the exchange between blood and body tissues.

Respiratory rate The number of breaths in 1 minute.

Resting position The first stroke of the massage; the simple laying on of hands.

Reticular fibers Delicate, connective tissue fibers that occur in networks and support small structures, such as capillaries, nerve fibers, and the basement membrane. Reticular fibers are made of a specialized type of collagen called reticulin.

Retraction Backward movement in a horizontal plane.

Rhythm The regularity of application of a technique. If the method is applied at regular intervals, it is considered even or rhythmic. If the method is choppy or irregular, it is considered uneven or not rhythmic.

Ribonucleic acid Nucleic acids that transfer genetic information and control cellular chemical activities. Abbreviated RNA.

Right of refusal The entitlement of the client and the professional to stop the session.

Rocking Rhythmic movement of the body.

Root word The part of a word that provides the fundamental meaning.

Rotation Partial turning or pivoting in an arc around a central axis.

Rupture The tearing or disruption of connective tissue fibers that takes place when they exceed the limits of the plastic range.

Saddle joint Joint that is convex in one plane and concave in the other with the surfaces fitting together like a rider on a saddle.

Safe touch Secure, respectful, considerate, sensitive, responsive, sympathetic, understanding, supportive, and empathetic contact.

Sanitation The formulation and application of measures to promote and establish conditions favorable to health, specifically public health.

Schwann cell A specialized cell that forms myelin.

Science The intellectual process of understanding through observation, measurement, accumulation of data, and analysis of findings.

Scoliosis A lateral curvature of the spine.

Scope of practice The knowledge base and practice parameters of a profession.

Sebaceous glands The oil glands found in the skin.

Sebum The oily substance secreted by sebaceous glands that prevents dehydration, softens skin and hair, and slows the growth of bacteria.

Self-employment To work for oneself rather than another.

Serotonin A neurotransmitter that works primarily as an inhibitor in the central nervous system and is synthesized into melatonin and affects our sleep and moods. The neurochemical that regulates mood in terms of appropriate emotions, attention to thoughts, calming, quieting, and comforting effects; it also subdues irritability and regulates drive states.

Service An action performed for another person that results in a specific outcome.

Sesamoid bones Round bones that often are embedded in tendons and joint capsules.

Seven Emotions The Asian concept that joy, anger, fear, fright, sadness, worry, and grief are emotional responses that may trigger disharmony in the body, mind, or spirit under certain conditions.

Sexual misconduct Any behavior that is sexually oriented in the professional setting.

Shaking A technique in which the body area is grasped and shaken in a quick, loose movement; sometimes classified as rhythmic mobilization.

Shiatsu An acupressure and meridian-focused bodywork system from Japan.

Shock An inadequate blood supply to vital organs, causing reduced function in these organs.

Side-lying The position in which the client is lying on his or her side.

Signs Objective changes that someone other than the client or patient can observe and measure.

Sinus Four groups of air-filled spaces that open into the internal nose. They are located in the frontal, ethmoid, sphenoid, and maxillary bones of the skull. Sinuses are lined with mucosa and function to lighten the weight of the skull, making it easier to hold the head up and help in the production of sound.

Six Pernicious Influences The Asian concept that heat, cold, wind, dampness, dryness, and summer heat, which are natural climate changes, may induce disease under certain conditions.

Skeletal muscle fibers Large, cross-striated cells that are connected to the skeleton and under voluntary control of the nervous system.

Skin rolling A form of massage that lifts skin.

Slapping A form of tapotement that uses a flat hand.

Smooth muscle fibers Muscle fibers that are neither striated nor voluntary. These muscle cells help regulate blood flow through the cardiovascular system, propel food through the gut, and squeeze secretions from glands.

SOAP charting A problem-oriented method of medical record keeping; the acronym SOAP stands for subjective, objective, assessment (analysis), and plan.

SOAP notes The acronym refers to subjective, objective, analysis or assessment, and plan, the four parts of the written account of record keeping.

Soft tissue The skin, fascia, muscles, tendons, joint capsules, and ligaments of the body.

Somatic Pertaining to the body.

Somatic nervous system A system of nerves that keeps the body in balance with its external environment by transmitting impulses between the central nervous system, skeletal muscles, and skin.

Somatic pain Pain that arises from the body as opposed to the viscera. Superficial somatic pain comes from the stimulation of receptors in the skin, whereas deep somatic pain arises from stimulation of receptors in skeletal muscles, joints, tendons, and fascias.

Spa treatments Various hydrotherapies, applications of preparations to the body, and massage applications found in the spa setting.

Spastic Term used to describe a muscle with excessive tone.

Speed Rate of application (i.e., fast, slow, or varied).

Spinal cord Portion of the central nervous system that exits the skull into the vertebral column. The two major functions of the spinal cord are to conduct nerve impulses and to be a center for spinal reflexes.

Spinal nerves Thirty-one pairs of mixed nerves, originating in the spinal cord and emerging from the vertebral column, that make sensation and movement possible.

Spindle cells Sensory receptors in the belly of the muscle that detect stretch.

Spongy (cancellous) bone The lighter-weight portion of bone made up of trabeculas.

Stabilization Holding the body in a fixed position during joint movement, lengthening, and stretching.

Stabilizer A force or an object that helps maintain a position. Stabilization is essential to assess movement patterns accurately.

Standard precautions Safety measures established by the Centers for Disease Control and Prevention. The precautions were instituted to prevent the spread of bacterial and viral infections by setting up specific methods of dealing with human fluids and waste products. Standard precautions protect client and practitioner from pathogens.

Standards of practice The principles that form specific guidelines to direct professional ethical practice and quality care, including a structure for evaluating the quality of care. Standards of practice represent an attempt to define the parameters of quality care.

Start-up costs The initial expenses involved in starting a business.

State-dependent memory The encoding and storing of a memory based on the effects of the autonomic nervous system and the resulting chemical levels of the body. The memory is retrievable only during a similar physiologic experience in the body.

Static force Force applied to an object in such a way that it does not produce movement.

Sterilization The process by which all microorganisms are destroyed.

Stimulation Excitation that activates the sensory nerves.

Strain-counterstrain Using tender points to guide the positioning of the body into a space where the muscle tension can release on its own.

Strength testing Testing intended to determine whether a muscle is responding with sufficient strength to perform the required body functions. Strength testing determines the force of contraction of a muscle.

Stress Any external or internal stimulus that requires a change or response to prevent an imbalance in the internal environment of the body, mind, or emotions. Stress may be any activity that makes demands on mental and emotional resources. Some responses to stress may stimulate neurons of the hypothalamus to release corticotropin-releasing hormone.

Stressors Any internal perceptions or external stimuli that demand a change in the body.

Stretching Mechanical tension applied to lengthen the myofascial unit (muscles and fascia); two types are longitudinal and cross-directional stretching.

Stroke A technique of therapeutic massage that is applied with a movement on the surface of the body, whether superficial or deep.

Structural and postural integration approaches Methods of bodywork derived from biomechanics, postural alignment, and the importance of the connective tissue structures.

Subacute Diseases with characteristics between acute and chronic.

Subtle energies Weak electric fields that surround and run through the body.

Suffering An overall impairment of a person's quality of life.

Suffix A word element added to the end of a root to change the meaning of the word.

Superficial fascia The subcutaneous tissue that composes the third layer of skin, consists of loose connective tissue, and contains fat or adipose tissue.

Superficial pressure Pressure that remains on the skin.

Supervision Support from more experienced professionals.

Supination External rotary movement of the radius on the ulna that results in the hand moving from the palm-down to the palm-up position.

Supine Lying horizontal with the face up.

Surface anatomy The study of internal organs and structures as they can be recognized and related to external features.

Suture A synarthrotic joint in which two bony components are united by a thin layer of dense fibrous tissue.

Sweat glands The sudoriferous glands in the skin; they are classified as apocrine or eccrine based on their location and structure.

Symmetrical stance The position in which body weight is distributed equally between the feet.

Sympathetic autonomic nervous system The energy-using part of the autonomic nervous system, the division in which the fight-or-flight response is activated.

Sympathetic nervous system The part of the autonomic nervous system that provides for most of the active function of the body; when the body is under stress, the sympathetic nervous system predominates with fight-or-flight responses.

Symphysis A cartilaginous joint in which the two bony components are joined directly by fibrocartilage in the form of a disk or plate.

Symptoms The subjective changes noticed or felt only by the client or patient.

Synapse Spaces between neurons or between a neuron and an effector organ.

Synarthrosis A limited-movement, nonsynovial joint.

Synchondrosis A joint in which the material used for connecting the two components is hyaline growth cartilage.

Syndesmosis A fibrous joint in which two bony components are joined directly by a ligament, cord, or aponeurotic membrane.

Syndrome A group of different signs and symptoms that identify a pathologic condition, especially when they have a common cause.

Synergist A muscle that aids or assists the action of the agonist but is not primarily responsible for the action; also known as a guiding muscle.

Synergistic The interaction of medication and massage to stimulate the same process or effects.

Synovial fluid A thick, colorless lubricating fluid secreted by the joint cavity membrane.

Synovial joint A freely moving joint allowing motion in one or more planes.

System A group of interacting elements that function as a complex whole.

Systemic anatomy The study of the structure of a particular body system.

Systemic massage Massage structured to affect one body system primarily. This approach usually is used for lymphatic and circulation enhancement massage.

Tao An ancient philosophic concept that represents the whole and its parts as one and the same.

Tapotement Springy blows to the body at a fast rate to create rhythmic compression of the tissue; also called percussion.

Tapping A type of tapotement that uses the fingertips.

Target muscle The muscle or groups of muscles on which the response of the methods is focused specifically.

Techniques Methods of therapeutic massage that provide sensory stimulation or mechanical change of the soft tissue of the body.

Tendon organs Structures found in the tendon and musculotendinous junction that respond to tension at the tendon. Articular (joint) ligaments contain receptors that are similar to tendon organs and adjust reflex inhibition of the adjacent muscle when excessive strain is placed on the joints.

Tendonitis Inflammation of a tendon.

Tenosynovitis Inflammation of a tendon sheath.

Tensegrity An architectural principle developed in 1948 by R. Buckminster Fuller. The tensegrity principle underlies geodesic domes. A tensegrity system is characterized by a continuous tensional network (tendons, ligaments, and fascial structures) connected by a discontinuous set of compressive elements, or struts (bones).

Therapeutic applications Healing or curative powers.

Therapeutic change Beneficial change produced by a bodywork process that results in a modification of physical form or function that can affect a client's physical, mental, and/or spiritual state.

Therapeutic relationship The interpersonal structure and professional boundaries between professionals and the clients they serve.

Thermal receptors Sensory receptors that detect changes in temperature.

Thorax Also known as the chest cavity, the thorax is the upper region of the torso enclosed by the sternum, ribs, and thoracic vertebrae and contains the lungs, heart, and great vessels.

Threshold stimulus The stimulus at which the first observable muscle contraction occurs.

Tissue A group of similar cells combined to perform a common function.

Tone The state of tension in resting muscles.

Tonic vibration reflex Reflex that tones a muscle with stimulation through vibration methods at the tendon.

Touch Contact with no movement.

Touch technique The basis of soft tissue forms of bodywork methods.

Toughening/hardening The reaction to repeated exposure to stimuli that elicit arousal responses.

Trabecula An irregular meshing of small, bony plates that makes up spongy bone; its spaces are filled with red marrow.

Traction Gentle pull on the joint capsule to increase the joint space.

Tracts Collections of nerve fibers in the brain and spinal cord with a common function.

Training stimulus threshold The stimulus that elicits a training response.

Transference The personalization of the professional relationship by the client.

Trauma Physical injury caused by violent or disruptive action, toxic substances, or psychic injury resulting from a severe long- or short-term emotional shock.

Trigger point An area of local nerve facilitation; pressure on the trigger point results in hypertonicity of a muscle bundle and referred pain patterns. A hyperirritable area within a taut band of skeletal muscle, located in the muscular tissue and/or its associated fascia. The spot is painful on compression and can cause characteristic referred pain and autonomic phenomena.

Trochanter One of two large bony processes found only on the femur.

Tropic (or trophic) hormones Hormones produced by the endocrine glands that affect other endocrine glands.

Tubercle A small rounded process on a bone.

Tuberculosis An infection caused by bacteria that usually affects the lungs but may invade other body systems.

Tuberosity A large rounded protuberance on a bone.

Tumor Also referred to as a neoplasm, a tumor is a growth of new tissues that may be benign (nonthreatening or noncancerous) or malignant (cancerous).

Ulcer A round, open sore of the skin or mucous membrane.

Upper respiratory tract The nasal cavity and all its structures and the pharynx.

Upward rotation Scapular motion that turns the glenoid fossa upward and moves the inferior angle superiorly and laterally away from the spinal column.

Vector The direction of force.

Veins Blood vessels that collect blood from the capillaries and transport it back to the heart. Seventy-five percent of the blood in the body is in the venous system. Larger veins often contain a set of valves that ensure that blood flows in the correct direction to the heart and also prevents backflow.

Vena cava One of two large arteries that returns poorly oxygenated blood to the right atrium of the heart.

Ventral root One of two roots that attaches a spinal nerve to the spinal cord.

Ventricles The two large, lower chambers of the heart; they are thick-walled and are separated by a thick interventricular septum.

Venules The smallest veins.

Vibration Fine or coarse tremulous movement that creates reflexive responses.

Virulent A quality of organisms that readily causes disease.

Viruses Microorganisms that invade cells and insert their genetic code into the genetic code of the host cell. Viruses use the host cell nutrients and organelles to produce more virus particles.

Visceral pain Pain that results from the stimulation of receptors or an abnormal condition in the viscera (internal organs).

Viscoelasticity The combination of resistance offered by a fluid to a change of form and the ability of material to return to its original state after deformation. This term describes connective tissue.

Wellness The efficient balance of body, mind, and spirit, all working in a harmonious way to provide quality of life.

Whiplash An injury to the soft tissues of the neck caused by sudden hyperextension and/or flexion of the neck.

Word elements The parts of a word; the prefix, root, and suffix.

Yang The portion of the whole realm of function of the body, mind, and spirit in Eastern thought that corresponds with sympathetic autonomic nervous system functions.

Yellow elastic cartilage Cartilage that is more opaque, flexible, and elastic than hyaline cartilage and is distinguished further by its yellow color. The ground substance is penetrated in all directions by frequently branching fibers that give all of the reactions for elastin.

Yin The portion of the whole realm of function of the body, mind, and spirit in Eastern thought that corresponds with parasympathetic autonomic nervous system functions.

Yin/yang Yin and yang are terms used to describe polar relationships. Yin/yang refers to the dynamic balance between opposing forces and the continual process of creation and destruction. Yin/yang reflects the natural order and duality of the whole universe and everything in it, including the individual.